AMERICAN CANCER SOCIETY'S

Complementary and Alternative Cancer Methods Handbook

Books published by the American Cancer Society

A Breast Cancer Journey: Your Personal Guidebook

American Cancer Society's Guide to Complementary and Alternative Cancer Methods

American Cancer Society's Guide to Pain Control

Cancer in the Family: Helping Children Cope with a Parent's Illness, Heiney et al.

Caregiving: A Step-By-Step Resource for Caring for the Person with Cancer at Home, Houts and Bucher

Colorectal Cancer: A Thorough and Compassionate Resource for Patients and Their Families, Levin

Coming to Terms with Cancer: A Glossary of Cancer-Related Terms, Laughlin

Consumers Guide to Cancer Drugs, Wilkes et al.

Crossing Divides: A Couple's Story of Cancer, Hope, and Hiking Montana's Continental Divide, Bischke

Good For You! Reducing Your Risk of Developing Cancer

Informed Decisions: The Complete Book of Cancer Diagnosis, Treatment, and Recovery, 2nd Edition, Eyre et al.

Our Mom Has Cancer, Ackermann and Ackermann

Prostate Cancer: What Every Man—and His Family—Needs to Know, Revised Edition, Bostwick et al.

Women and Cancer: A Thorough and Compassionate Resource for Patients and Their Families, Runowicz et al.

Cookbooks published by the American Cancer Society

American Cancer Society's Healthy Eating Cookbook: A Celebration of Food, Friends, and Healthy Living, 2nd Edition

Celebrate! Healthy Entertaining for Any Occasion

Kids' First Cookbook: Delicious-Nutritious Treats to Make Yourself!

AMERICAN CANCER SOCIETY'S

COMPLEMENTARY AND ALTERNATIVE CANCER METHODS HANDBOOK

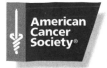

Published by American Cancer Society
    Health Content Products
    1599 Clifton Road NE
    Atlanta, Georgia 30329, USA

MANAGING EDITOR
Katherine Bruss, PsyD

EDITOR
Anneke Smith

EDITORIAL REVIEW
Terri Ades, RN, MS, AOCN
Ted Gansler, MD, MBA

EDITORIAL DIRECTOR
Chuck Westbrook

PUBLISHING DIRECTOR
Diane Scott-Lichter

BOOK PUBLISHING MANAGER
Candace Magee

COVER AND INTERIOR DESIGN
Mouse Design Studio, Atlanta

Printed in the United States of America

5 4 3 2 1   02 03 04 05 06

LIBRARY OF CONGRESS CATALOGING-IN-PUBLICATION DATA
American Cancer Society's complementary and alternative cancer methods handbook.
        p. ; cm.
    Includes bibliographical references and index.
    ISBN 0-944235-40-9 (pbk.)
            1. Cancer—Alternative treatment—Handbooks, manuals, etc.
        [DNLM: 1. Alternative Medicine—methods—Handbooks. WB 39
A5115 2002] I. Title: Complementary and alternative cancer methods handbook.
    II. American Cancer Society.
    RC271.A62 A46 2002
    616.99'406—dc21   2001006462

A NOTE TO THE READER

The information contained in this book is not intended as medical advice and should not be relied upon as a substitute for consulting with your physician. This information may not address all possible actions, precautions, side effects, or interactions. All matters regarding your health require the supervision of a physician who is familiar with your medical needs. For more information, contact your American Cancer Society at 1-800-ACS-2345 (www.cancer.org).

Contents

Acknowledgments
vi

HOW TO USE THIS BOOK
vii

OVERVIEW
OF COMPLEMENTARY AND ALTERNATIVE METHODS
1

CHAPTER 1
MIND, BODY, AND SPIRIT METHODS
15

CHAPTER 2
MANUAL HEALING AND PHYSICAL TOUCH METHODS
55

CHAPTER 3
HERB, VITAMIN, AND MINERAL METHODS
95

CHAPTER 4
DIET AND NUTRITION METHODS
196

CHAPTER 5
PHARMACOLOGICAL AND BIOLOGICAL TREATMENT METHODS
228

Resource Guide
268

Index
272

Acknowledgments

WE ARE GRATEFUL TO the following individuals who contributed to the development of the *American Cancer Society's Guide to Complementary and Alternative Cancer Methods*, which was used to create this handbook: Emily Pualwan, Katherine Bruss, PsyD, Christina Salter, MA, Esmeralda Galán, Steve Frandzel, Dennis Connaughton, Lynne Camoosa, Jeff Clements, Ryan Siemers, MPH, Dorothy Breckner, MPH, Leah Tuzzio, MPH, Robert Stephan, PhD, Suzanne Cassidy, Tom Gryczan, Jennifer Miller, Stuart J. Birkby, Melissa Kulick, PhD, Peter Dakutis, Steve Lewis, Lynn Yoffee, and Carol Carter.

We are also indebted to the following individuals who were instrumental in reviewing the content for the *American Cancer Society's Guide to Complementary and Alternative Cancer Methods*: Terri Ades, RN, MS, AOCN, Ted Gansler, MD, MBA, David Rosenthal, MD, Richard H. Lange, MD, FACP, Mary Ann Richardson, DrPH, John J. Lynch, MD, FACP, Muriel J. Montbriand, PhD, RN, Connie Henke Yarbro, RN, MS, FAAN, William T. Jarvis, PhD, Freddie Ann Hoffman, MD, Abby S. Bloch, PhD, RD, MaryBeth Augustine, RD, CDN, Carol A. Balmer, PharmD, Dan Nixon, MD, Daniel D. Anthony, MD, Susan Paulsen, PharmD, LaMar McGinnis, MD, and William Faire, MD.

How to Use This Book

This book begins with a basic overview of complementary and alternative methods, including information on commonly used terms, how to identify fraudulent products, potential dangers, and guidelines for use. The methods are organized into the 5 categories listed below and alphabetized within each category. Each method has been classified into one of the categories based on similar characteristics and how the treatment is administered or performed. The methods that are included have been promoted for conditions related to cancer, its consequences, or effects related to treatment. There is also a resource guide at the end of the book that provides standards for finding reliable sources of information.

This book is intended to serve as a reference tool, not to be read from beginning to end. If you do not find a particular method in the section you would expect, please consult the index to see if it is included elsewhere. In some cases, methods have been grouped together into broader categories that you may not immediately consider. If, however, an entire category interests you, you may want to read through all of the entries contained in that section to gain a better understanding of that area of complementary or alternative care. Some entries contain only a few lines, or short paragraphs, because they have limited information, or are not widely available. In these cases, there was not enough scientific information to evaluate the evidence, so only a brief description is provided.

CATEGORIES OF METHODS

MIND, BODY, AND SPIRIT METHODS
This chapter includes methods that focus on the connections between the mind, body, and spirit, and their power for healing.

MANUAL HEALING AND PHYSICAL TOUCH METHODS
Treatment methods in this chapter involve touching, manipulation, or

movement of the body. These techniques are based on the idea that problems in one part of the body often affect other parts of the body.

HERB, VITAMIN, AND MINERAL METHODS
This chapter contains information about plant-derived preparations that are used for therapeutic purposes, as well as everyday vitamins and minerals. It is noted when there are instances where chemicals extracted from plants are used rather than the plant components.

DIET AND NUTRITION METHODS
This chapter includes dietary approaches and special nutritional programs related to prevention and treatment.

PHARMACOLOGICAL AND BIOLOGICAL TREATMENT METHODS
This chapter provides information about substances that are synthesized and produced from chemicals or concentrated from plants and other living things. Extracted chemicals are not the same as the raw plant or plant in its natural state.

SAMPLE BOOK ENTRY

◣ ENTRY NAME
OTHER COMMON NAMES
Following the list of other common names is a synopsis of whether or not the method is effective based on scientific findings, and if any serious side effects may occur.

DESCRIPTION
This section includes a description of the method, components, and claims.

USE
This section explains what the treatment method involves and how it is administered.

EFFECTS
This section provides information about the scientific evidence regarding the effectiveness of the method. It also describes any possible problems or complications that may develop.

AMERICAN CANCER SOCIETY'S

Complementary and Alternative Cancer Methods Handbook

OVERVIEW
OF COMPLEMENTARY AND ALTERNATIVE METHODS

EACH YEAR, AMERICANS SPEND more than $34 billion on complementary and alternative treatment methods, and visit alternative practitioners more often than they see primary care doctors. It has been reported that up to 50% of people with cancer use some type of complementary and/or alternative medicine.

Herbal remedies and megavitamins are selling fast in health food stores and pharmacies, making promises of relief from common complaints and long-term illnesses, despite being virtually unregulated for safety, effectiveness, quality, and actual content. This trend of using complementary and alternative treatments is predicted to grow even more in the 21st century.

Defining Complementary and Alternative Therapies

The words complementary and alternative are often mistakenly used interchangeably; however, there are important distinctions between the two terms. *Complementary therapies* are those that are used along with conventional medicine. Some of these therapies can help relieve symptoms and improve the quality of life by reducing the side effects of conventional treatments or by providing psychological benefits.

Alternative therapies are treatments that have not been proven to be effective, and are used *instead of* conventional therapy to attempt to prevent, lessen, or cure disease. Alternative therapies may be harmful in and of themselves. They may also be dangerous because they are used instead of conventional medicine, which delays treatments that have been proven to be helpful. The term *alternative* was generally used in the past to describe most of the therapies that were not part of conventional medicine.

Proven treatments refer to evidence-based, conventional, mainstream, or standard medical treatments that have been tested following a strict set of guidelines and found to be safe and effective. The results of such clinical studies have been published in peer-reviewed journals—meaning that other doctors or scientists in the field evaluate the quality of the research and decide whether the article will be published. These treatments have been approved by the Food and Drug Administration (FDA).

Research or **investigational treatments** are therapies being studied in a clinical trial. Clinical trials are controlled research projects that determine whether a new treatment is effective and safe for patients. Before a drug or other treatment can be used regularly to treat patients, it is studied and tested carefully, first in laboratory test tubes and then in animals. After these studies are completed and the therapy is found safe and promising, it is tested to see if it helps patients. After careful testing among patients shows the drug or other treatment is safe and effective, the FDA may approve it for regular use. Only then does the treatment become part of the standard, conventional collection of proven therapies used to treat disease in human beings.

Complementary refers to supportive methods that are used to *complement*, or add to, conventional treatments. Complementary therapies may lessen the side effects of standard treatments or provide mental and physical benefits to the person with cancer. Examples of complementary methods include meditation (to reduce stress), peppermint tea (to relieve nausea), and acupuncture (to relieve chronic back pain). Methods now called complementary, such as massage therapy, yoga, and meditation, have actually been referred to as supportive *therapies* in the past.

Integrative therapy refers to the combined use of evidence-based proven therapies and complementary therapies. This is the term that many people in the field are using more frequently. In fact, integrative medicine services are becoming part of cancer centers and hospitals across the country.

Alternative treatments are unproven because they have not been scientifically tested, or they were tested and found to be ineffective.

Alternative treatments are used *instead of* conventional treatment. They may cause the patient to suffer, either from lack of or delay in helpful treatment or because the alternative treatment is actually harmful. They were also called *questionable therapies* in the past.

Quackery refers to the promotion of methods that claim to prevent, diagnose, or cure cancers that are known to be false or that are unproven. These methods are often based on the use of patient testimonials as evidence of their effectiveness and safety. Many times the treatment is claimed to be effective against other diseases as well as cancer.

Nontraditional is used in the same way as unconventional to describe complementary and alternative therapies; however, some therapies that seem nontraditional to modern American or European doctors may have been used in certain cultures for thousands of years, such as traditional Chinese medicine or traditional Native American medicine. These traditional native medicines are often used in complementary or alternative therapies.

How to Evaluate Claims

The claims about the effectiveness of these therapies range from the reasonable to the extraordinary. The most outrageous claim that some promoters make is that any alternative therapy can actually cure people with cancer. Even conventional cancer therapies, such as surgery, chemotherapy, and radiation therapy, cannot guarantee a cure. If certain cancers are diagnosed early enough in their development, conventional therapies may completely remove or destroy the cancer. Many cancer specialists do not even like to use the term *cure*, but prefer to say that a cancer is in *remission*. **Alternative therapies cannot cure cancer, and any claims for a cure should be treated with skepticism.**

The main appeal of many alternative cancer therapies is the promise of a cure. Another attraction is the claim that the alternative therapy not only cures cancer or prolongs the survival time of a person living with cancer but also has no bad side effects. People should also be skeptical of these claims. Promoters usually have no evidence to back up these claims, except, perhaps, testimonials from some people who have used the therapies. **The reality is that some alternative therapies can actually cause serious side effects, including allergic reactions, liver toxicity, heart problems, nutritional deficiencies, and harmful interactions with medications including cancer drugs** (see pages 8–10 for potential dangers). Other promoters of alternative therapies may claim their treatments can reduce the risk of developing cancer, stop the progression of cancer once it has occurred, or prevent cancer recurrences.

All claims should be evaluated on the basis of available scientific evidence to support them. Is there solid scientific evidence based on clinical trials to support the claim, or is the claim based solely on the word of the manufacturer, promoter, or certain people who have tried the therapy? Controlled human clinical trials of complementary and alternative cancer therapies are needed to evaluate the therapies. These studies are the gold standard, which provide scientific evidence about the effectiveness of a treatment in humans. Animal and laboratory studies may show that a certain therapy holds promise as an effective treatment, but further studies are necessary to determine if the results apply to humans.

Laws prohibit manufacturers and marketers of dietary supplements (such as vitamins, minerals, and herbal medicines) from claiming that their products can cure or prevent disease; however, companies are allowed to make claims that are not directly related to disease. For example, some state that their products "boost the immune system" to help the body fight disease naturally. This commonly used phrase leads one to believe that the product will increase the function of the immune

SIGNS OF POSSIBLE FRAUDULENT PRODUCTS

Claims that promote the product with such terms as *miracle cure, breakthrough,* or *new discovery.*

Claims that the product has benefits, but no side effects.

Claims that the product can be used for a wide variety of unrelated illnesses.

Claims that the treatment is safe and effective based solely on testimonials.

Claims that the treatment is based on a secret ingredient or method.

system. Yet, these statements are not evaluated by the FDA and are often made without any evidence to back them up. The same standard of proof should be held for claims that an herbal product or other type of complementary or alternative cancer therapy can inhibit the growth or spread of tumors or actually destroy cancer cells. In some cases, these claims may be based on solid evidence; in many other instances, they are not.

Dietary Supplements

Dietary supplements have received a great deal of attention over the past decade, but many people do not know much about them. If you take a vitamin pill regularly, you are taking a dietary supplement. That is, you are adding something to your diet of foods, most likely in an attempt to make up for a less-than-perfect diet, to promote good health, or to help speed healing when illness strikes.

The term *dietary supplement* includes vitamins, minerals, herbs, amino acids, and other products that are not already approved as drugs. Dietary supplements are sold through grocery stores, health food shops, drugstores, national discount chain stores, mail-order catalogs, television programs, the Internet, and direct sales. Vitamins are the supplements most often purchased in this country.

Dietary ingredients used in dietary supplements are not subject to the premarket safety evaluations required of other new food ingredients, such as "food additives." It is up to the manufacturer to ensure that the dietary supplement is safe and properly labeled before marketing. Dietary supplements can make claims regarding effects on nutrition (eg, works as an antioxidant), body function (eg, maintains a healthy circulatory system), and well-being (eg, helps you relax). Because these statements are not reviewed by the FDA prior to being sold to the public, manufacturers are required to include a disclaimer on the label: "This statement has not been evaluated by the FDA. This product is not intended to diagnose, treat, cure, or prevent any disease." Claims regarding effects on treating or preventing disease (eg, vitamin C prevents scurvy) require testing and approval by the FDA.

GUIDELINES FOR THE SAFE USE OF DIETARY SUPPLEMENTS

Rule One: Investigate before you buy or use. There are many resources in libraries and on the Internet; however, much of this information is produced by promoters and it contains biased or incorrect information. Rely on materials by reputable organizations, a recognized expert, or government agencies with which you are familiar.

Rule Two: Check with your doctor before you try a dietary supplement. He or she may or may not be thoroughly versed in all of the product areas, but hopefully your doctor will prevent you from making a dangerous mistake.

Rule Three: Do not take any self-prescribed remedy instead of the medicine prescribed by your doctor without discussing it first.

Rule Four: Introduce one product at a time. Be alert to any negative effects you experience while taking the product. Any product that produces a rash, sleeplessness, restlessness, anxiety, gastrointestinal disturbance (nausea, vomiting, diarrhea, or constipation), or severe headache should immediately be stopped, and the reaction should be reported to your doctor.

Rule Five: Avoid any dietary supplements not prescribed by a licensed doctor during pregnancy, or if you are breast-feeding. Few, if any, of these products have been studied for safety, and their effects on the growing fetus are largely unknown.

Rule Six: Don't depend on any nonprescription product to cure cancer or any other serious disease. Regardless of the claims you might hear, the old adage rings true: "If it sounds too good to be true, it probably is."

Rule Seven: Never give a supplement to a person younger than 18 years without consulting your doctor first. Their bodies metabolize nutrients and drugs differently from an adult's body, and the effects of many of these products in children are not known.

Rule Eight: Always follow the dosage recommendations on the label. Overdosage could be deadly. Do not take a dietary supplement any longer than experts recommend.

Rule Nine: Try to avoid mixtures. The more ingredients, the greater the possibility for harmful effects.

Botanicals as Medicine

The use of botanicals as medicine has been flourishing over the past 5 years. It is estimated that at least 4 billion people (80% of the world's population) use them for some aspect of primary health care. The term *botanical* includes plant materials, algae, macroscopic fungi, and any combination of these. Botanicals may consist of whole plants, mixtures of many plants, or specific plant parts, including roots, stems, flowers, leaves, pollen, and juices. The term *herbal* refers specifically to the leafy part of a plant. Depending on their intended use, botanical products may be considered food (including dietary supplements), drugs, medical devices, or cosmetics.

Buyer Be Aware

Labels can be confusing, and it is easy to misunderstand manufacturers' product claims. It is up to consumers to educate themselves. We are in a "let the buyer beware" mode when it comes to nutritional dietary supplements and herbal medicines. There are currently no requirements for proof of safety, accurate labeling, or proof of a health benefit for dietary supplements sold in the United States. Congress has seen the need to protect the public against harmful prescription medications, but this protection is not extended to dietary supplements sold directly to consumers.

The FDA has permission to stop production of a product only when the FDA proves that the product is dangerous to the health of Americans. Manufacturers still are not required to show that their products are safe or effective prior to marketing. The public has only limited protection against the marketing of products that often promise much and produce little if any benefit. Indeed, some products marketed in health food stores have recently been removed from shelves only after serious harm and even death from those products were reported.

The challenge to consumers is to determine which products are safe and which are not. Consumers should read the product label to be sure they are purchasing what they think they are. Some botanicals contain ingredients that can interact with conventional products or treatments or may interact with other dietary supplements or food products. **If a label on a dietary supplement makes a claim that the product can diagnose, treat, cure, or prevent disease, such as "cures cancer," the product is being sold illegally as a drug.**

Consumers should be aware of the ingredients in the herbal medicines and other dietary supplements they take and be wary of false claims. To help protect consumers, the FDA recommends that they:

- Look for products with the USP notation, indicating that the manufacturer of the product followed standards set by the *US Pharmacopoeia* in formulating the product.

- Realize that the use of the term *natural* on an herbal product is no guarantee that the product is safe. For example, poisonous mushrooms are natural but not safe.

- Take into account the name and reputation of the manufacturer or distributor. Herbal products and other dietary supplements made by nationally known food or drug manufacturers are more likely to have been made under tight quality controls because these companies have a reputation to uphold.

- Write to the manufacturer for more information than what is on the label of the supplement. Ask about the company's manufacturing practices and the quality-control conditions under which the product was made.

Potential Dangers

While some complementary and alternative treatments may be harmless and can restore feelings of hopefulness, not all of them are safe. Just because a practice is natural or legal does not mean it is harmless. Some treatments can interfere with the effectiveness of conventional medical therapies, including medications and anesthesia. There are very few scientific studies to guide us. More information is needed on the safety of these therapies. Some diet therapies actually cause nutritional deficiencies that interfere with the body's ability to heal and withstand the side effects of conventional treatment. Others may involve procedures that can lead to serious injury or infection. Many botanicals contain ingredients that can cause side effects, hazardous drug interactions, and allergic reactions. The possibility of drug supplement interactions is so high that cancer experts recommend that patients undergoing surgery, chemotherapy, or radiation therapy avoid taking dietary supplements at the same time.

GUIDELINES FOR USING COMPLEMENTARY AND ALTERNATIVE METHODS OF CANCER MANAGEMENT

Many people with cancer use one or more kinds of alternative or complementary therapies. They are often reluctant to tell their doctors or nurses about their decision. The best approach is to look carefully at your choices. When evaluating any complementary or alternative method, ask yourself the following questions.

- What claims are made for the treatment: To cure the cancer? To enable the conventional treatment to work better? To relieve symptoms or side effects?

- What are the credentials of those supporting the treatment? Are they recognized experts in cancer treatment? Have they published their findings in trustworthy medical journals?

- How is the method promoted? Is it promoted only in the mass media (books, magazines, TV, and radio talk shows) rather than in scientific journals?

- What are the costs of the therapy?

- Is the method widely available for use within the health care community, or is it controlled with limited access to its use?

- If used in place of conventional therapies or clinical trials, will the ensuing delay in conventional treatment affect any chances for cure or advance the cancer stage?

In addition, use the checklist below to spot those approaches that might be open to question. If you are not sure, talk to your doctor or nurse before moving ahead.

- Is the treatment based on an unproven theory?

- Does the treatment promise a cure for all cancers?

- Are you told not to use conventional medical treatment?

- Is the treatment or drug a secret that only certain people can give?

- Is the treatment or drug offered by only one individual?

- Does the treatment require you to travel to another country?

- Do the promoters attack the medical or scientific establishment?

It is very difficult for the public to know which of the many widespread alternatives are safe or provide any benefits at all. Laws and regulations protecting people from unsafe practices are sometimes vague, and few attempts are made to enforce those that do exist. Certainly, there is no law against traveling to another country for a treatment that is illegal or not available in the United States. Indeed, several treatments that are not considered effective by American doctors are used in conventional practice in European countries, which only increases the confusion for someone with cancer.

SUPPLEMENTS AND SURGERY

A number of ingredients sold in supplements can produce severe swings in blood pressure and other dangerous interactions with anesthetics and, therefore, should not be taken before surgery. In fact, the American Society of Anesthesiologists advises that patients stop taking herbal medications at least 2 to 3 weeks before surgery to allow enough time for the herbals to clear from the body. If the patient does not have enough time to stop taking herbal medicines before surgery, he or she should bring the product to the hospital and show the anesthesiologist what it is.

It is also unfortunate when those with very advanced disease turn to unconventional therapy because they believe they have "nothing to lose." People have been known to spend their remaining weeks receiving ineffective and expensive treatments overseas. Family members later report regretting the decisions that they made as they reflect on the suffering of their loved one.

The promises made by the proponents of some of these treatments create false hope and can cost a significant amount of money. What often causes so much dismay among conventional practitioners is that alternative therapies sometimes steer people away from treatment that would have been effective had it not been delayed. The greatest danger in alternative medicine for people with cancer lies in losing the best opportunity to help treat cancer and prolong survival with conventional therapy. **Unnecessary delays and interruptions in conventional therapies are dangerous.**

Talking with Your Health Care Team

About 60% of all people who use complementary or alternative therapies do not tell members of their health care team they are trying these treatments. Many people feel uncomfortable asking their doctor or nurse about complementary or alternative treatments. But most health care professionals understand that patients and caregivers want to do all they can to improve their quality of life or improve the quality of life for their loved ones. Although people may be reluctant to share their complementary or alternative therapy interests with their health care team, it could be dangerous to the health of the person with cancer to withhold information.

Talk to your health care team about any methods you are considering. Consider the risks and benefits of using any complementary or alternative methods and make an informed decision in an atmosphere of shared decision-making. There are many complementary methods you can safely use along with conventional treatment to help relieve symptoms or side effects, to ease pain, and to help you enjoy life more.

If you are considering using complementary or alternative therapies, here are some tips for your discussion with your doctor and other members of your health care team:

Educate yourself first. Before beginning a conversation with them, research the proven conventional treatment for your disease. It is important to be as informed as possible before the office visit. Then, find out as much as you can about the alternative method that you wish to discuss. Some questions for patients to ask the doctor are: What do you know about this alternative? Can you give me additional sources of information? Do you know someone who tried the alternative method? What was their experience?

When looking at information (especially on the Internet), try to determine whether or not the information is provided by someone selling a product. If a product is being promoted for sale, then the information will likely be slanted toward helping to sell the product. The objectivity and accuracy of the information may not be reliable.

Let your health care team know before beginning an alternative. Tell them that you are thinking about taking an alternative therapy but that you want to make sure it does not interfere with the prescribed treatment. Once the treatment is recorded in your medical record, your doctor will be able to watch for potential drug interactions and/or harmful effects.

Ask questions. It can be helpful to write down a list of questions for your health care team and bring in any literature you want to discuss. Let them know you are an educated consumer—even though you may be apprehensive about what you are facing, you are seeking as much information as you can. Let them know you want them to be supportive partners in your education and treatment process.

Bring someone with you to the doctor's office. A friend or relative can help you retain information, ask questions, and remain more objective than you may be able to alone. Support from your loved ones will not only help you communicate but can also help lessen the stress of making decisions alone.

Understand your health care team's perspective. If you take herbs or megadoses of vitamins or start on a special diet, they need to know. Some therapies are considered alternative because they have not been proven to be safe and effective in controlled scientific studies. People with cancer who rely on alternative therapies may run the risk of jeopardizing their primary treatment because of possible drug interactions, or they may harm themselves with unsafe methods. If your health care team has not heard of the particular method, don't become discouraged. Ask them to help you find out more about it.

Don't delay or forego conventional therapy. If you are considering stopping or not taking current conventional treatment, discuss the implications of this decision with your health care team. You may be giving up the only proven treatment for your cancer.

If you're taking dietary supplements, review your usage. Whenever you receive new medication or there is a change in medication or medical history, review the list of supplements you are taking with your doctor or nurse. Also, let your health care team know if you change or add any dietary supplements. By telling your health care providers about supplement use, the medical record can be used to analyze the risks, benefits, and interactions with medications.

Ask about the use of alternative therapies if you are pregnant or breast-feeding. Most herbalists advise not using alternative medicines if you are. Do not give alternative medicine to children.

Ask your health care team to help you identify possible fraudulent products.

Follow up with your health care team. On your next office visit, be sure to continue your conversation about your use of any alternative therapies. Discuss any decision you have reached about using an alternative method. They may or may not agree with your decision, but it's important that they know if you're planning to use alternative therapies so that they can provide you with the best possible care.

Be open to change. Realize that new studies may yield new information about complementary and alternative methods of managing cancer that may change your treatment plan.

The Position of the American Cancer Society (ACS)

The ACS believes that all cancer interventions must withstand the scrutiny of scientific evaluation before they can be recommended for the prevention, diagnosis, or treatment of cancer. The following are questions that researchers, doctors, and other health care professionals use when evaluating treatment:

- Has the method been objectively demonstrated in peer-reviewed scientific literature to be more effective than doing nothing?

- Has the method shown a potential for benefit that clearly exceeds the potential for harm?

- Have objective studies been conducted properly, appropriately evaluated by other qualified scientists, and approved by responsible human studies committees to answer these questions?

The ACS urges individuals with cancer to remain in the care of doctors who use standard, conventional therapies for cancer and approved clinical trials of promising new treatments. The ACS also encourages patients to talk openly with their health care providers about any other therapy they are considering, and to seek information from unbiased and reliable sources.

Open, trusting, noncritical communication is essential in making health care decisions. In this way, you will be able to make informed decisions by selecting methods most likely to be safe and effective in relieving symptoms and improving your well-being. You will also be able to avoid methods that are dangerous, likely to interfere with conventional treatments, and known to be ineffective. Contact the ACS at 1-800-ACS-2345 (www.cancer.org) for the latest information about treatment and complementary or alternative medicine.

CHAPTER ONE

MIND, BODY, AND SPIRIT METHODS

THIS CATEGORY INCLUDES METHODS that focus on the connections between the mind, body, and spirit, and their power for healing.

▄ AROMATHERAPY

OTHER COMMON NAME(S): Holistic Aromatherapy, Aromatic Medicine

There is no scientific evidence that aromatherapy is effective in preventing or treating cancer, but it can be used to enhance quality of life. Early clinical trials suggest aromatherapy may have some benefit as a complementary treatment in reducing stress, pain, and depression.

DESCRIPTION: Aromatherapy is the use of fragrant substances distilled from plants, called essential oils, to alter mood or improve health. These highly concentrated aromatic substances are either inhaled or applied as oils during massage. There are approximately 40 essential oils commonly used in aromatherapy; among the most popular are lavender, rosemary, eucalyptus, chamomile, marjoram, jasmine, peppermint, and geranium.

Aromatherapy is promoted as a natural way to help patients cope with chronic pain, depression, and stress and produce a feeling of well-being. There is some evidence suggesting this may be true. Proponents also claim aromatherapy can help relieve bacterial infections; stimulate the immune system; fight colds, flu, and sore throats; improve urine production; increase circulation; and cure cystitis, herpes simplex, acne, headaches, indigestion, PMS, muscle tension, and even cancer. However, there is no scientific evidence to support these further claims. Fragrances from different oils are promoted to have specific health benefits. For example, lavender oil is promoted to relieve muscular tension, anxiety, and insomnia.

USE: Aromatherapy is either self-administered or applied by a practitioner. Many aromatherapists in the United States are trained as massage therapists, psychologists, social workers, or chiropractors and use the oils as part of their practices.

The essential oils, which are used individually or in combination, may be inhaled or applied to the skin. For inhalation, a few drops of the essential oil are placed in steaming water, diffusers, or humidifiers that are used to spread the steam/oil combination throughout the room.

Essential oils can be applied to the skin during massage, or they can be added to bathwater. For application to the skin, the oils are combined with a carrier, usually vegetable oil. Some people also apply drops of certain essential oils on their pillows.

EFFECTS: There is no scientific evidence that aromatherapy cures or prevents disease; however, a few clinical studies suggest aromatherapy may be a beneficial complementary therapy. In Britain, there are reports of the successful use of aromatherapy massage as a complementary treatment for people with cancer to reduce anxiety, depression, tension, and pain. There are also reports that inhaled peppermint, ginger, and cardamom oil seem to relieve the nausea caused by chemotherapy and radiation; however, these reports have not been scientifically proven.

Essential oils should never be taken internally, as many of them are poisonous. Also, people should avoid exposure for a long time, because some may have allergic reactions to the oils.

▚ ART THERAPY

OTHER COMMON NAME(S): None

Many clinicians have observed and documented significant benefits among people who have participated in art therapy. Art therapy has not undergone rigorous scientific study to determine its therapeutic value for people with cancer.

DESCRIPTION: Art therapy is a form of treatment used to help people with physical and emotional problems by using creative activities to express emotions. It provides a way for people to come to terms with emotional conflicts, increase self-awareness, and express unspoken and often unconscious concerns about their disease.

Art therapy has been used to treat burn patients, people with eating disorders, emotionally impaired young people, people with disabilities, the chronically ill, chemically addicted individuals, sexually abused adolescents, and others. Art therapy may also be used to distract patients whose diseases or treatments cause pain.

Proponents use artwork as a diagnostic tool, particularly with children, who often have difficulty talking about painful events or emotions. Art therapists say that often children can express difficult emotions or relay information about traumatic times in their lives more easily through drawings than in conventional therapy.

USE: People involved in art therapy are provided with the tools necessary to produce paintings, drawings, sculptures, and other types of artwork. Art therapists work with patients individually or in groups. The job of the art therapist is to help patients express themselves through their creations and to discuss patients' emotions and concerns as they relate to their art. For example, an art therapist may encourage a person with cancer to create an image of themselves with cancer and in this way express feelings about the disease that may be difficult to verbalize or may be unconscious.

In another form of art therapy, patients view pieces of art, often in photographs, and then talk with a therapist about what they have seen. A caregiver or family member can also gather artwork in the form of photographs, books or prints and give the patient an opportunity to look at and enjoy the art.

Many medical centers and hospitals include art therapy as part of inpatient care. It can be practiced in many other settings, such as schools, psychiatric centers, drug and alcohol rehabilitation programs, prisons, day care treatment programs, nursing homes, hospices, patients' homes, and art studios.

EFFECTS: Numerous case studies have reported art therapy benefits patients with both emotional and physical illnesses. Case studies have involved many areas, including burn recovery in adolescent and young children, eating disorders, emotional impairment in young children, reading performance, chemical addiction, childhood grief, and sexual abuse in adolescents. Some of the potential uses of art therapy to be researched include reducing anxiety levels, improving recovery times, decreasing hospital stays, and pain control.

Art therapy is considered safe and may be useful as a complementary therapy to help people with cancer deal with their emotions. Although uncomfortable feelings may be stirred up at times, this is considered part of the healing process.

⬛ AYURVEDA

OTHER COMMON NAME(S): Ayurvedic Medicine

Ayurveda is one of several ancient Asian healing systems that have recently gained popularity in the West. While the effectiveness of many aspects of Ayurveda has not been scientifically proven, some preliminary research suggests certain components may offer potential therapeutic value.

DESCRIPTION: Ayurveda (pronounced eye-yer-vay-duh), meaning knowledge of life, is an ancient Indian system of medicine that has an integrated approach to the prevention and treatment of disease, which tries to maintain or reestablish the harmony between the mind, body, and forces of nature. It combines a variety of interventions, such as changes in lifestyle, herbal remedies, exercise, and meditation.

A central idea in Ayurveda is that disease occurs when a person's physical, emotional, and spiritual forces are out of balance with each other, resulting in disharmony with the natural environment. One of the primary goals of Ayurveda is to restore this balance and invigorate the body's biological and spiritual forces. Practitioners claim certain combinations of Ayurvedic interventions, matched to a patient's unique physical and emotional needs and personal medical history, increase physical vitality, foster spiritual well-being, bring individuals into harmony with the world, and even prevent and cure disease.

USE: Practitioners of Ayurveda may combine dietary programs, herbal remedies, intestinal cleansing preparations, yoga, meditation, massage, breathing exercises, and visual imagery to treat their patients (see Massage, Meditation, Imagery, and Yoga). Ayurvedic herbal preparations often consist of complex mixtures of plants. An estimated 1250 plants are used by practitioners. Some of the more controversial and less common practices of Ayurveda include bloodletting, bowel purging, and inducing vomiting.

To diagnose disease, Ayurveda practitioners closely observe a patient's tongue, nails, lips, and body's 9 "doors": both eyes, ears, and nostrils, and the mouth, genitalia, and anus. They also listen carefully to the lungs, check the pulse, and take a detailed history of the patient's life and health. Through these observations, practitioners claim to evaluate a patient's *doshas*. According to Ayurveda practitioners, doshas not only enable the various organs of the body to work together, they also establish a person's connection to the environment and the cosmos.

When formulating a plan of treatment, Ayurveda practitioners consider the state of a patient's doshas and the complex relationship between the doshas and other factors such as emotions, disease, physical activity, lifestyle, diet, relationships with other people, and even the four seasons, colors, and the time of day. Practitioners strive to harmonize all of these factors so that their patients can attain health and well-being.

EFFECTS: Although Ayurveda has been largely untested by Western researchers, there is a growing interest in integrating some components of the system into modern medical practice. Some preliminary studies suggest Ayurveda may have potential therapeutic value.

According to a report of a panel convened by the National Institutes of Health, one clinical study showed that in 79% of cases, the health of patients with various chronic diseases improved measurably after Ayurvedic treatment. Laboratory and clinical studies have suggested that some Ayurvedic herbal preparations may have the potential to prevent and treat certain cancers, including breast, lung, and colon cancers; however, further study is needed to make conclusions about the role of Ayurveda in cancer prevention and treatment. The National Cancer Institute has funded a series of laboratory studies to evaluate Ayurvedic herbal remedies.

Some aspects of Ayurveda, such as bloodletting and inducing vomiting, can be harmful. Many people with cancer already have low blood cell counts as a consequence of the disease itself, and removing additional blood can worsen fatigue and other symptoms. Inducing vomiting can cause imbalances of electrolytes (salt and minerals) in the blood. In addition, the potential interactions between Ayurvedic herbal preparations and conventional drugs and other herbal medications should be taken into consideration. Some of these combinations may be dangerous. Relying on this type of treatment alone, and avoiding conventional medical care, may have serious health consequences.

■ BIOENERGETICS

OTHER COMMON NAME(S): Bioenergetic Therapy, Bioenergetic Medicine, Bioenergetic Analysis

There is no scientific evidence that bioenergetics is effective in treating cancer; however, some patients report it is useful as a relaxation method.

DESCRIPTION: Bioenergetics is a complementary therapy that involves psychotherapy, relaxation techniques, and gentle touch to relieve muscle tension. Proponents believe the body "records" negative emotional reactions and stores them in the form of muscle tension and stiffness, poor posture, and low energy levels. To release these trapped emotions and return the body and mind to a balanced, healthy, peaceful state, they say patients must first release muscle tension and correct physical imbalances. Proponents further claim bioenergetics can offer relief from the side effects of cancer treatment and even strengthen the body's ability to fight disease, although there is no scientific evidence to support this claim.

They also believe disease is a part of the life process and that serious diseases, including cancer, are symptoms of underlying imbalances caused by factors such as poor diet, exposure to toxins, genetic history, and repressed emotions. They claim that by balancing electrical and energy disturbances within the patient and eliminating toxins, the body will heal itself (see Electromagnetic Therapy).

USE: Therapists of bioenergetics use a combination of psychotherapy, gentle body movements, massage, deep breathing, and exercises that involve crying, screaming, and kicking in an effort to help patients "release" their emotional memories. They claim they can "read" a patient's muscular movements, tone of voice, breathing, posture, and emotions to determine his or her physical and psychological problems. The therapy may also incorporate aspects of traditional Chinese medicine, biofeedback, herbal medicine, homeopathy, and nutrition (see Acupuncture, Biofeedback, Chinese Herbal Medicine, and Homeopathy).

EFFECTS: Some patients may feel more relaxed and at ease after a bioenergetics therapy session; however, there is no scientific evidence that bioenergetics is useful in treating cancer or any other disease. No studies have been published in medical journals to show that it offers any long-term physical or psychological benefits.

People with cancer and chronic conditions, such as arthritis and heart disease, should consult their doctor before undergoing any type of therapy that involves the manipulation of joints and muscles. Relying on this type of treatment alone, and avoiding conventional medical care, may have serious health consequences.

▮ BIOFEEDBACK

OTHER COMMON NAME(S): None

Biofeedback is one of several relaxation methods that has been approved by an independent panel, convened by the National Institutes of Health (NIH), as a useful complementary therapy for treating chronic pain and insomnia. There is no scientific evidence that biofeedback can influence the development or progression of cancer; however, it can help to improve the quality of life for some people with cancer.

DESCRIPTION: Biofeedback is a treatment method that uses monitoring devices to help people consciously regulate physiological processes that are usually controlled automatically. Through changing autonomic processes such as heart rate, skin temperature, breathing rate, muscle control, and other physiological activity in the body, biofeedback can reduce stress and muscle tension from a variety of causes. It can promote relaxation, correct urinary incontinence, treat migraines, and lessen serious headaches. It helps people with Raynaud's disease (a blood circulation condition that causes the fingers and toes to feel very cold) increase the temperature of their hands and toes. Biofeedback is also useful in retraining muscles after injury or teaching new muscles to take over.

USE: Various monitoring devices are used to provide biofeedback information so that mental processes can be adjusted to control bodily functions. Under the guidance of a biofeedback therapist, the patient concentrates on changing a specific physiological process. A monitor hooked via electrodes to the patient's skin measures changes in whichever function is to be altered. Tones or images produced by the monitor inform the patient when the desired results have been achieved. The process is repeated as often as necessary until the patient can reliably use conscious thought to change physical functions.

There are at least 5 different ways to measure body functions for biofeedback purposes. An electromyogram (EMG) measures muscle tension. It is used to help heal muscle injuries, relieve chronic pain, and control some types of incontinence. Thermal biofeedback provides information about skin temperature, which is a good indicator of blood flow. Several health problems are related to blood flow, such as migraine headaches, Raynaud's disease, anxiety, and high blood pressure. Electrodermal activity (EDA) shows changes in perspiration rates, which is used in treating anxiety. Finger pulse measurements are used to reflect high blood pressure, heartbeat irregularities, and anxiety. Breathing rate is also monitored, which is used to treat asthma and hyperventilation and to promote relaxation.

EFFECTS: Although biofeedback has no direct effect on the development or progression of cancer, it can improve the quality of life for some people with cancer. Research has found that biofeedback can be helpful for patients in regaining urinary and bowel continence following surgery. In one well-controlled human study, relaxation therapy was more effective than biofeedback in reducing some side effects of chemotherapy.

After examining data on biofeedback, an NIH panel found the technique to be moderately effective for relieving many types of chronic pain, particularly tension headaches, and that it alleviates some types of insomnia. The panel also found that biofeedback was better than relaxation therapy for treating migraine headaches. The effects of biofeedback vary significantly from person to person.

Biofeedback is considered a safe technique. It is noninvasive and requires little effort, although a trained and certified professional is necessary to control monitoring equipment and interpret changes. Battery-operated devices sold for home use have not been found to be reliable.

BREATHWORK

OTHER COMMON NAME(S): None

Breathwork is the general term used to describe a variety of breathing techniques that are implemented in many relaxation exercises and spiritual healing methods. Focused, deep breathing exercises, such as exaggerating the way a person naturally inhales and exhales, is said to promote relaxation, awareness, and emotional release. Shallow breathing is an indicator of stress, so the goal in breathwork is to take long, deep breaths. These breaths are said to be "cleansing," freeing both the body and mind from toxins that prohibit a healthy state. There is no scientific evidence to support this claim; however, breathwork may help in relaxation and stress reduction (see Imagery and Meditation).

CRYSTALS

OTHER COMMON NAME(S): Crystal Healing

There is no scientific evidence that crystals are effective in treating cancer or any other disease; however, there are some anecdotal reports that crystals can be used as a method to promote relaxation and relieve stress.

DESCRIPTION: Crystals such as quartz, malachite, and other gemstones are used to treat a wide variety of physical and emotional conditions including bursitis, headaches, indigestion, insomnia, hemorrhages, rheumatism, thrombosis, forgetfulness, anxiety, depression, Parkinson's disease, blindness, and cancer. Proponents claim certain gemstones or crystals contain special energy that can be transferred to an individual to provide protection against disease, restore health, and provide spiritual guidance. There is no scientific evidence to support these claims.

Most supporters do not claim that stones or crystals can cure disease directly. They say certain stones and crystals emit vibrations that can correct underlying problems. It is thought that disease occurs when an individual is misaligned with the divine energy (or light) believed to be the foundation of all creation. The application of stones or crystals within specific energy centers, called *chakras*, creates a flow of energy that promotes healing by clearing, balancing, and re-energizing the body's energy fields (called auras; see Electromagnetic Therapy).

USE: Crystal therapists claim to intuitively determine where "blockages" of energy are located and then place particular stones or crystals on specific parts of the body. Different types and colors of stones or crystals are promoted to have different healing powers. For example, amethysts are thought to calm the mind, red-orange agates are thought to energize, and bloodstones are thought to purify the blood. Each one is chosen based on the individual's needs and energy fields.

Some people carry crystals in their pockets, wear them on a chain, or place them in the house to bring the power of healing within reach. Crystals are sometimes used along with other methods such as acupuncture, meditation, and polarity therapy (see Acupuncture, Meditation, and Polarity Therapy).

EFFECTS: There is no scientific evidence that crystals are useful in promoting healing. Some crystals have the ability to bend light, which creates a rainbow effect. Phosphorescent crystals can hold light for a short time, but they do not have their own energy source or special powers. Some people believe that crystals or gemstones are helpful as a complementary treatment to promote relaxation and reduce stress. This may occur as a result of the "placebo effect" in which believing that something can or will happen generates a positive result.

Crystals are considered relatively safe; however, relying on this type of treatment alone, and avoiding conventional medical care, may have serious health consequences.

▨ CURANDERISMO

OTHER COMMON NAME(S): Curanderos, Latin American Healing

There is no scientific evidence that curanderismo is effective in treating cancer or any other disease; however, there are some anecdotal reports that curanderismo helps to improve physical ailments, reduce pain, and relieve stress.

DESCRIPTION: Curanderismo is a form of folk healing that includes various techniques such as herbal medicine, healing rituals, elements of spiritualism, and psychic healing (see Homeopathy, and Spirituality and Prayer). It is a system of traditional beliefs that are common in Hispanic-American communities, particularly those in the southwestern United States.

Proponents claim folk illnesses such as *mal de ojo* (the evil eye), *susto* (fright), and *empacho* (blockage of the digestive tract) can be treated by curanderismo. In these cases, the curandero may perform *barridas*, a ritual cleansing, to rebalance the body and soul of the sick person. They also claim curanderismo can be used to treat a wide range of physical complaints, including headache, gastrointestinal distress, back pain, and fever, as well as emotional problems such as anxiety, irritability, fatigue, and depression. There is no scientific evidence to support these claims.

USE: While some aspects of curanderismo are practiced at home for mild cases of illness, most people seek out specially trained folk healers called *curanderos* who believe their healing powers are gained through divine inspiration. They believe good health is achieved by maintaining a balance of hot and cold. In order to treat a person, curanderos often classify that person's physical activities, food intake, drugs consumed, and diseases as hot or cold and treat the person to restore a balance of both. The healing often involves others in the family and community.

The treatments given by curanderos can vary widely depending upon the nature of the disease or complaint. The techniques can involve the use of herbs, massage, manipulation of body parts, spiritual rituals, and prayer, either in combination or by themselves. For example, one cure for a headache is to place a slice of raw potato over each temple. Dandruff is treated by rinsing hair with juice from the olivera plant, a type of cactus. To reduce the size of an overly large "energy field," the curandero may beat the air around the patient's head with a large feather, then roll an egg around the patient's face before cracking it open into a glass.

EFFECTS: There is no scientific evidence that curanderismo cures cancer or any other disease, although some people report it helps to reduce pain, relieve stress, and promote spiritual peace. A study in 1977 that looked at the relationship between Mexican-American populations and folk medicine suggested that curanderismo should be looked at more closely by conventional medicine. Researchers proposed that a better understanding of folk medicine, such as curanderismo, might help doctors treat their patients more effectively and understand patient fears and beliefs. A more recent study found that patients often seek treatment by curanderismo alongside conventional medical treatment.

There are no known harmful effects of curanderismo; however, some treatment by curanderos may involve the ingestion of unregulated herbs and teas. Relying on this type of treatment alone, and avoiding conventional medical care, may have serious health consequences.

▚ CYMATIC THERAPY

OTHER COMMON NAME(S): None

Cymatic therapy is a form of sound therapy developed by Sir Peter Guy Manners, MD, DO, PhD, from England. According to practitioners, disease appears when the rhythms of the heart, brain, and other organs are not working harmoniously. Although no sounds can be heard by those treated with this method, hand-held instruments are used to transmit sound waves through the skin. The signals passed through these cymatic devices are supposed to restore synchronous rhythms and boost the body's regulatory and immunologic systems. There is no scientific evidence to support this claim (see Music Therapy).

▚ DANCE THERAPY

OTHER COMMON NAME(S): Movement Therapy

There have been few scientific studies conducted to evaluate the effects of dance therapy on health, prevention, and recovery from illness. Clinical reports suggest dance therapy is effective in improving self-esteem and reducing stress. As a form of exercise, dance therapy can be useful.

DESCRIPTION: Dance therapy is the therapeutic use of movement to improve the mental and physical well-being of a person. It focuses on the connection between the mind and body to promote health and healing. Through dance, it is thought that people can identify and express their innermost emotions, bringing those feelings to the surface. Some people claim this can create a sense of renewal, unity, and completeness.

Dance therapy is offered as a health promotion service for healthy people and as a complementary method of reducing the stress of caregivers and people with cancer and other chronic diseases. Physically, dance therapy can provide exercise, improve mobility and muscle coordination, and reduce muscle tension. Emotionally, dance therapy is reported to improve self-awareness, self-confidence, and interpersonal interaction and is an outlet for communicating feelings. Some promoters claim that dance therapy may strengthen the immune system through muscular action and physiological processes and even help prevent disease. There is no scientific evidence to confirm the effects of dance therapy on prevention and recovery from illness.

USE: Dance therapists help people develop a nonverbal language that offers information about what is going on in their bodies. The therapist observes a person's movements to make an assessment and then designs a program to help the specific condition. The frequency and level of difficulty of the therapy are usually tailored to meet the needs of the participants.

Dance therapy is used in a variety of settings with people who have social, emotional, cognitive, or physical concerns. It is often used as a part of the recovery process for people with chronic disease. Dance therapists work with both individuals and groups, including entire families.

EFFECTS: Although anecdotal accounts provide support for the value of dance therapy, few studies evaluating the effects of dance therapy on health have been published. Clinical reports suggest that dance therapy helps in developing body image; improving self-concept and self-esteem; reducing stress, anxiety, and depression; decreasing isolation, chronic pain, and body tension; and increasing communication skills and feelings of well-being. Well-controlled research is needed to confirm the effects of dance therapy on prevention and recovery of illness or disease.

Some of the physical motions of dance therapy can be useful exercises that provide similar health benefits gained through exercise. Physical activity has been shown to increase special neurotransmitter substances in the brain (endorphins) that create a state of well-being. And total body movement enhances the functions of other body systems, such as circulatory, respiratory, skeletal, and muscular systems. Dance therapy can help people stay physically fit and enjoy the pleasure of creating rhythmic motions with their bodies.

People with cancer and chronic conditions such as arthritis and heart disease should consult with their doctor before undergoing any type of therapy that involves manipulation of joints and muscles.

■ FAITH HEALING

OTHER COMMON NAME(S): Spiritual Healing

There is no scientific evidence that faith healing can cure cancer or any other disease. Even the "miraculous" cures at the French shrine of Lourdes, after careful study by the Catholic Church, do not outnumber the spontaneous remissions seen among people with cancer; however, faith healing may promote peace of mind, reduce stress, relieve pain and anxiety, and strengthen the will to live.

DESCRIPTION: Faith healing is founded on the belief that certain people or places have the ability to cure and heal—that someone or something can eliminate disease or heal injuries through a close connection to a higher power. Faith healing can involve prayer, a visit to a religious shrine, or simply a strong belief in a supreme being.

According to proponents, there is little that faith healing cannot do. They claim it can cure blindness, deafness, cancer, AIDS, developmental disorders, anemia, arthritis, corns, defective speech, multiple sclerosis, rashes, and total body paralysis and heal various injuries. Christian Scientists claim that disease is an illusion caused by bad thoughts. The disease can be healed or made to leave the sick person's body by trained practitioners through prayer. There is no scientific evidence to support these claims.

USE: Faith healing is practiced either at a distance from or in close proximity to the patient. When practiced from afar, it can involve a single faith healer or a group of individuals praying for the patient. When near to the patient, as in revivalist tent meetings, the healer touches, or "lays hands on," the patient while invoking a supreme being. Faith healing can also involve a pilgrimage to a religious shrine, such as the French shrine at Lourdes, in search of a miracle. Christian Scientists train and use their own practitioners to heal sick persons through prayer.

EFFECTS: Although it is known that a small percentage of people with cancer experience remissions of their disease that cannot be explained, there is no scientific evidence that faith healing can actually cure physical ailments. When a person has a strong belief that a healer can create a cure, a placebo effect can occur, which makes the person feel better. The placebo effect is an improvement that occurs because of a powerful belief in the treatment. The patient usually credits the improvement to the healer. Taking part in faith healing can evoke the power of suggestion, promoting peace of mind. This can help people cope more effectively with their disease.

One review published in 1998 looked at 172 cases of fatalities among children treated by faith healing instead of conventional methods. These researchers found that if conventional treatment had been given, the survival rate for these children could have exceeded 90%, with the remainder of the children also having a good chance of survival. There are some organizations working towards creating laws to protect children from inappropriate treatment by faith healers.

People who seek help through faith healing and are not cured can develop feelings of hopelessness, failure, guilt, worthlessness, and depression. Relying on this type of treatment alone, and avoiding conventional medical care, may have serious health consequences.

█ FENG SHUI

OTHER COMMON NAME(S): None

The ancient Chinese art of feng shui rests on placement of things so that they are in harmony with one another and with the environment. There is no scientific evidence to support the claim that feng shui can influence health.

DESCRIPTION: Feng shui (pronounced fung-shway) is the ancient Chinese philosophy and art of placing objects, ornaments, furniture, rooms, buildings, and even towns in positions that promote the beneficial flow of vital energy or life force called *qi* (or *chi*). The words *feng shui* literally mean wind and water. Adherents to feng shui hold that the same natural elements that form the earth, such as wind and water, can bring healthy energy into homes, buildings, and cities if the placement of these man-made elements permits energy to flow through the environment.

By extension, some believe that living and work environments that are out of balance may promote disease, including cancer, and prevent those who live in the environment from responding to treatment. Changes in the environment, proponents claim, may help prevent disease and promote healing. For example, simply placing the bed of a person with cancer, or at risk of cancer, in a new position is thought to prevent the development or progression of the disease.

USE: The idea behind feng shui is to orient physical objects to allow humankind to live in harmony with the environment and the universe. To accomplish this goal, a feng shui practitioner will first study the physical environment outside a person's home to make sure the house is positioned in a way that will promote a positive flow of energy. Next, the inside of the house is examined. Furniture may be moved or set at angles until rooms are more open and free of clutter or obstacles that may hinder energy from flowing around the house. A feng shui practitioner will also analyze the electromagnetic energy in a person's home, sometimes using a specialized compass, and in the surrounding property to make sure the energy is balanced in order to promote good health and well-being.

EFFECTS: There is no scientific evidence that feng shui has any effect on cancer or any other disease. No adverse effects have been reported with the use of feng shui; however, consultants in feng shui are not licensed, and relying on this type of treatment, and avoiding conventional medical care, may have serious health consequences.

▨ HOLISTIC MEDICINE

OTHER COMMON NAME(S): Holistic Health, Holism

There is no scientific evidence that holistic medicine alone is effective in treating cancer or any other disease; however, many health professionals promote healthy lifestyle habits such as exercising, eating a nutritious diet, and not smoking as important in maintaining good health. Holistic methods can be used as complementary therapy.

DESCRIPTION: Holistic medicine focuses on how the physical, mental, emotional, and spiritual elements of the body are interconnected to maintain wellness (holistic health). When one part of the body is not working properly, it is believed to affect the whole person. The treatment concentrates on the whole body rather than focusing narrowly on the disease or part of the body that is not healthy.

Holistic medicine approaches health and disease from several angles and suggests that a person should not only treat the disease but the whole self—to reach a higher level of wellness. For example, patients treat disease by changing diet and behavior, taking botanical supplements, and undergoing various complementary therapies (see Acupuncture, Aromatherapy, Art Therapy, Hypnosis, Psychotherapy, Spirituality and Prayer, and Yoga). These approaches can be used along with conventional medicine such as chemotherapy, surgery, radiation therapy, and hormone therapy. By combining these different techniques, a person can take control of the disease and obtain a feeling of total wellness—spiritually, physically, and mentally.

Some proponents claim that conventional medicine does not work and that only the holistic approach to cancer and other diseases is effective. They offer not just a treatment but a "cure" for many different kinds of cancer based on anecdotal reports or personal experience. There is no scientific evidence to support these claims.

USE: The field of holistic medicine is very diverse. Some providers define holistic oncology as care that doesn't ignore emotional and spiritual aspects, while others focus on these aspects to the exclusion of the physical. There are many different techniques and approaches in holistic medicine, depending on the person and the disease. In any case, all styles stress the use of treatments that encourage the body's natural healing system and take into consideration the person as a whole.

Holistic medicine can involve the use of conventional and alternative therapies but focuses mostly on lifestyle changes. Holistic medicine can also include natural supplements that cause the same changes as conventional drugs. The American Holistic Association says that healthy lifestyle habits will improve a person's energy and vitality. Those habits might include exercising, eating a nutritious diet, getting enough sleep, learning how to breath properly, taking antioxidants and supplements, acupuncture, and other methods.

EFFECTS: Some doctors suggest that cancer pain and some side effects of treatment can be managed by incorporating different aspects of holistic medicine that include the physical, psychological, and spiritual factors involved with each individual. Increasingly, the health care team, such as nurses, psychiatrists, social workers, dieticians, clergy, and others, plays an important role in the treatment provided by many research centers and hospitals. Health professionals realize that a person's health depends on the balance of physical, psychological, social, and cultural forces. Adopting healthy habits related to diet, exercise, and emotional and spiritual well-being are considered important to maintaining good health.

Although there has been research on various complementary methods that may be considered part of a holistic approach, there is no research focusing on holistic medicine by itself as a cure for cancer or any other disease. Relying on this type of treatment alone, and avoiding conventional medical care, may have serious health consequences.

▨ HUMOR THERAPY

OTHER COMMON NAME(S): Laugh Therapy

Although there is no scientific evidence that laughter can cure cancer or any other disease, it can reduce stress, promote health, and enhance the quality of life. Humor has physiological effects that can stimulate the circulatory system, immune system, and other systems in the body.

DESCRIPTION: Humor therapy is the use of humor or laughter for the relief of physical and emotional difficulties. It is used as a complementary tool to promote health and cope with disease, improve quality of life, provide some pain relief, encourage relaxation, and reduce stress. Researchers have described different types of humor. For example, passive humor is created by observing a comic film or reading a book. Humor production is a type of humor that involves creating or finding humor in stressful situations. It is thought that being able to find humor in everyday events can be helpful.

USE: The physical effects of laughter on the body involve increased breathing, oxygen use, and heart rate, which stimulate the circulatory system. Many hospitals and ambulatory care centers have incorporated special rooms where humorous materials, and sometimes people, are there to help make people laugh. Materials commonly used include movies, audio and videotapes, books, games, and puzzles. Many hospitals use volunteer groups who visit patients for the purpose of providing opportunities for laughter.

EFFECTS: There is no scientific evidence that humor is effective in treating cancer or any other disease; however, laughter has many clinical benefits that include positive physiological changes and an overall sense of well-being. Humor therapy is considered safe when used as a complementary therapy.

Research has been done on the effects of humor on pain and stress relief. One study found the use of humor led to an increase in pain tolerance. It is thought laughter stimulates the release of special neurotransmitter substances in the brain (endorphins) that help control pain. Another study demonstrated neuroendocrine and stress-related hormones decreased during episodes of laughter, which provides support for the claim that humor can relieve stress. More studies are needed to clarify the impact of laughter on health.

■ HYPNOSIS

OTHER COMMON NAME(S): Hypnotherapy, Hypnotic Suggestion

Hypnosis is one of several relaxation methods that has been approved by an independent panel, convened by the National Institutes of Health (NIH), as a useful complementary therapy for treating chronic pain. The technique may also be effective in reducing fear and anxiety, treating pain and duration of labor and delivery, and controlling bleeding and pain during dental procedures. There is no scientific evidence that hypnosis can influence the development or progression of cancer; however, it can help to improve the quality of life for some people with cancer.

DESCRIPTION: Hypnosis is a state of restful alertness during which a person enters into a trance-like state, becomes more aware and focused, and is more open to suggestion. It is commonly used to reduce stress and anxiety and create a sense of well-being. It can also be used to change undesirable behaviors, such as smoking, alcohol dependency, and bedwetting, and to overcome common fears, such as the fear of flying or meeting people. Hypnosis is occasionally substituted for anesthetic drugs during minor surgical and dental procedures and during childbirth. Some supporters also believe hypnosis not only accelerates recovery after an operation but also reduces the amount of surgical bleeding and enhances the body's immune system. Some claim that hypnosis can be used to reduce chronic and acute pain. Hypnosis may be used to relieve pain caused by cancer. Proponents do not claim that hypnosis can cure cancer or any other disease or that it always results in the desired effects; however, they say that it can be a useful addition to conventional therapy for some conditions.

USE: There are many different hypnotic techniques. One method involves leading patients into a state of hypnosis by talking in gentle, soothing tones and describing images meant to create a sense of relaxation, security, and well-being. People under hypnosis may appear to be asleep, but they are actually in an altered state of concentration and can focus intently when asked to do so by the hypnotherapist. While a patient is under hypnosis, the hypnotherapist may suggest particular goals, such as controlling pain, stabilizing emotions, and reducing stress, fear, or anxiety.

Contrary to what many believe, people under hypnosis are not under the control of the hypnotherapist nor can they be made to do something they do not want. Quite the opposite is true. Hypnosis is used to help patients gain more control over their behavior, emotions, and even physiological processes that cause undesired consequences. People cannot be hypnotized involuntarily, and not everyone can be put into a hypnotic trance. Success depends upon the patient's willingness and receptivity to the idea of undergoing hypnosis. Some people can learn to hypnotize themselves.

EFFECTS: Numerous reports demonstrate that hypnosis can help patients reduce blood pressure, stress, anxiety, and pain; create relaxing brain wave patterns; modify negative behaviors such as smoking, alcohol consumption, and overeating; and eliminate or decrease the intensity of phobias. Some research has also demonstrated that hypnosis can be used to control nausea and vomiting caused by chemotherapy. According to a report from the NIH, there is strong evidence that hypnosis can relieve some pain associated with cancer. When conducted under the care of a trained hypnotherapist, hypnosis is considered safe as a complementary method.

▨ IMAGERY

OTHER COMMON NAME(S): Guided Imagery, Visualization

Imagery involves the use of visualization techniques that are used as complementary therapies in people with cancer and other diseases. The techniques can help to reduce stress, anxiety, and depression; manage pain; lower blood pressure; ease some of the side effects of chemotherapy; and create feelings of being in control. There is no scientific evidence that imagery can influence the development or progression of cancer.

DESCRIPTION: Imagery involves mental exercises designed to enable the mind to influence the health and well-being of the body. It is said to be a relaxation technique, similar to meditation, which has physical and psychological effects (see Meditation). Imagery is also used in biofeedback, hypnosis, and neuro-linguistic programming (see Biofeedback, Hypnosis, and Neuro-Linguistic Programming). Promoters claim it can relax the mind and body by decreasing heart rate, lowering blood pressure, and altering brain waves. Some proponents also claim that imagery can relieve physical pain and emotional anxiety, improve the effectiveness of drug therapies, and provide emotional insights. It is used to treat people with phobias and depression, reduce stress, increase motivation, promote relaxation, increase control over one's life, improve communication, and even to help people quit smoking.

For people with cancer, some supporters of imagery have found the techniques can alleviate nausea and vomiting associated with chemotherapy, relieve stress associated with having cancer, enhance the immune system, facilitate weight gain, combat depression, and lessen pain.

USE: There are many different imagery techniques. One popular method is known as guided imagery, which involves visualizing a specific image or goal to be achieved and then imagining achieving that goal. Athletes use this technique to improve their game. One type of guided therapy used for cancer patients is called the Simonton method, which was developed in the 1970s by O. Carl Simonton, a radiation oncologist, and Stephanie Matthews-Simonton, a psychotherapist. In the Simonton method, people with cancer are asked to imagine their bodies fighting cancer cells and winning the battle. The Simontons used their method as complementary therapy with conventional cancer treatments.

Another example of an imagery technique is palming, which involves placing the hands (the palms) over the eyes and imagining a color associated with anxiety or stress (such as red), and then a color associated with relaxation or calmness (such as blue). Such techniques can be done as self-taught therapy with the help of one of a number of books or learning tapes published on the subject, or they can be practiced under the guidance of a trained therapist. Imagery is used in clinics at medical centers and local hospitals. It is often combined with other behavioral treatments. Imagery sessions with a health professional may last 20 to 30 minutes.

EFFECTS: Research has found that guided imagery is effective in managing stress, anxiety, and depression and lowering blood pressure, pain, and the side effects of chemotherapy. According to some studies, guided imagery may help reduce some of the side effects of conventional cancer treatment, as well as ease anxiety related to radiation therapy, including fears about the equipment, surgical pain, and recurrence of cancer. Some studies also suggest that imagery can directly affect the immune system. Although one uncontrolled, exploratory study suggested that guided imagery can increase survival rates for people with cancer, there is no scientific evidence that these techniques can cure cancer or any other disease. More research is needed to determine how guided imagery can be most effectively used.

Imagery techniques are considered safe, especially under the guidance of a trained health professional. They are best used as complementary therapy along with conventional treatment.

▨ KIRLIAN PHOTOGRAPHY

OTHER COMMON NAME(S): None

Kirlian photography involves recording the responses of high-voltage electricity passed through a metal plate onto a piece of photographic paper. There is no evidence that Kirlian photography is useful in diagnosing cancer or any other disease.

DESCRIPTION: Kirlian photography advocates believe that all objects, including humans, emit auras that represent the body's energy fields, or life forces. These auras are invisible, believers say, but Kirlian photography captures them on film. Proponents claim Kirlian photographs of the human body carry information about the subject's physiological, psychological, and psychic state. The various colors of the photographs are said to reflect the subject's mood, energy level, and health. For example, they say that predominantly red auras indicate repressed anger; green auras suggest drug or alcohol addiction; gray or brown auras are signs of emotional or physical deficiency. The photographs are used to diagnose problems with specific organs such as kidney disorders, nutritional deficiencies, substance abuse, mental illness, anxiety, confusion, and even cancer. There is no scientific evidence to support these claims.

USE: Kirlian photography does not actually involve a photographic lens or camera. The apparatus to produce a Kirlian photograph consists of a high-voltage electrical source that is attached to a metal plate. A glass plate sits on top of the metal plate, and a piece of photographic paper is laid on top of the glass plate. The object being photographed, such as a hand or foot, is placed directly on the photographic paper. A Kirlian photograph emerges consisting of jagged, colored lines that outline the shape of the photographed object. The resulting image is said to represent an aura, or outline of the body's life force.

EFFECTS: There is no scientific evidence demonstrating that Kirlian photographs can be used to diagnose physical or psychological problems. Research has shown that the images are caused by a variety of factors, none of which are an indication of health problems.

Scientists explain that Kirlian film images reflect differences in skin temperature, position and pressure of the finger or object on the plate, air temperature, moisture levels, and other physiologic changes, rather than auras. Changes in voltage and length of exposure can also affect images captured in the films.

Kirlian photography is generally considered safe; however, relying on this method alone for diagnosis, and avoiding conventional medical care, may have serious health consequences.

▨ LABYRINTH WALKING

OTHER COMMON NAME(S): Labyrinths

Labyrinth walking is a form of meditation that may be helpful as a complementary method to decrease stress and create a state of relaxation.

DESCRIPTION: Labyrinth walking involves walking on labyrinths (winding pathways drawn or laid on the ground). These labyrinths have only one path from start to finish and can be found indoors and outdoors. In fact, it is described by many as walking meditation. People walk through labyrinths to reach any number of goals, such as inner peace, heightened spirituality, personal insight, prayer, relaxation, stress relief, or just "letting go" (see Meditation).

USE: Labyrinth walkers follow the labyrinth path from a specified beginning, through a well-defined central area, and continue on to the exit. They might pray, reflect on life, consider a particular problem, and let the mind wander while seeking spiritual awakening and unity as they move along the twisting trail. Their aim is not to reach the end, but to become immersed in all aspects of the labyrinth walking process, and potentially to experience some degree of personal transformation.

EFFECTS: There is no scientific evidence that labyrinth walking can be used to treat cancer or any other disease. Many doctors consider any activity that promotes relaxation and relieves stress beneficial to overall health. Labyrinth walking should not be used to prevent or treat cancer, but it is generally considered safe as a complementary therapy.

▨ MEDITATION

OTHER COMMON NAME(S): Transcendental Meditation®

Meditation is one of several relaxation methods approved by an independent panel, convened by the National Institutes of Health (NIH), as a useful complementary therapy for treating chronic pain and insomnia. There is no scientific evidence that meditation is effective in treating cancer or any other disease; however, it can help to improve the quality of life for people with cancer.

DESCRIPTION: Meditation is a mind-body process that uses concentration or reflection to relax the body and calm the mind in order to create a sense of well-being. Practitioners claim meditation improves mood, strengthens immune functioning, and enhances fertility. They further claim that meditation increases mental efficiency and alertness and raises self-awareness that contributes to relaxation.

There are different forms of meditation. Meditation is usually done while sitting, but there are also moving forms of meditation, like tai chi, walking in Zen Buddhism, and the Japanese martial art aikido (see Tai Chi). Meditation can be self-directed or guided by doctors, psychiatrists, other mental health professionals, and yoga masters.

The NIH National Center for Complementary and Alternative Medicine reports that regular meditation can increase longevity and quality of life, as well as reduce chronic pain, anxiety, high blood pressure, cholesterol, health care use, substance abuse, post-traumatic stress syndrome in Vietnam War veterans, and blood cortisol levels initially brought on by stress.

USE: Self directed meditation is done by selecting a quiet place free from noise and distraction, sitting or resting quietly with eyes closed (usually on a floor), and trying to achieve a feeling of peace. The person achieves a relaxed yet alert state by concentrating on a pleasant idea or thought, chanting a phrase or special sound, or focusing on the sound of his or her own breathing. The ultimate goal of meditation is to separate oneself mentally from the outside world. Some practitioners recommend two 15 to 20 minute sessions a day.

EFFECTS: In the last 15 years, meditation has been studied in clinical trials as a way of reducing stress on both the mind and body. Research shows that meditation can reduce anxiety, stress, blood pressure, chronic pain, and insomnia. An NIH panel found evidence that regular meditation can also reduce cholesterol, post-traumatic stress syndrome in Vietnam War veterans, substance abuse, and health care use and increase longevity and quality of life.

Most experts agree that the positive effects of meditation outweigh any negative reactions. Complications are rare; however, a small number of people who meditate have become disoriented and experienced some negative feelings.

◾ MUSIC THERAPY

OTHER COMMON NAME(S): Sound Therapy

There is some evidence that when used along with conventional treatment, music therapy can help to reduce pain and relieve chemotherapy-induced nausea and vomiting. It may also relieve stress and provide an overall sense of well-being. Some studies have found that music therapy can lower heart rate, blood pressure, and breathing rate.

DESCRIPTION: Music therapy is a method that consists of the active or passive use of music to promote healing and enhance quality of life. Because of its soothing quality, proponents use music therapy for a variety of physical, emotional, and psychological symptoms. There is some evidence that music therapy reduces high blood pressure, rapid heartbeat, depression, and sleeplessness. Music therapy is often used in cancer treatment to help reduce pain, anxiety, and nausea caused by chemotherapy. Some proponents believe music therapy may enhance the health care of pediatric oncology patients by promoting social interaction and cooperation.

There are no claims music therapy can cure cancer or other diseases, but medical experts do believe it can reduce some symptoms, aid healing, improve physical movement, and enrich a patient's quality of life.

USE: Music therapists design music sessions for individuals and groups based on individual needs and tastes. Some aspects of music therapy include music improvisation, receptive music listening, song writing, lyric discussion, imagery, music performance, and learning through music. Individuals can also perform their own music therapy at home by listening to music or sounds that help relieve their symptoms. Music therapy can be conducted in a variety of places, including hospitals, cancer centers, hospices, at home, or anywhere people can benefit from its calming or stimulating effects.

A related practice called music thanatology is sometimes used at the end of a patient's life to ease the person's passing. It is practiced at home and in hospices or nursing homes.

EFFECTS: Scientific studies have shown the positive value of music therapy on the body, mind, and spirit of children and adults.

Researchers have found that music therapy used along with anti-emetic drugs (drugs that relieve nausea and vomiting) for patients receiving high-dose chemotherapy can be effective in easing the physical symptoms of nausea and vomiting.

A number of clinical trials have shown the benefit of music therapy for acute pain, including pain from cancer. When used in combination with pain-relieving drugs, music has been found to decrease the overall intensity of the patient's experience of pain. Music therapy can sometimes result in a decreased use of pain medication. Other clinical trials have revealed a reduction in heart rate, blood pressure, breathing rate, insomnia, depression, and anxiety with music therapy. In general, music therapy has a positive effect on people and is considered safe when used as a complementary therapy.

◾ NATIVE AMERICAN HEALING

OTHER COMMON NAME(S): None

There is no scientific evidence that Native American healing can cure cancer or any other disease; however, the communal support provided by this approach to health care can have some worthwhile physical, emotional, and spiritual benefits.

DESCRIPTION: Native American healing combines religion, spirituality, herbal medicine, and rituals to treat medical and emotional problems. Proponents claim it can help cure physical diseases (such as heart disease, diabetes, thyroid problems, rashes, asthma, and cancer), injuries, and emotional problems. There is no scientific evidence to support these claims.

Native American healing is based on the belief that health is interconnected with morality, spirituality, and harmonious relationships with community and nature. The goal is to find balance and wholeness in an individual to restore one to a healthy and spiritually pure state. Practitioners of Native American healing presume disease stems from spiritual problems. They believe a person under psychological distress cannot be healed. They also claim that diseases are more likely to invade the body of a person who is imbalanced, has negative thinking, and lives an unhealthy lifestyle.

USE: Native American healing practices vary greatly because there are about 500 Native American Nations (commonly called tribes);

however, they do have some basic rituals and healing practices in common. Some of the most common aspects include the use of herbal remedies (teas, tinctures, and salves), purifying rituals, shamanism, and spiritual healing to treat diseases of both the body and spirit.

Purifying and purging the body is also an important technique used in Native American healing. Sweat lodges (similar to a steam bath) and special teas that induce vomiting are used for this purpose. Smudging (cleansing a place or person with the smoke of sacred plants) is also used to bring about an altered state of consciousness and sensitivity, making a person more open to the healing techniques. Because some diseases are believed to come from angry spirits, shamans are sometimes used to invoke the healing powers of spirits or to help appease the angered spirits (see Shamanism).

Another practice of Native American healing, symbolic healing rituals, can involve a shaman and even entire communities. These rituals use ceremonies that can include chanting, singing, body painting, dancing, exorcisms, sand paintings, and even the use of mind-altering substances (like peyote) to persuade the spirits to heal the sick person. Rituals can last minutes or weeks. Prayer is also an essential part of all Native American healing techniques (see Spirituality and Prayer).

EFFECTS: Although Native American healing has not been shown to cure disease, anecdotal reports suggest that it can reduce pain and stress and improve quality of life. The communal support provided by this type of healing could have beneficial effects. Prayers, introspection, and meditation can be calming and can help to reduce stress.

Because Native American healing is based on spirituality and mysticism, there are very few scientific studies to support the validity of the practices. It is difficult to study Native American healing under accepted scientific standards because practices differ among various Nations, shamans, and diseases. Many Native Americans do not want their practices studied because they believe sharing such information exploits their culture and weakens their power to heal.

Like other complementary therapies, Native American healing practices may be used in relieving certain symptoms of cancer and side effects of cancer treatment. People with cancer and other chronic conditions should consult their doctor before pursuing purification rituals or herbal remedies. Relying on this type of treatment alone, and avoiding conventional medical care, may have serious health consequences.

▌ NATUROPATHIC MEDICINE

OTHER COMMON NAME(S): Naturopathy, Natural Medicine

There is no scientific evidence that naturopathic medicine can cure cancer or any other disease. Specific methods within naturopathic medicine vary in effectiveness. Some methods, such as homeopathy, may be of little value (see Homeopathy). Other methods have shown some evidence of effectiveness in prevention and symptom management, such as the importance of diet in lowering the risk of severe diseases such as heart disease and cancer and the usefulness of acupuncture to reduce pain.

DESCRIPTION: Naturopathic medicine integrates a wide range of complementary approaches, such as nutrition, herbal medicine, physical manipulation, exercise, stress reduction, and acupuncture with conventional medicine. It is a holistic approach (designed to treat the whole person) that enlists the healing power of the body and nature to fight disease (see Holistic Medicine). It is promoted for the treatment of migraine headaches, chronic lower back pain, enlarged prostate, menopause, AIDS, and cancer.

Proponents claim naturopathic medicine uses the healing power of nature to maintain and restore health. The whole person is supported to create a healthy environment inside and outside the body. Supporters claim naturopathic medicine prevents disease because people are taught to incorporate healthy diets and lifestyles to avoid disease. Diagnosis and treatment are focused on the cause of the disease, rather than on the symptoms. Naturopaths diagnose disease with many of the same methods used in conventional medicine. They use x-rays, lab tests, and physical examinations. In contrast, naturopathic treatment does not involve the use of drugs, modern medical technology, or major surgery. Practitioners often refer complicated cases or people needing major treatment to conventional medical professionals.

USE: Naturopathic medicine uses many different techniques and methods. Practitioners act mostly as teachers. They decide how to treat a particular patient based on case history, observation, medical records, clinical nutrition information, and previous experience. Naturopathic treatment can include acupuncture; nutritional medicine and therapeutic fasting; herbs, minerals, and vitamins; homeopathy; hypnotherapy; and a variety of other therapies. For more information about some of the treatments involved in naturopathic medicine, see Acupuncture,

Homeopathy, Hypnosis, Colon Therapy, and chapters on Herb, Vitamin, and Mineral Methods, and Diet and Nutrition Methods.

Counseling or behavioral medicine is an important part of naturopathic medicine. Practitioners are trained in counseling, biofeedback, stress reduction, and other means to improve mental health (see Biofeedback and Psychotherapy). They may also use other unproven techniques, such as ozone therapy, for people with cancer and AIDS.

Chiropractors, massage therapists, holistic nurses, and nutritionists offer naturopathic remedies but may not have educational training in naturopathic medicine. Treatment by naturopathic doctors is not covered by Medicare or most insurance policies.

EFFECTS: There have been no controlled clinical studies showing the effectiveness of naturopathic medicine. Most of the documentation of treatment includes case history observations, medical records, and summaries of practitioners' clinical experiences. Naturopathic medicine uses several methods that have been shown to vary in how effective they are.

It involves the use of several unproven methods (eg, homeopathy and colonic irrigation), while other aspects (eg, proper diet and nutrition) are accepted practices used to lower the risk of severe conditions such as heart disease and cancer. Some aspects of naturopathic medicine may be useful as complementary methods to conventional medical treatment.

Most naturopathic methods are not harmful, although some herbal preparations can be toxic (see specific herbs for more information). Excessive fasting, dietary restrictions, or use of enemas may be dangerous. Relying on this type of treatment alone, and avoiding conventional medical care, may have serious health consequences.

▨ NEURO-LINGUISTIC PROGRAMMING
OTHER COMMON NAME(S): NLP

Some smaller studies have reported positive effects of neuro-linguistic programming (NLP) in such areas as increasing relaxation and treating phobias; however, there is no scientific evidence that NLP is effective in treating cancer or any other disease.

DESCRIPTION: NLP uses a number of techniques or tools to teach people to identify personal goals, change unhelpful beliefs, reach a higher level of achievement, and communicate better with others. Special attention is paid to the relationship between language, thoughts, and behavior.

Practitioners of NLP claim it is used to identify and change unconscious patterns of thinking and behavior to help treat a wide range of physical conditions. They also claim NLP can be used to help people with phobias, allergies, arthritis, migraines, Parkinson's disease, AIDS, and cancer. There is no scientific evidence to support these claims.

NLP is based on the belief that the brain (ie, neuro-) controls how the body functions, language (ie, -linguistic) determines how people communicate, and programming is used to develop models for interaction. NLP involves studying the relationship between all 3 parts. Practitioners claim people who have problems healing from physical conditions often have negative beliefs about their health.

USE: NLP practitioners may ask a person questions about his or her life or physical condition, then analyze eye movements, body posture, voice tone, muscle tension, gestures, and language to understand and correct problems. This observational information is used to show how people are consciously and unconsciously relating to their life and condition and what limiting beliefs may exist. Practitioners claim some diseases or other problems can be cured with one NLP session, although some conditions may require a few repeated sessions.

EFFECTS: Although there have been anecdotal and case reports of the effectiveness of NLP, there have been no large-scale controlled clinical trials of the method. Several reviews of the literature have reported there is little or no evidence to support the effectiveness of NLP. A recent survey of 139 psychologists listed in the National Register of Health Service Providers in Psychology found that the soundness of NLP was questionable. More scientific research is needed to determine if NLP holds any benefit for any medical condition.

Not all NLP practitioners have a background in medical settings, and some may not even be properly trained. Someone without training or experience in the field may not be skilled enough or sensitive to the needs and issues important to someone living with cancer and could cause psychological harm.

PSYCHOTHERAPY

OTHER COMMON NAME(S): Therapy, Counseling, Psychological Intervention, Psychotherapeutic Treatment

Research has shown that psychotherapy may improve a patient's quality of

life. It can help reduce the anxiety and depression that sometimes occur in people with cancer. Psychotherapy has not been demonstrated to increase survival in people with cancer.

DESCRIPTION: Psychotherapy covers a wide range of approaches designed to help people change their ways of thinking, feeling, or behaving. The idea of the existence of a mind-body connection has been around for a very long time and has received more support and attention in recent years. Psychotherapists believe that what a person experiences mentally and emotionally affects his or her body. They also believe psychotherapy can help people, including those with cancer, find the inner strength they need to improve their coping skills, allowing them to more fully enjoy their lives. Psychotherapy can be used to help people deal with the diagnosis and treatment of cancer. It can also be useful in overcoming depression and anxiety, which many people with cancer experience.

USE: Psychotherapy is available in many forms and settings. It is offered individually as well as in couples, families, and groups (see Support Groups). There are a wide range of psychotherapeutic approaches and techniques used, such as behavioral therapy (behavior modification), client-centered therapy, body-oriented therapy, cognitive therapy, psychodynamic therapy, family/couples therapy, and group therapy. Whatever approach is used, when a person has a serious physical condition such as cancer, the therapy is likely to focus on the emotional stress resulting from the disease. It will also focus on depression and anxiety if present, as well as exploring past or present issues that may affect the person's adjustment to the disease. Attention may be paid to the person's previous experiences with loss in general, as well as with the specific disease now being faced.

People can get referrals by asking members of their health care team or by contacting professional organizations for names of psychotherapists who specialize in the area. Oncology units of hospitals sometimes have departments that staff therapists. Most individual psychotherapy is held in the therapist's office, but there are situations when different arrangements can be made (eg, the hospital or person's home). Sessions typically last 50 minutes and occur at a frequency determined by the client and therapist, although most are weekly and only short-term (3 to 4 months).

EFFECTS: Research has generally shown that psychotherapy can be beneficial to people with cancer in a variety of ways, such as helping to reduce anxiety and depression, improving quality of life, teaching ways of managing time more effectively, and helping people return to work. Psychotherapy can also help people learn to communicate better with their doctors and be more compliant with medical instructions because they feel their own needs are being recognized.

Research has not clearly shown, however, that individual psychotherapy can prolong the life of cancer patients. Few controlled studies of this nature have been conducted. Additionally, it is not clear whether support groups or group counseling actually leads to a longer life. Research has revealed contradictory results about the ability of support groups or group therapy to extend life (see Support Groups).

Psychotherapists vary in the amount of their training and experience in dealing with issues relevant to the treatment of people with cancer. Difficult personal issues that arise from psychotherapy can be emotionally upsetting or uncomfortable. Some doctors have raised a concern that an "alternative" method such as psychotherapy may lead to a delay of conventional treatment, although most now view psychotherapy as complementary to standard medical intervention.

▌ QIGONG

OTHER COMMON NAME(S): Chi-kung

There is no scientific evidence showing that qigong is effective in treating cancer or any other disease; however, it may be useful to enhance quality of life. According to limited scientific literature, qigong may reduce chronic pain for a short time and relieve anxiety.

DESCRIPTION: Qigong (pronounced chee-gong) is a Chinese system of self-care designed to enhance the natural flow of vital energy called *qi* (or *chi*) in the body. The process of working toward a regulated, smooth flow of qi is called "gong." Proponents of qigong believe disease, injury, and stress can disrupt the vital energy or life force of the body (qi). By correcting these disruptions, individuals can lead healthier, less stressful lives (see Electromagnetic Therapy).

Qigong is promoted to strengthen the body or to enhance other conventional health care treatments, not to cure existing disease. Practitioners claim it may be helpful in managing pain and reducing anxiety. There is some limited evidence for these claims. Some promoters also claim that qigong can help to prevent cancer by improving the oxygen supply to the body and regulating the autonomic nervous system. They further claim qigong can be used to treat hypertension, stroke, heart and other circulatory diseases, abnormal sex hormone levels, low bone density, and senility. Some qigong masters even claim they can cure a person with the energy released from their fingertips. There is no scientific evidence to support any of these claims.

USE: Qigong consists primarily of meditation, physical movements, and breathing exercises (see Meditation). Internal qigong involves exercises that individuals can do on their own. External qigong involves skilled masters who claim to use their own qi to help heal other people. The qigong master does not have to touch a person in order to promote healing.

A typical qigong session might require a person to sit or stand quietly while thinking about the qi flowing through his or her body and performing breathing and movement exercises at the same time. The breathing and movements used in qigong are slow, deliberate, and controlled. Qigong can also be used to target specific areas of the body where problems may exist.

EFFECTS: While some scientists believe that qigong may be useful as a form of exercise to help to relieve stress, improve coordination, and generally improve a person's quality of life, there is no scientific evidence that qigong can cure cancer or any other disease.

One study recently published in the United States found that for people with chronic pain, qigong training resulted in a short-term reduction of pain and a long-term reduction in anxiety. It was a small study, and more well-controlled clinical research, using larger groups of patients, is needed to determine what effect qigong may have in treating various medical conditions.

Qigong is generally considered safe because of the slow, deliberate exercises involved. Those with a history of muscle aches and joint pain should realize that the deliberate, slow movement of qigong may cause muscle fatigue and joint pain if overdone. People with cancer and chronic conditions such as arthritis and heart disease should consult with their doctor before undergoing any type of therapy that involves manipulation of joints and muscles.

SHAMANISM

OTHER COMMON NAME(S): Shaman

Although anecdotal stories have existed for centuries and many people around the world continue to practice shamanism today, there is no scientific evidence that it can cure cancer or any other disease. Some key elements of shamanism, such as the use of imagery, have been shown to reduce stress and anxiety (see Imagery).

DESCRIPTION: Shamanism is a form of folk medicine that uses spiritual healing and is performed by a *shaman*, an individual recognized by a people or a tribe who is believed to have special religious and/or magical powers of healing (see Native American Healing). It is based on the belief that healing has a spiritual dimension that must be addressed before healing can begin. The goal of shamanism is to help people discover meaning within themselves, as well as in society and nature. Proponents claim that shamanism can heal both the body and soul, as well as restore harmony to the community and nature. Shamans claim they communicate with the spirits to help heal. Some shamans claim they can heal spiritual, psychic, and physical wounds, as well as communities and global conditions.

Not all shamans claim the ability to cure every disease. Many shamans are very selective in choosing which people they will treat because if they fail to cure someone, they may be punished by the tribe. For example, shamans who believe that their brand of healing will not influence the course of cancer are not likely to work with a person who has been diagnosed with cancer.

USE: The shaman enters a trance, either self-induced or through the aid of hallucinogens or fasting, and then prays, sings, chants, dances, and/or beats drums around the patient. Storytelling and other art forms may also be used. During the trance, the shaman's soul is believed to travel in the quest to help the sick individual. The soul is said to leave the body and ascend to the spiritual world. This is where the shaman communicates with the evil spirits thought to be responsible for the disease. Although the shaman is in a state of trance, he is still conscious, which enables him to bargain with the spirits that are responsible for the patient's disease. Successful bargaining is thought to result in a cure. Today, some shamans also use herbal medicine or even conventional medicine in an effort to heal.

Each shaman must complete rigorous training, especially in the ability to achieve the trance required for communication with the spirits. Shamans work both with individual patients and with groups.

EFFECTS: There are many stories about the success of shamans throughout history. Most of these stories are not unlike the reports of religious "miracles" at shrines such as Lourdes in France. There is no scientific evidence that demons exist, that a shaman can communicate with and influence them, or that disease is caused by spirits. There is no proof of shamanic ability to cure disease; any results are most likely due to the placebo effect, in which believing that something can or will happen generates a positive result. Some key elements of shamanism, such as the use of imagery, have been shown to reduce stress and anxiety; however, there is no scientific evidence that shamanism is effective in treating cancer or any other disease.

Shamanism is generally considered safe and may be useful as a complementary therapy to help people with cancer deal with their emotions, certain symptoms of cancer, and side effects of cancer treatment. Relying on this type of treatment alone, and avoiding conventional medical care, may have serious health consequences.

▪ SPIRITUALITY AND PRAYER

OTHER COMMON NAME(S): Religion

Studies have found that spirituality and religion are very important to the quality of life for some people with cancer. Although research has not shown that spirituality can cure cancer or any other disease, some studies have found intercessory prayer (praying for others) to be an effective addition to conventional medical care. The psychological benefits of prayer may include reduction of stress and anxiety, promotion of a more positive outlook, and the strengthening of the will to live.

DESCRIPTION: Spirituality is generally described as an awareness of something greater than the individual self and is usually expressed through religion and/or prayer. Proponents of spirituality claim that prayer can decrease the negative effects of disease, speed recovery, and increase the effectiveness of medical treatments. Many people believe the spiritual dimension in healing is important, especially for coping with serious disease. Religious attendance has been associated with improvement of various health conditions, such as heart disease, hypertension, stroke, colitis, cancer, and overall health status; however, the scientific evidence is mixed.

Some religious groups, such as Christian Scientists, claim prayer can cure any disease. These groups often rely entirely on prayer in place of conventional medicine. This belief is based on a spiritual rather than a biological explanation of how disease develops. There have been some reported cases that prayer has lead to tumor regression. There is no scientific evidence to support these claims.

Use: Spirituality has many forms and can be practiced in several ways. Prayer, for example, may be silent or spoken out loud and can be done alone or in a group in any setting (as in a church or temple). Regular attendance at a church or temple may involve prayer that focuses on one's self (supplication) or on others (intercessory prayer). In this type of setting, the entire congregation of a church may be asked to pray for a sick person or the person's family.

Some religions set aside certain times of the day and special days of the week for praying. Standard prayers written by religious leaders are often memorized and repeated during private sessions and in groups. Prayers often ask a higher being for help, understanding, wisdom, or strength in dealing with life's problems.

Many medical institutions and practitioners include spirituality and prayer as important components of healing. In addition, hospitals have chapels and contracts with ministers, rabbis, and voluntary organizations to serve their patients' spiritual needs.

Effects: Studies done on the impact of prayer and spirituality generally focus on the effect of religious beliefs and behavior on health, survival, and quality of life and the effects of intercessory prayer. The results of many of these studies have been mixed. Although some research has found that religious groups with orthodox beliefs and behavior have lower cancer death rates, other studies have not found any health benefits related to religion and health. Patient consent is important before conducting any activity that may impact health. Those who do not believe in prayer and those who do not wish to be healed are among those who may object to being the object of intercessory prayer. Relying on this type of treatment alone, and avoiding conventional medical care, may have serious health consequences.

▌ SUPPORT GROUPS

Other common name(s): Group Therapy, Group Psychotherapy, Psychosocial Interventions, Psychosocial Treatment

Preliminary research has shown that many support groups can enhance quality of life. There is no scientific evidence, however, that support groups can actually extend the survival time of people with cancer.

Description: Support groups present information, provide comfort, teach coping skills, help reduce anxiety, and provide a place to share common concerns and emotional support. Participants believe that people can live healthier, happier lives in the company of others. They believe that when relatives and friends lend support, it is easier for people to deal with their health and social problems. Some proponents claim the bonds formed between members of support groups help them feel stronger. They further claim that sharing feelings and experiences within support groups can reduce stress, fear, and anxiety and help to promote healing. Evidence suggests that support groups can improve quality of life for people with cancer.

USE: Support groups are composed of education, behavioral training, and group interaction. Behavioral training can involve muscle relaxation or meditation to reduce stress or the effects of chemotherapy or radiation therapy (see Meditation). People with cancer are often encouraged by doctors to seek support from groups of individuals that have direct or indirect experiences with the same type of cancer.

Many different kinds of support groups are available, and they vary in their structure, location, and activities. Some are time-limited, while others are ongoing. There are also support groups composed of people with the same type of cancer. Others are composed of people who are undergoing the same kind of treatment. Support groups are available for patients, family members, and other caregivers of people with cancer. The format of different groups varies from lectures and discussions to exploration and expression of feelings. Topics discussed by support groups are those of concern among the members and those considered of value by a therapist who may lead the group.

Support groups are different from group therapy in that sessions may be led by survivors, group members, or trained professionals, while therapy groups are always facilitated by licensed counselors. Group therapy is generally longer and more involved and focuses on in-depth personal growth (see Psychotherapy). Support groups focus on learning to manage current concerns and situations. Most support groups involve little or no cost to the participants, while there is usually a fee for group therapy.

EFFECTS: The scientific community believes that support groups can enhance the quality of life for people with cancer by providing information and support to overcome the feelings of helplessness that sometimes accompany a diagnosis of cancer. Research has shown that people with cancer are better able to deal with their disease when supported by others in similar situations.

One clinical trial found that support groups helped in reducing tension, anxiety, fatigue, and confusion. Some research has shown that there is a link between group support and greater tolerance of cancer treatment and treatment compliance; however, research has shown contradictory results about the ability of groups to extend life. Although more research is needed to determine what types of groups are most effective with what type of people, support groups may be useful as a complementary therapy for people with cancer and other diseases.

Support groups vary in quality. People with cancer may find that the support group they have joined does not discuss topics relevant to their personal situation. Some people may find a support group upsetting because it stirs up too many uncomfortable feelings or because the leader is not skilled. Internet support groups should be used with caution. This method cannot always ensure confidentiality, and the people involved may have no special training or qualifications, especially if found in unmonitored chat rooms.

▧ TAI CHI

OTHER COMMON NAME(S): T'ai Chi, Tai Chi Chuan, Tai Chi Chih, Tai Ji Juan, Tai Ji Quan, Tai Ji, Shadow Boxing

Research has shown tai chi is useful as a form of exercise that may improve posture, balance, muscle mass and tone, flexibility, stamina, and strength in older adults. Tai chi is also recognized as a method to reduce stress that can provide the same cardiovascular benefits as moderate exercise, such as lowered heart rate and blood pressure.

DESCRIPTION: Tai chi (pronounced tie-chee) is an ancient Chinese form of martial arts. It is a mind-body, self-healing system that uses movement, meditation, and breathing to improve health and well-being. People who practice the deep breathing and physical movements of tai chi report it makes them feel more relaxed, younger, and agile and helps their circulation. Its slow, graceful movements, accompanied by rhythmic breathing, relax the body as well as the mind. Research has found that tai chi can reduce stress, lower blood pressure, and reduce the risk of heart disease. (See Qigong and Yoga for other Eastern methods of exercise.) There is also evidence that tai chi is particularly suited for older adults or for others who are not physically strong or healthy.

Proponents claim tai chi balances the flow of vital energy or life force called *qi* (or *chi*). This balance serves to prevent illness or disease, improve general health, and extend life. It is also based on the theory of *yin* and *yang* (interaction of opposite forces). Practitioners claim tai chi is designed to balance yin and yang forces to achieve inner harmony.

USE: Tai chi students begin by learning a series of gentle, deliberate movements called *forms*. Each form contains between 20 to 100 moves and requires up to 20 minutes to complete. Each form derives its name from nature, for example, "Wave Hands Like Clouds" or "Grasping the Bird's Tail." In order to balance the yin and yang, the movements are practiced in pairs of opposites; for example, a turn to the right follows one to the left. While performing these exercises, the individual is urged to pay close attention to his or her breathing, which is centered in the diaphragm. Tai chi relies entirely on technique rather than strength or power. Meditative concentration is focused on a point just below the navel, from which it is believed qi radiates throughout the body.

EFFECTS: Researchers have focused on studying the benefits of relaxation and exercise that result from practicing tai chi. Clinical trials found that tai chi improves posture, balance, flexibility, muscle mass and tone, stamina, and strength in older adults and may help prevent falls and fractures. It has also been found to improve overall well-being in older adults and encourages exercise. As an exercise, the benefits have also been noted for older individuals with chronic diseases such as arthritis, osteoporosis, and chronic obstructive pulmonary disease. Research has found that tai chi can reduce stress and provide the same cardiovascular benefits as moderate exercise, such as reduced heart rate and blood pressure. There is no scientific evidence that tai chi cures cancer or any other disease, although it may be useful as a complementary therapy to conventional treatment.

Tai chi is considered to be a relatively safe, moderate physical activity. As with any form of exercise, it is important to be aware of physical limitations. People with cancer and chronic conditions such as arthritis and heart disease should consult with their doctor before undergoing any type of therapy that involves manipulation of joints and muscles.

YOGA

OTHER COMMON NAME(S): Hatha Yoga

Yoga can be a useful method to help relieve some symptoms associated with chronic diseases, such as cancer, arthritis, and heart disease, and can lead to increased relaxation and physical fitness. There is no scientific evidence that yoga is effective in treating cancer or any other disease; however, it may enhance quality of life.

DESCRIPTION: Yoga is a form of nonaerobic exercise that involves a program of precise posture and breathing activities. It is promoted as a system of personal development. It is a way of life based on the Hindu philosophy that combines ethical standards, dietary guidelines, physical exercise, and meditation to create a union of mind, body, and spirit. Yoga is said to cultivate *prana*, which is similar to *qi* (or *chi*) in traditional Chinese medicine, meaning vital energy or life force. People who practice yoga claim it leads to a state of physical health, relaxation, happiness, peace, and tranquility. There is some evidence that shows that yoga can lower stress, increase strength, and provide a good form of exercise.

Proponents also claim yoga can be used to stop smoking, eliminate insomnia, and increase stamina. They further claim that the mastery of yoga can give people extraordinary mental and physical powers. *Yogis*, who are masters and teachers of yoga, claim they can obtain heightened senses, overcome hunger and thirst, and develop almost complete control over physiological processes such as heartbeat and respiration.

USE: There are different variations, types, and aspects of yoga. The most common form of yoga involves the use of movement, breathing exercises, and meditation to achieve a connection with the mind, body, and spirit. The goal of yoga is perfect concentration to attain the ancient Hindu ideal of *samadhi*—separation of pure consciousness from the outside world through the development of intuitive insight.

Practitioners say yoga should be done either at the beginning or the end of the day. A typical session can last between 20 minutes and 1 hour. A yoga session starts with the person sitting in an upright position and performing gentle movements, all of which are executed very slowly while taking slow, deep breaths from the abdomen. A session may also include guided relaxation, meditation, and sometimes visualization (see Imagery). It often ends with the chanting of a *mantra* (a meaningful word or phrase) to achieve a deeper state of relaxation. Yoga requires several sessions a week in order to become proficient. Yoga can be practiced at home without an instructor, in adult education classes, or in classes usually offered at health clubs and community centers. There are also numerous books and videotapes available on yoga.

EFFECTS: Research has shown that yoga can be used to control physiological functions such as blood pressure, heart rate, respiration, metabolism, body temperature, brain waves, skin resistance, and other bodily functions. This can result in improved physical fitness, lower levels of stress, and increased feelings of relaxation and well-being.

According to a report to the National Institutes of Health, there is also some evidence to suggest yoga may be useful as a complementary therapy to conventional medical treatment to help relieve symptoms associated with cancer, asthma, diabetes, drug addiction, high blood pressure, heart disease, arthritis, and migraine headaches. Yoga may also help to reduce cholesterol levels when used with diet and exercise.

Some yoga postures are difficult to achieve. People with cancer and chronic conditions, such as arthritis and heart disease, should consult their doctor before undergoing any type of therapy that involves manipulation of joints and muscles.

CHAPTER TWO

MANUAL HEALING AND PHYSICAL TOUCH METHODS

TREATMENT METHODS IN THIS CATEGORY INVOLVE touching, manipulation, or movement of the body. These techniques are based on the idea that problems in one part of the body often affect other parts of the body.

▌ ACUPUNCTURE

OTHER COMMON NAME(S): Acupuncture Therapy, Zhenjiu

Although there is no evidence that acupuncture is effective as a treatment for cancer, clinical studies have found it to be effective in treating nausea caused by chemotherapy drugs and surgical anesthesia and in relieving pain following dental surgery. The technique may also assist people who are trying to stop addictive behaviors, such as smoking or alcoholism, and may be useful for treating headaches, helping in rehabilitation from strokes, and treating a number of musculoskeletal conditions.

DESCRIPTION: Acupuncture is a technique in which very thin needles of varying lengths are inserted through the skin in specific locations called acupoints to treat a variety of conditions. There is evidence that acupuncture eases nausea caused by chemotherapy and surgical anesthesia and relieves postoperative dental pain. It may also assist withdrawal from addiction to drugs and alcohol and help relieve headaches, menstrual cramps, tennis elbow, lower back pain, carpal tunnel syndrome, and asthma.

In China, acupuncture is used as an anesthetic during surgery and is believed to have the power to cure diseases and relieve the symptoms of various conditions. The teachings of traditional Chinese medicine explain that acupoints lie along invisible meridians, which are channels for the flow of vital energy or life force called *qi* (or *chi*) that is present in all living things. Meridians also represent an internal system of communication that is said to connect specific organs or networks of organs.

USE: In traditional acupuncture, needles are inserted at specific locations (acupoints), just deep enough into the skin to keep them from falling out in order to restore balance and a healthy energy flow to the body. They are usually left in place for less than half an hour. Skilled acupuncturists cause virtually no pain. The acupuncturist may twirl the needles and apply heat or a weak electrical current to enhance the effects of the therapy. Acupuncture is sometimes accompanied by less well-known traditional healing techniques (see Moxibustion and Cupping).

In acupressure, a popular variation of acupuncture, therapists press on acupoints with their fingers instead of using needles. This technique is used by itself or as part of an entire system of manual healing such as in shiatsu (see Bodywork).

EFFECTS: There is no scientific evidence that acupuncture is effective as a treatment for cancer, but it appears to be useful as a complementary method for relieving some symptoms related to cancer and other conditions. Acupuncture has been the subject of numerous clinical studies. According to a National Institutes of Health expert panel consisting of scientists, researchers, and health care providers, acupuncture is an effective treatment for nausea caused by chemotherapy drugs and surgical anesthesia and for dental pain following surgery.

Acupuncture may also be useful by itself or combined with conventional therapies to treat headaches, menstrual cramps, tennis elbow, arthritis, lower back pain, asthma, and other conditions and to assist in the rehabilitation of stroke patients. There is also some evidence that acupuncture may lessen the need for conventional pain-relieving drugs.

When conducted by a trained professional, acupuncture is generally considered safe. The number of complications reported has been relatively few, but there is a risk that a patient may be harmed if the acupuncturist is not well trained. When performed improperly, acupuncture can cause fainting, local internal bleeding, convulsions, hepatitis B, dermatitis, and nerve damage. Acupuncture also poses risks such as infection from contaminated needles or improper delivery of treatment. Relying on this type of treatment alone, and avoiding conventional medical care, may have serious health consequences.

█ APPLIED KINESIOLOGY

OTHER COMMON NAME(S): Muscle Testing, AK

There is no scientific evidence that applied kinesiology can diagnose or treat cancer. Muscle-testing methods appear to have no health benefits.

DESCRIPTION: Applied kinesiology is a technique used to diagnose disease by testing muscles for strengths and weaknesses. Practitioners claim that by discovering the weak muscle, they can identify the underlying disease and make decisions about subsequent treatment. They claim strengthening the weak muscles will restore the health of internal organs. Applied kinesiology is usually used for evaluation purposes, but claims have been made that after undergoing an AK session, it is possible to observe the "spontaneous remission" of cancer. There is no scientific evidence to support these claims.

Kinesiologists claim muscle weakness may be caused by a number of internal energy disruptions, such as nerve damage, drainage impairment of the lymph system, reduced blood supply, chemical imbalances, or organ and gland dysfunction. Practitioners usually recommend people confirm the diagnosis with conventional diagnostic techniques, such as laboratory testing and x-rays.

USE: Applied kinesiologists assess their patients by observing posture, gait, muscle strength, and range of motion and by palpation (touching). These observations may be combined with more conventional methods of diagnosis, such as a clinical history, a routine physical examination, and laboratory tests. They may also test for environmental or food sensitivities.

During the therapy, the patient might be asked to hold his or her arm parallel to the floor and resist the downward push of the practitioner, then repeat the exercise with the other arm. The relative strength differences supposedly help the kinesiologist diagnose internal imbalances. The practitioner might also press on key "trigger points" to detect muscle weakness.

To restore muscle strength, the kinesiologist may apply manual stimulation and relaxation techniques to key muscles. The therapy can include joint manipulation or mobilization, dietary management, reflex procedures, and cranial manipulation.

EFFECTS: A few researchers have investigated kinesiology muscle-testing procedures in controlled clinical studies. The results showed that applied kinesiology was not an accurate diagnostic tool and that muscle response was not any more useful than random guessing. In fact, one study found that applied kinesiologists made very different assessments regarding nutrient status for the same patients. Some anecdotal accounts of successful applied kinesiology treatments do exist; however, there is no scientific evidence that kinesiology cures cancer or any other disease. Applied kinesiology is considered relatively safe, although relying on this diagnostic method alone, and avoiding or delaying conventional medical diagnosis and treatment, may have serious health consequences.

▨ BIOLOGICAL DENTISTRY

OTHER COMMON NAME(S): None

There is no scientific evidence that removing teeth or fillings can prevent cancer or any other disease. In 1987, the American Dental Association declared that the unnecessary removal of silver amalgam is improper and unethical.

DESCRIPTION: Biological dentistry is the removal or replacement of dental fillings or teeth claimed to contain toxins (such as mercury), which may cause systemic diseases or pain. Proponents of biological dentistry claim dental health has an impact on the health of the entire body. They claim the toxins in ordinary fillings can escape, travel to distant organs, and contribute to the development of diseases, including cancer. They also say replacing metal fillings with synthetic, nontoxic compounds will eliminate toxins from the body and increase resistance to disease. Some also claim decaying teeth and root canal procedures increase the risk of disease in other parts of the body.

USE: Practitioners approach their patients holistically, meaning they consider the entire body rather than just the diseased area (see Holistic Medicine). A biological dentist may also prescribe other remedies or diets that claim to detoxify the body and strengthen the immune system. Biological dentistry can also involve oral acupuncture, surgical scraping, chelation therapy, neural therapy, laser therapy, and "mouth balancing," which is the attempt to improve structural deformities in the mouth and jaw (see Chelation Therapy and Neural Therapy).

EFFECTS: The few clinical studies that have been published in peer-reviewed medical journals found no association between teeth fillings and the development of cancer. The amount of mercury absorbed by the body from amalgams is so small it is considered harmless. Typical dental fillings do contain materials such as mercury, copper, and silver, but there is no solid evidence showing that the presence of these metals in teeth fillings causes disease in other parts of the body.

Many dentists and other health experts believe the removal of healthy teeth or fillings is improper and unethical and should be avoided. Relying on this treatment alone, and avoiding conventional medical care, may have serious health consequences.

▨ BODYWORK

OTHER COMMON NAME(S): Movement Therapy, Rolfing®, Alexander Technique®, Feldenkrais Method, Trager Approach, Shiatsu Massage

There is no scientific evidence that bodywork is effective in treating cancer, but it can be used to enhance quality of life. Many forms of bodywork have the potential to bring pain relief and stress reduction, although the effectiveness of these techniques has not yet been proven scientifically.

DESCRIPTION: Bodywork refers to a variety of physically oriented techniques. Some forms of bodywork involve hands-on manipulation of joints or soft tissue, realignment of the body, and correction of posture imbalances. Others focus on increasing a person's awareness of their own body through gentle, deliberate movement and breathing exercises.

Various forms of bodywork are generally promoted to relieve pain, reduce stress, soothe injured muscles, stimulate blood and lymphatic circulation, and promote relaxation. Practitioners also claim that through bodywork, their patients become more comfortable with their bodies by learning how to move more freely, gracefully, and efficiently.

Some practitioners claim bodywork and movement therapy are effective treatments for many conditions, including cancer, circulation problems, colic, depression, headaches, heart problems, high blood pressure, hyperactivity, insomnia, sinus infections, and tension. There is no scientific evidence to support these claims.

USE: Many of the most commonly used bodywork therapies resemble traditional massage, but each differs from massage in one or more notable ways. *Rolfing* is a form of myofascial massage guided by the contours of the body (see Myotherapy). Rolfers use their fingers, hands, elbows, and knees to place deep pressure and shift bones into proper alignment to increase range of motion and make movement easier. *Shiatsu* consists of pressing with the fingers on acupuncture points (see Acupuncture and Ohashiatsu®) to stretch and open pathways for the body's flow of vital energy or life force called *qi* (or *chi*). The *Feldenkrais Method* involves a slow and gentle sequence of movements to help people develop a heightened awareness of their bodies, improve mobility, and break habits of poor posture and inefficient motion that can cause pain and discomfort. The *Alexander Technique* involves gently mobilizing parts of a patient's body that appear to be strained to improve movement. Therapists also explain how to relax and move the body properly. The *Trager Approach* uses gentle, rhythmical touch combined with movement exercises. The therapist feels how the client is holding his or her body, then applies various rocking, pulling, and rotational movements to the head, neck, torso, arms, and legs.

EFFECTS: Very little scientific research has been done to find out what positive effects these treatments can offer; however, many people who undergo one or more of these techniques enthusiastically report they feel more relaxed or can move with greater ease or less pain. Some people with cancer may find that these therapies help to relieve certain symptoms of cancer and side effects of treatments, but the evidence is anecdotal or based on very small research studies. There is no scientific evidence that any of these techniques are effective in treating cancer or any other disease.

There are types of bodywork that can sometimes be quite painful. One concern for people with cancer is that therapies involving bodywork might increase the risk that tissue manipulation will cause cancer cells to travel to other parts of the body; however, there is no research to indicate that this will happen. People with rheumatoid arthritis, cancer that has spread to the bone, spine injuries, or bone diseases that could be aggravated by physical manipulation should avoid therapies that involve body manipulation because these conditions could worsen.

Manipulation of a bone where cancer metastasis is present could result in a bone fracture. People with cancer and chronic conditions, such as arthritis and heart disease, should consult their doctor before undergoing any type of therapy that involves manipulation of joints and muscles.

■ CANCER SALVES

OTHER COMMON NAME(S): Black Salve, Escharotics, Escharotic Therapy, Botanical Salve, Curaderm

There is no scientific evidence that salves are effective in treating cancer or tumors. In fact, some ingredients may cause great harm to the body. There have been numerous reports of severe burns and permanent scarring.

DESCRIPTION: Cancer salves are pastes, salves, or poultices applied to external tumors or on the skin above internal tumor sites. There are many variations in the formulas, which can contain 10 or more ingredients in bases of olive oil, beeswax, and pine tar. Ingredients may include chaparral, DMSO (dimethyl sulfoxide), chickweed, Indian tobacco, comfrey, myrrh, and other herbs, oils, and chemicals.

Practitioners claim cancer salves have the power to kill cancer cells or draw them out of the body and that salves can cure any type of cancer. Some of the companies that sell cancer salves claim their products can heal cancer without the need for conventional treatments, such as surgery, chemotherapy, or radiation. One manufacturer claims the company's salves are successful at curing from 75% to 80% of cancer cases and even 99% of one type of skin cancer. Other proponents claim their cancer salves have antitumor properties that cause no damage to healthy skin. There is no scientific evidence to support these claims.

USE: For skin cancers, the salves are rubbed directly onto the tumor. For other types of cancers, the salves are rubbed on the skin above the internal location of the tumor. Because the salves are widely available, some people apply them at home, while others receive salve treatments from naturopaths (see Naturopathic Medicine).

EFFECTS: All claims that cancer salves cure cancer are based on anecdotal reports and testimonials. There have been no clinical studies of cancer salves, and there is no scientific evidence that cancer salves cure cancer or any other disease.

There have been numerous reports of severe scarring and burns associated with the use of cancer salves. The Food and Drug Administration does not regulate cancer salves. The contents of different cancer salves vary and can contain potentially dangerous substances. Women who are pregnant or breast-feeding should not use cancer salves.

■ CASTOR OIL

OTHER COMMON NAME(S): Castor, Castor Bean, Palma Christi

There is no scientific evidence that castor oil is effective in preventing or treating cancer; however, researchers are currently studying castor oil as a vehicle for delivering chemotherapy drugs to cancerous tumors.

DESCRIPTION: Castor oil is extracted from the seeds of *Ricinus communis*, an herb considered native to Africa and India. It is used as a laxative in conventional medicine and may also be used to treat some eye irritations and skin conditions. It is also an ingredient in some hair conditioners and skin products. There have been no scientific studies to support any other claims.

Alternative practitioners claim castor oil boosts the immune system by increasing lymphocytes (white blood cells that help the body fight infection) and other immune cells. They also claim castor oil helps dissolve cysts, warts, and tumors, as well as soften bunions and corns. Other claims for castor oil include treating lymphoma, bacterial and viral diseases (including HIV), arthritis, skin and hair conditions, eye irritations, diseases of the colon and gallbladder, bursitis, multiple sclerosis, and Parkinson's disease. There is no scientific evidence to support these claims.

USE: Treatment involves massaging castor oil into the body or using a warm or hot castor oil pack or compress. The castor oil is massaged along the problem region, spine, abdomen, and lymph drainage pattern. Promoters say application of castor oil should continue until the problem is healed.

EFFECTS: There is no scientific evidence that castor oil cures cancer or any other disease; however, researchers are currently studying the possibility of using castor oil as a vehicle for delivering chemotherapy drugs to cancerous tumors. Castor oil shows promise as a carrier of Taxol®, a drug used to treat metastatic breast cancer and other tumors. However, a study on high-intensity focused ultrasound therapy for liver cancer found castor oil did not work as well as iodized oil in producing a higher and faster temperature rise in the area of the tumor.

Castor oil is considered safe in proper doses for conventional uses as a laxative. Side effects can include abdominal pain or cramping, colic, nausea, vomiting, and diarrhea. Long-term use of castor oil can lead to fluid and electrolyte loss. Women who are pregnant or breast-feeding should not use castor oil, as well as people with intestinal obstruction, acute inflammatory intestinal disease, appendicitis, or abdominal pain.

Castor beans are extremely poisonous and can lead to death if chewed or swallowed. Also, handling the seeds over time can lead to allergic reactions.

▚ CHIROPRACTIC

OTHER COMMON NAME(S): Chiropractic Techniques, Spinal Manipulation

There is no scientific evidence that chiropractic treatment cures cancer or any other disease. It has been shown, however, to be effective in treating lower back pain and other pain due to muscle or bone problems. It can also promote relaxation and stress reduction. Complications may occur in a few cases.

DESCRIPTION: Chiropractic is a treatment involving manipulation (moving) of the spine to correct medical problems. It is most commonly used to treat lower back pain and other pain due to muscle or bone problems. While there is evidence that it is effective for this use, there is no scientific evidence for other health claims. For example, some chiropractors claim to be able to treat health problems such as heart disease, epilepsy, impotence, and allergies, among other conditions. They claim the spine plays a vital role in nearly all health problems.

Chiropractic is based on the idea that the human body has the ability to heal itself and that the body always seeks to maintain a balance among its systems and organs. Disease is thought to result from a blockage of nerve impulses. Chiropractors claim manipulating the spine is designed to correct these blockages or other unnatural relationships between bones and nerves.

USE: The chiropractor first diagnoses the person's ailment through a personal interview, visual and touch examination, and x-rays of the spine. Electrical activity of the nerves and muscles may be measured. The examination is designed to pinpoint the source of the symptoms; for example, if a person complains of a pain in the shoulder, the chiropractor will search for the cause of the pain in the spinal column. Then the chiropractor will try to restore proper realignment and nerve function through manipulation of the vertebrae.

To receive treatment, a person lies face down on a specially designed treatment table. The chiropractor stands to the side and uses the hands, elbows, and special equipment to manipulate the spine, working to correct misalignments or other irregularities. Some chiropractors may also prescribe exercises to correct health problems, especially those that involve the skeletal and nervous systems.

EFFECTS: Chiropractic has been shown to be effective in treating short-term lower back pain and other pain due to muscle or bone problems.

Chiropractors have also treated headaches, sports injuries, and carpal tunnel syndrome with some success; however, two major reviews of the literature concluded that there is not enough information to determine if chiropractic has any long-term benefits for lower back pain.

Chiropractic is considered relatively safe, but there have been some reported cases of complications and even death following chiropractic care, as well as misdiagnoses of patients' conditions. Several people with cancer developed leg and even full-body paralysis after manipulation of the spine when cancer had spread to the bones. People with cancer and chronic conditions, such as arthritis and heart disease, should consult their doctor before undergoing any type of therapy that involves manipulation of joints and muscles.

COLD LASER THERAPY

OTHER COMMON NAME(S): None

Cold laser therapy is similar to acupuncture, but it involves the use of laser beams to stimulate the body's acupoints rather than needles (see Acupuncture). The term cold laser refers to the use of low-intensity, or low levels of, laser light. This treatment regimen appeals to those who fear the pain of needles. Proponents claim that cold laser therapy can reduce pain and inflammation. There is no scientific evidence to support these claims. This method should not be confused with conventional laser surgery, which involves vaporizing tissue with hot lasers and is used as a valid treatment for some cancers.

COLON THERAPY

OTHER COMMON NAME(S): Colonic Irrigation, High Colonic, Detoxification Therapy, Colon Hydrotherapy, Coffee Enemas, Enema Irrigation, Hydro-Colon Therapy, High Enema

There is no scientific evidence that colon therapy is effective in treating cancer or any other disease. Colon therapy can be dangerous and can cause infection or death.

DESCRIPTION: Colon therapy is the cleansing of the large intestine (colon) through the administration of water, herbal solutions, or other substances such as coffee. Proponents of colon therapy consider it to be a method of detoxifying the body through the removal of accumulated waste from the colon. Because they claim detoxification increases the efficiency of the body's natural healing abilities, it is sometimes promoted as a treatment for disease or illness. Practitioners often promote it as a general preventive health measure or as part of a routine internal hygiene regimen.

Coffee enemas have been promoted as part of several controversial cancer treatment regimens. People who promote the use of coffee enemas to detoxify the body claim that an "unpoisoned" body or a "clean" colon has the ability to recognize and destroy cancer cells. There is no scientific evidence to support these claims.

USE: Colon therapy is administered by a colonic hygienist or colon therapist and is accomplished through the use of plastic tubes inserted through the rectum and into the colon. A machine or gravity-driven pump sends large quantities of liquid (up to 20 gallons) into the large intestine. In contrast, regular enemas only flush out the rectum, and generally use about a quart of fluid. After filling the colon with fluid, the therapist massages the abdomen to facilitate the removal of waste material from the colon wall. Fluid and waste are carried out of the body through another tube. The procedure is generally repeated several times, and the average session lasts from 45 to 60 minutes.

EFFECTS: There is no scientific evidence supporting the claims on which colon therapy is based. It is known that most digestive processes take place in the small intestine, where nutrients are absorbed into the body. What remains enters the large intestine, where it passes to the rectum for elimination after water and minerals are extracted. There is no scientific evidence that toxins accumulate on intestinal walls or that toxicity results from poor elimination of waste from the colon.

The machines used for colon therapy are illegal unless used during conventional medical treatment. Colon therapy can be dangerous, leading to death from contaminated equipment, electrolyte (salt and mineral) depletion, or perforation of intestinal walls. Relying on this type of treatment alone, and avoiding conventional medical care, may have serious health consequences.

▧ CRANIOSACRAL THERAPY

OTHER COMMON NAME(S): Cranial Balancing, Cranial Osteopathy, Cranial Sacral Manipulation, Craniopathy

There is no scientific evidence that craniosacral therapy is effective in treating cancer or any other disease; however, it may help people with cancer

feel more relaxed. The gentle, hands-on method is noninvasive and may offer some relief for symptoms of stress, headaches, and muscle tension.

DESCRIPTION: Craniosacral therapy involves the gentle massage of bones in the skull (including the face and mouth), spinal column, and pelvis to ease stress in the body and improve physical movement. It is a variation of chiropractic and osteopathy (see Chiropractic and Osteopathy). Promoters believe that gentle massage of the bones of the head, spine, and pelvis increases the flow of cerebrospinal fluid, which can cure any number of ailments. They say it normalizes, balances, and eliminates obstructions in various systems throughout the body. By removing obstructions, they claim the body can function in a healthy manner. Practitioners claim craniosacral therapy can be used to help relieve headaches, neck and back pain, chronic fatigue, coordination difficulties, eye problems, depression, hyperactivity, attention deficit disorder, and many other conditions. They also claim the birthing process can have a negative effect on growth of the cartilage and membranes surrounding an infant's skull and offer this treatment to fix this problem. There is no scientific evidence to support these claims.

USE: Craniosacral therapy is usually performed by osteopaths, chiropractors, and massage therapists. The treatment involves either gentle massage or manipulation of the bones of the skull. Sessions last from 30 minutes to 1 hour.

EFFECTS: There are only anecdotal reports of successful treatment with craniosacral therapy. Some patients report that it helps to reduce stress, tension, and headaches; however, there have been no controlled clinical studies of this method. In a report to the National Institutes of Health Office of Alternative Medicine, it was stated that successes have not been documented in formal studies.

Craniosacral therapy should not be used on children younger than 2 years because the bones of the skull are not fully developed. People with cancer and chronic conditions, such as arthritis and heart disease, should consult their doctor before undergoing any type of therapy that involves manipulation of joints and muscles.

▨ CUPPING

OTHER COMMON NAME(S): Fire Cupping, Body Vacuuming, The Horn Method

There is no scientific evidence that cupping leads to any health benefits.

DESCRIPTION: Cupping involves warming the air inside a glass, metal, or wooden cup and inverting it over a part of the body to treat various health conditions. Proponents use cupping to realign and balance the flow of vital energy or life force called *qi* (or *chi*). In the presence of disease or injury, proponents say the qi is disturbed and may become excessive or deficient at certain points. The practitioner diagnoses any imbalances in the qi and attempts to restore them.

Cupping is a practice of Chinese medicine recommended primarily for treating bronchial congestion, arthritis, and pain. It is also promoted to ease depression and reduce swelling. Although not widely used as an alternative method of treatment for cancer, some practitioners may use it to rebalance energy in the body that has been blocked by certain tumors. There is no evidence to support these claims.

USE: A flammable substance, such as alcohol, herbs, or paper, is placed in a cup made of glass, metal, wood, or bamboo. The material inside the cup is set on fire. As the fire goes out, the cup is placed upside down over qi pathways associated with the patient's disease, where it remains for 5 to 10 minutes.

As the air inside the jar cools, it creates a vacuum, causing the skin to rise. This is supposed to open up the skin's pores and create a route for toxins to escape the body. The skin under the cup reddens as blood vessels expand. In a more modern version of cupping, a rubber pump attached to the jar is used to create the vacuum.

In "wet" cupping, the skin is punctured before treatment. When the cup is applied, blood flows out of the punctures, supposedly carrying along harmful substances and toxins. In "dry" cupping, the skin is left intact. Some practitioners sterilize the cups in an autoclave, which heats the cups to more than 250°F.

EFFECTS: No research or clinical studies have been done on cupping. Any reports of successful treatment with cupping are anecdotal. There is no scientific evidence that cupping can cure cancer or any other disease.

Cupping is considered relatively safe; however, the treatment may be uncomfortable and slightly painful. Cupping also leaves purplish marks on the skin, which heals after several days and can cause swelling due to the accumulation of excess fluid around the cupped area.

ELECTROACUPUNCTURE

OTHER COMMON NAME(S): None

Electroacupuncture, considered an enhanced version of traditional acupuncture, involves applying electrical stimulation, with or without needles, to the acupoints that are targeted during traditional acupuncture. Controlled human studies have shown that this treatment method can benefit some people with postoperative pain, nausea associated with chemotherapy, and kidney colic (see Acupuncture).

ELECTRODERMAL SCREENING

OTHER COMMON NAME(S): None

Electrodermal screening is used to diagnose disease by detecting energy imbalances along acupuncture meridians (see Acupuncture and Electromagnetic Therapy). It involves the use of devices to monitor energy signals from the skin. Proponents claim the devices can help select specific treatments, measure the progress of therapy, and even detect disease before it becomes apparent. There is no scientific evidence to support these claims.

ELECTROMAGNETIC THERAPY

OTHER COMMON NAME(S): Electromagnetism, Bioelectricity, Black Boxes, Energy Medicine, Electronic Devices, Electrical Devices, Zapping Machine, Rife Machine, Cell Com System, BioResonance Tumor Therapy

There is no scientific evidence that electromagnetic therapy is effective in diagnosing or treating cancer or any other disease. There are some medically approved uses for some electronic devices, such as the electroencephalogram (EEG), electrocardiogram (EKG), and transcutaneous electrical nerve stimulation units (TENS), which are used to diagnose nervous system and heart problems (see Transcutaneous Electrical Nerve Stimulation). Many of the alternative electronic devices promoted to cure disease have not been scientifically proven to be effective.

DESCRIPTION: Electromagnetic therapy involves the use of electrical and magnetic energy to diagnose or treat disease. Practitioners claim that when electromagnetic frequencies or fields of energy within the body go out of balance, disease and illness occur. They claim these imbalances disrupt the body's chemical makeup. By applying electrical energy from outside the body, usually with electronic devices, practitioners claim they can correct the imbalances in the body. Claims include the treatment of ulcers, headaches, burns, chronic pain, nerve disorders, spinal cord injuries, diabetes, gum infections, asthma, bronchitis, arthritis, cerebral palsy, heart disease, and cancer. There is no scientific evidence to support any of these claims made for the electronic devices.

USE: Electromagnetic therapy encompasses several different kinds of electronic devices that use an energy field—electrical, magnetic, microwave, or infrared—to diagnose or treat disease by detecting imbalances in the body's energy fields and then correcting them. These devices emit some form of low-voltage electrical current or radio frequency. Magnets and other unconventional treatments may also be a part of electromagnetic therapy (see Bioenergetics, Crystals, Magnetic Therapy, Polarity Therapy, Qigong, Reiki, and Therapeutic Touch).

EFFECTS: Science has established that electrical energy and magnetic energy exist in the human body. Electrical energy is used by doctors to restart the heart after heart attacks and is even applied to promote bone growth. Some accepted electrical devices commonly used in hospitals include EEGs to measure electrical activity in the brain and EKGs to measure electrical patterns of heartbeats. There is no relationship between these conventional uses of electrical energy and the alternative devices or methods that use externally applied electrical forces. There is no scientific evidence that electromagnetic therapies are effective in diagnosing or treating cancer or any other disease. Low-level electrical impulses or radio waves are not strong enough to produce a biological effect. There is no evidence that radio waves destroy bacteria or any living cells.

Untested, unproven electrical devices may pose some risk. There have been reports of injuries due to faulty electrical wiring, power surges during lightning storms, and misuse of equipment. Relying on this type of treatment alone, and avoiding conventional medical care, may have serious health consequences.

▨ HEAT THERAPY

OTHER COMMON NAME(S): Hyperthermia, Heat Treatment

Although not part of routine cancer treatment, local and regional heat therapy is being studied as part of conventional treatment for some cancers. Whole-body heat therapy is currently investigational, and clinical trials are underway to study its use along with radiation and chemotherapy. The use of heat therapy outside clinical trials remains questionable and is an alternative treatment. There are some serious complications associated with whole-body heat therapy. More research is needed to determine the full benefits of heat therapy in cancer treatment.

DESCRIPTION: Heat therapy involves exposing part or all of the body to high temperatures, usually to enhance other forms of therapy (eg, radiation and chemotherapy). There is some evidence that local and regional heat therapy may stop cancers from growing and increase the effectiveness of radiation and chemotherapy in some cases. It seems to work by increasing blood flow, which can make the cancer cells more responsive to conventional treatment.

Proponents of the alternative use of heat therapy claim it reduces or even eliminates the need for conventional treatment. They say it decreases the number of invading organisms, so the immune system can handle them, acting much like a fever helping the body fight off disease. There is no scientific evidence for this theory.

USE: There are 3 major types of heat therapy: local, regional, and whole-body. Local heat therapy involves applying heat to a very small area, such as a tumor. The area may be heated externally with high-frequency waves or internally using one of several types of sterile probes (thin, heated wires or hollow tubes filled with warm implanted microwave antennae) and radiofrequency electrodes. In regional heat therapy, an organ or limb is heated. Whole-body heat therapy is used to treat metastatic cancer (cancer that has spread). It involves the use of warm blankets, hot wax, inductive coils (similar to those in electric blankets), or thermal chambers (similar to large incubators).

EFFECTS: Numerous laboratory and clinical studies have demonstrated that heat therapy can enhance the effectiveness of radiation therapy in local and regional tumor control and the effectiveness of chemotherapy in some cancers.

Whole-body heat therapy is currently under investigation as a method to treat system-wide diseases. A small, well-controlled human study found that there were some positive effects of using the combination of whole-body heat therapy and melphalan (a chemotherapy drug), but more research is needed. The National Cancer Institute is currently sponsoring 3 advanced clinical trials using whole-body heat therapy in combination with chemotherapy drugs in treating patients with advanced melanoma, advanced sarcoma, and metastatic and recurring lymphoma.

Heat therapy can cause internal bleeding. The high death rate and labor-intensive methods associated with whole-body heat therapy have also caused concerns. Heat therapy should only be administered under the careful supervision of a qualified doctor. It should also be used with caution in people who have anemia, heart disease, diabetes, seizure disorders, and tuberculosis, as well as women who are pregnant and people who are sensitive to the effects of heat. Relying on this type of treatment alone, and avoiding conventional medical care, may have serious health consequences.

■ HYDROTHERAPY

OTHER COMMON NAME(S): Water Therapy

Hydrotherapy is beneficial as a means of physical therapy, promoting relaxation, and relieving minor aches and pains. There is no evidence that any form of hydrotherapy is effective in preventing or treating cancer.

DESCRIPTION: Hydrotherapy is the use of water as a medical treatment, either internally or externally. There are many medically accepted uses of hydrotherapy. Each involves water in the form of ice, liquid, or steam. Some of the more common examples of hydrotherapy include using water to clean wounds, warm water compresses, ice packs, whirlpool or steam baths, and drinking liquids to reduce dehydration. It is also used in physical rehabilitation, exercise, and child birthing. When performed in water, these activities can be more effective and cause less strain on the skeleton and joints.

Some proponents claim one form of hydrotherapy that involves frequent enemas cleanses the bowels and helps cure cancer (see Colon Therapy). There is no scientific evidence to support this claim, and serious side effects may occur.

USE: In most types of hydrotherapy, either water is directly applied to the desired area in the form of an ice pack or a warm compress, or the body is immersed in water, such as a hot tub or bath. Hydrotherapy includes the use of warm compresses, which expand blood vessels and increase circulation to relax muscles, reduce pain, and speed rehabilitation. Warm water in a bath, Jacuzzi, or hot tub also provides relaxation and stress relief. The steam used in a humidifier can reduce the discomfort of minor sore throats and colds. Steam used in a sauna or sweat lodge causes perspiration, which helps rid the body of waste products. Hydrotherapy in the form of ice packs is used to reduce inflammation and swelling. The coldness constricts blood vessels and reduces circulation to the applied area, thereby decreasing fluid and swelling.

Internal means of hydrotherapy range from drinking the recommended amount of water daily or receiving an intravenous (IV) infusion (directly into a vein through a needle) to getting a water enema. Dehydration, which can be a serious medical problem, is treated through the administration of water or liquids, either by drinking or intravenously.

EFFECTS: Hydrotherapy is an accepted, useful form of symptom treatment for many conditions. The ability to promote relaxation in its many forms is well established. Certain types of hydrotherapy are proven to be effective, such as ice packs for slight sprains and hot compresses for sore muscles. Water immersion is effectively used in physical therapy. Hydrotherapy is also useful for patients with severe burns, rheumatoid arthritis, spinal cord injuries, and bone injuries.

Hydrotherapy has not been proven effective in slowing the growth or spread of cancer. There is no scientific evidence that alternative uses of hydrotherapy, such as colon therapy, can cure cancer or any other disease. Most forms of hydrotherapy are safe; however, colon therapy can cause perforation of the colon, which can lead to death. Cases of bacterial infection due to improperly cleaned whirlpools and hot tubs have also been reported. Excessively hot or cold water applied directly to the skin for a long time may cause pain and tissue damage.

◾ HYPERBARIC OXYGEN THERAPY

OTHER COMMON NAME(S): Hyperbaric Medicine, Hyperbarics, HBOT

Research has shown that hyperbaric oxygen therapy (HBOT) is effective when used in addition to conventional therapy for the prevention and treatment of osteoradionecrosis (bone damage caused by radiation therapy). There is also some evidence suggesting HBOT may be helpful as an additional therapy for soft-tissue injury caused by radiation. There is no evidence that HBOT cures cancer or any other disease.

DESCRIPTION: HBOT involves the breathing of pure oxygen that has been pressurized 1.5 to 3 times normal atmospheric pressure. HBOT is used in conventional treatment for decompression sickness and severe carbon monoxide poisoning. Decompression sickness, commonly known as "the bends," is an extremely painful and potentially dangerous condition that strikes scuba divers who surface too quickly and, occasionally, fighter pilots who ascend very quickly.

Claims about the alternative use of HBOT include that it destroys disease-causing microorganisms, cures cancer, alleviates chronic fatigue syndrome, and decreases allergy symptoms. A few proponents also claim HBOT helps patients with arthritis, multiple sclerosis, cyanide poisoning, autism, stroke, cerebral palsy, senility, cirrhosis, and gastrointestinal ulcers. There is no scientific evidence to support these claims.

Use: HBOT can be conducted in a sealed chamber with a single person, called a *monoplace*, or one that can accommodate more than a dozen people at a time, called a *multiplace*. A monoplace chamber consists of a clear plastic tube about 7 feet long. The patient lies on a padded table that slides into the tube. The chamber is gradually pressurized with pure oxygen. Patients are asked to relax and breathe normally during treatment. Due to chamber pressures that are 2.5 times normal atmospheric pressure, patients may experience ear popping or mild discomfort, which usually disappears if the pressure is lowered a bit. At the end of the session, which can last from 30 minutes to 2 hours, technicians slowly depressurize the chamber and patients often feel light-headed and tired.

Effects: There is strong scientific evidence showing that HBOT is an effective treatment for decompression sickness, arterial gas embolism, and severe carbon monoxide poisoning. It may also be useful as an additional therapy for the prevention and treatment of osteoradionecrosis and clostridial myonecrosis (a life-threatening bacterial infection that invades the muscle) and for assisting skin grafts and flap healing. Other evidence suggests HBOT may be helpful for less severe carbon monoxide poisoning and as a complementary therapy for radiation-induced, soft-tissue injury; anemia due to severe blood loss (when transfusions are not an option); or crushing injuries, poor wound healing, and refractory osteomyelitis (chronic bone inflammation). There is conflicting evidence about whether HBOT is helpful in treating thermal burns and rapidly growing infections of the skin and underlying tissues.

The lack of controlled clinical studies makes it difficult to judge the value of HBOT for many of its claims. There is no scientific evidence that HBOT stops the growth of cancer cells, destroys disease-causing microorganisms, decreases allergy symptoms, or helps patients who have chronic fatigue syndrome, arthritis, multiple sclerosis, cyanide poisoning, autism, stroke, cerebral palsy, senility, cirrhosis, or gastrointestinal ulcers.

HBOT is a relatively safe method for approved medical treatments. Complications can be minimized if pressures within the hyperbaric chamber remain below 3 times normal atmospheric pressure and sessions last no longer than 2 hours. Milder problems associated with HBOT include claustrophobia in monoplace chambers, fatigue, and headache. More serious complications include myopia (short-sightedness) that can last for weeks or months, sinus damage, ruptured middle ear, and lung damage. A complication called *oxygen toxicity* can result in convulsions, fluid in the lungs, and even respiratory failure. Pregnant women should not be treated with HBOT. Hyperbaric chambers may also present a fire hazard. Fires or explosions in hyperbaric chambers have caused about 80 deaths worldwide.

▨ LIGHT THERAPY

OTHER COMMON NAME(S): Light Boxes, Ultraviolet (UV) Light Therapy, Chromatotherapy, Colored Light Therapy, Ultraviolet Blood Irradiation

There is no evidence that the alternative use of light therapy is effective in treating cancer. Some forms of light therapy are used in conventional medicine, such as in the medical treatment for seasonal affective disorder (SAD). Moreover, UV light therapy is currently used to treat psoriasis and cutaneous T-cell lymphoma, a type of cancer that first appears on the skin. A special form of UV blood irradiation, called photopheresis, may inhibit T-cell lymphoma.

DESCRIPTION: Light therapy involves the use of visible or UV light to treat a variety of conditions. Light boxes contain lights that approximate the wavelength of light produced by the sun. Conventional medical professionals may recommend light boxes, photopheresis, or UV light therapy for the treatment of a few conditions for which studies have shown these methods to be safe and effective.

Several forms of light therapy are promoted for alternative uses. For example, proponents claim that light box therapy relieves high blood pressure, insomnia, premenstrual syndrome, migraines, carbohydrate cravings, and hyperactivity in children and improves sexual functioning. Proponents of UV light therapy claim that it neutralizes toxins in the body and cures or weakens disorders of the immune system, bacterial infections, and cancer. Supporters of colored light therapy claim the therapy relieves sleep disorders, shoulder pain, diabetes, impotence, and allergies. Practitioners of one system called chromatotherapy believe that shining colored lights on the body will harm cancer cells. Proponents of UV blood irradiation claim that UV light exposure kills infectious organisms, such as viruses, bacteria, and fungi, and that it neutralizes toxins in the blood. They claim when the blood re-enters the circulatory system of the patient, it stimulates the immune system and increases attacks against invading organisms, including cancer cells. There is no scientific evidence to support these claims.

USE: Patients undergoing light box therapy sit in front of a light box for a prescribed amount of time each day. In UV light therapy, patients are exposed to UVA, UVB, and UVC light. Psoriasis treatment may involve the use of UVB and UVA light along with drugs, which make the skin sensitive to the light. Colored light therapy involves the use of colored lights such as blue, red, and violet that the practitioner shines directly on the patient. Sometimes the lights flash in patterns.

Ultraviolet blood irradiation (photopheresis) as a conventional treatment involves a procedure that uses a patient's blood to stimulate an immunological response. This treatment is approved by the Food and Drug Administration for T-cell lymphoma involving the skin. It is also used in clinical trials for the treatment of immune system diseases, such as multiple sclerosis, rheumatoid arthritis, lupus, and graft-versus-host disease (a complication related to stem cell transplants).

EFFECTS: There is no scientific evidence that light box therapy can cure cancer; however, it does have some medically accepted uses. Light box therapy has been shown to be effective in treating SAD, a type of depression caused by insufficient exposure to bright light, and UV light therapy is commonly used to treat psoriasis. There is also evidence that UVB light therapy inhibits the growth of cutaneous T-cell lymphoma. Other claims for UV light therapy have not been scientifically proven. While there is no evidence to support the use of colored light therapy, ultraviolet blood irradiation is currently under study at a number of institutions.

Light therapy that involves primarily visible light (light boxes and colored light therapy) is considered safe. Light box therapy should not be confused with a tanning bed, which is not a medical therapy and is dangerous due to high levels of UV radiation. Any treatment that exposes the patient to UV radiation presents some danger, including premature aging of the skin and an increased risk for skin cancer. Patients undergoing long-term UV light treatment for psoriasis may experience a greater-than-average number of skin-related problems.

◼ MAGNETIC THERAPY

OTHER COMMON NAME(S): Magnetic Field Therapy, Magnet Therapy

Although there are anecdotal reports of healing with magnetic therapy, there is no scientific evidence to support these claims. The Food and Drug Administration (FDA) considers magnets harmless and of no use for medical purposes.

DESCRIPTION: Magnetic therapy involves the use of magnets of varying sizes and strengths placed on the body in order to relieve pain and treat disease. Proponents claim magnetic therapy can relieve pain caused by arthritis, headaches, migraines, and stress and can also heal broken bones, improve circulatory problems, reverse degenerative diseases, and cure cancer. Practitioners also claim that placing magnets over areas of pain or disease intensifies the body's healing ability. They claim magnetic fields increase blood flow, alter nerve impulses, increase oxygen delivery to cells, decrease fatty deposits on artery walls, and realign thought patterns to improve emotional well-being.

Proponents of magnetic therapy assert that magnetic fields produced from the negative pole of the magnet have healing powers (see Electromagnetic Therapy). Negative magnetic fields presumably stimulate metabolism, increase the amount of oxygen available to cells, and create an alkaline (not acidic) environment within the body. Because they believe cancer cells cannot thrive when alkalinity is high, they claim the effects of negative magnetic fields can halt or reverse the spread of tumors. There is no scientific evidence to support these claims.

USE: Magnetic therapy involves the use of thin, metallic, wafer-like magnets attached to the body alone or in groups. They are sometimes mounted on bracelets and necklaces or attached to adhesive patches that hold them in place. Some magnets are placed in bands or belts that can be wrapped around the wrist, elbow, knee, ankle, foot, waist, or lower back. There are even magnetic insoles, blankets, and slumber pads. These magnets may be worn for a few minutes or for weeks, depending on the condition being treated and the practitioner.

EFFECTS: Magnetic therapy has undergone very little scientific investigation. Most of the success stories have come from a few isolated sources that have not provided proof that the treatment actually works. There is no scientific evidence that magnetic therapy cures cancer or any other disease.

According to the FDA, magnets used for magnetic therapy are generally considered safe. However, relying on this type of treatment alone, and avoiding conventional medical care, may have serious health consequences.

MASSAGE

OTHER COMMON NAME(S): Massage Therapy

Some recent studies show massage can decrease stress, anxiety, depression, and pain and increase alertness. Many doctors recognize massage as a useful addition to conventional medical treatment that is noninvasive and may offer some relief for these symptoms.

DESCRIPTION: Massage involves manipulation, rubbing, and kneading of the body's muscle and soft tissue. Some doctors recommend massage as a complementary therapy for people with serious diseases to reduce stress, anxiety, and pain. Many people find that massage brings a temporary feeling of well-being and relaxation. Massage is also used to relieve joint pain and stiffness, increase mobility, rehabilitate injured muscles, and reduce pain associated with headaches and backaches. Some researchers have found regular massage can help reduce blood pressure, insomnia, migraine headaches, and depression. There is also some evidence that massage can stimulate nerves, improve concentration, relax muscles, increase blood flow and the supply of oxygen to cells, and help circulation of the lymph system.

Some practitioners claim massage raises the body's production of endorphins (chemicals believed to improve overall mood) and flushes lactic acid (a waste product) out of muscles. Proponents also claim massage promotes recovery from fatigue produced by excessive exercise, breaks up scar tissue, loosens mucus in the lungs, promotes sinus drainage, and helps arthritis, colds, and constipation. There is no scientific evidence to support these claims.

USE: In all forms of massage, therapists use their hands (and sometimes forearms, elbows, and instruments such as rollers) to manipulate the body's soft tissue. Massage strokes can vary from light and shallow to firm and deep. The choice will depend on the needs of the individual and the style of the massage therapist. If a patient has a particular complaint, the therapist may focus on the area of pain or discomfort.

Massage usually takes place on a soft table covered with a clean sheet. Massage therapists often play soothing music and use dim lighting to increase relaxation and comfort. The client wears minimal clothing but is covered by a sheet or towel. Oils are often used to keep from irritating the skin. Typical massage therapy sessions last from 30 minutes to 1 hour.

EFFECTS: A growing number of doctors recognize massage as a useful addition to conventional medical treatment. While some evidence from research studies is positive, it is not clear whether massage therapy is responsible for measurable long-term physical or psychological benefits. Large, well-controlled human studies are needed to determine the long-term health benefits of massage.

Results from some recent studies indicate that massage may decrease stress, anxiety, depression, and pain and increase alertness. One review article reported massage helped improve migraines, blood pressure, postoperative pain, and chronic fatigue. One small study found that back massage helped critically ill patients sleep better, while another study found that 7 cancer patients felt more relaxed and had a reduction in pain and anxiety after getting massages. These potential benefits hold great promise for people with cancer, those who deal with the stresses of a serious disease, and patients who suffer from the unpleasant side effects of conventional medical treatment. However, there is no scientific evidence that massage slows or reverses the growth or spread of cancer.

Massage conducted by a trained, licensed professional is considered safe. One concern for people with cancer is that massage might increase the risk that tissue manipulation will cause cancer cells to travel to other parts of the body; however, there is no research to indicate that this will happen. People with cancer and chronic conditions, such as arthritis and heart disease, should consult their doctor before undergoing any type of therapy that involves manipulation of joints and muscles.

◾ MOXIBUSTION

OTHER COMMON NAME(S): Acumoxa, Auricular Moxibustion

There is no evidence that moxibustion is effective in preventing or treating cancer or any other disease. Oils from the herbs used in moxibustion are dangerous if consumed.

DESCRIPTION: Moxibustion is the application of heat resulting from the burning of a small bundle of tightly bound herbs, or moxa, to targeted acupoints. Used in conjunction with acupuncture, it is a practice of both traditional Chinese and Tibetan medicine that treats patients holistically, stimulating acupoints to promote the body's ability to heal itself (see Acupuncture and Holistic Medicine). Practitioners claim the radiant heat generated by moxibustion penetrates deeply into the body, restoring the balance and flow of vital energy or life force called *qi* (or *chi*).

Moxibustion is promoted for the advancement of general good health and for the treatment of chronic conditions, such as arthritis, digestive disorders, ulcers, and for cancerous lesions. There is no scientific evidence to support these claims.

USE: Moxibustion involves the use of a preparation created by gathering dried leaves from mugwort or wormwood plants, called a moxa, and forming it into a small cone (see Mugwort and Wormwood). In its earliest uses, direct moxibustion was most often applied over the acupuncture point, with the cone being placed directly on the skin, but this method produced pain and scarring. Those who still practice direct moxibustion will often place the moxa atop a thin layer of ginger and remove the cone as soon as it feels too warm to the patient.

Indirect moxibustion, most commonly used today, involves either placing the cone on top of an acupuncture needle and burning it or applying heat to needle points from an electrical source.

Another kind of moxibustion is *burnt match moxibustion*, in which the practitioner taps one or two auricular acupoints rapidly with the head of a burnt match. *Thread incense moxibustion* and *warm needle moxibustion* involve the use of heated needles.

EFFECTS: There have been no human studies on the effects of moxibustion and cancer; however, a recent study in Taiwan found that mice with tumors that had been treated with moxibustion lived longer than mice with tumors that had not. Further studies are necessary to determine if these animal study results apply to humans.

Direct moxibustion can burn the skin. Oils from mugwort and wormwood can cause toxic reactions if taken internally, although their toxicity is much lower when applied externally. Mugwort is on the

Commission E (Germany's regulatory agency for herbs) list of unapproved herbs. This means that it is not recommended for use because it has not been proven to be safe or effective. Relying on this type of treatment alone, and avoiding conventional medical care, may have serious health consequences.

■ MYOFASCIAL RELEASE

OTHER COMMON NAME(S): None

Myofascial release is based on the body's fascia system, which practitioners say is a tough connective tissue system that weaves through the entire body much like a spider web. Practitioners explain that fascia surrounds all the muscles, bones, nerves, blood vessels, and organs, and any kind of tension or pressure present in this system can cause the body to malfunction. A gentle form of stretching and manual compression is said to "heal" this connective tissue and provide relief from fascial restrictions and pain. There is no scientific evidence to support this claim.

■ MYOTHERAPY

OTHER COMMON NAME(S): Trigger Point Therapy, Pressure Point Therapy, Trigger Point Injections

Myotherapy appears to provide muscle-related pain relief; however, the effectiveness of myotherapy has not been proven scientifically. Other types of pain, such as cancer-related pain, are best treated by conventional therapies that have been proven to be safe and effective.

DESCRIPTION: Myotherapy is a form of massage that targets trigger points in soft tissues of the body to relieve pain and muscle tension and promote a sense of well-being (see Bodywork and Massage). Trigger points are abnormally sensitive, highly irritable spots found within muscles or around muscles that cause pain, limit range of joint motion, and constrict blood flow.

Proponents claim myotherapy can reduce 95% of all muscle-related pain and in some cases can replace the use of pain-relieving drugs. They say the techniques used in myotherapy relax muscles and improve muscle strength, flexibility, and coordination; relieve pain; reduce the need for pain medications; increase blood circulation; improve stamina and sleep patterns; and correct posture imbalances.

While most myotherapists do not claim they can cure disease, some claim it is effective for relieving pain in people with conditions such as rheumatoid arthritis, lupus, cancer, multiple sclerosis, and AIDS. There is no scientific evidence to support the claim that myotherapy can treat disease-related pain.

USE: After an initial evaluation, a myotherapy patient lies on a massage table and the therapist then probes muscles for active trigger points that have resulted from muscle damage or stress. Direct, firm, and rhythmical pressure is applied with fingers, hands, and elbows to trigger points. Patients typically wear loose clothing during a session.

The myotherapist may choose to employ a variety of techniques, including trigger point compression (direct pressure applied to irritable points along a muscle), myo massage (muscle massage to aid healing and circulation), passive stretch (assisted flexibility movements), and corrective exercise programs that can be done at home. Many myotherapists are also licensed massage therapists. Some nurses are trained to practice myotherapy. It can also be taught to caregivers who can perform it on patients at home.

EFFECTS: There is no scientific evidence to support the claims made for myotherapy, but many people who have undergone the treatment say they feel better and experience less pain after a myotherapy session. Trigger point therapy is not considered a long-term method of pain relief.

Some investigators have found that myotherapy does not interfere with other medical treatments and may be done safely without the pre-approval of a surgeon or attending doctor. One practitioner reported that myotherapy frequently provided temporary muscle pain relief for patients and that the technique could easily be taught to family members.

Myotherapy is generally considered safe; however, pressure applied to muscles improperly or in the wrong places may increase pain. Patients should choose a therapist who has undergone training from a reputable myotherapy school. People with cancer and chronic conditions, such as arthritis and heart disease, should consult their doctor before undergoing any type of therapy that involves manipulation of joints and muscles.

◼ NEURAL THERAPY

OTHER COMMON NAME(S): None

Research into neural therapy has been conducted mainly in Germany where the therapy is widely used. No research is currently underway in the United

States on the effectiveness of neural therapy for pain management or for any other health problems.

DESCRIPTION: Neural therapy involves the injection of anesthetics (drugs to reduce pain) into various sites of the body to eliminate pain and cure disease. The practice of neural therapy is based on the belief that energy flows freely through the body of a healthy person. Proponents claim injury, disease, malnutrition, stress, and even scar tissue disrupt this flow, creating energy imbalances called "interference patterns," which are responsible for chronic disease. Even those who practice neural therapy acknowledge that the process is not well understood.

Neural therapy is promoted mainly to relieve chronic pain. There are conflicting beliefs about its usefulness for easing cancer-related pain. Some proponents believe neural therapy can even cause reversal of cancer when applied at the right moment; however, they say if applied too early, it could cause cancer to spread. Practitioners also claim neural therapy is effective against allergies, arthritis, depression, emphysema, glaucoma, headaches, heart disease, prostate disorders, skin diseases, and ulcers. There is no scientific evidence to support any of these claims.

This method is not to be confused with the nerve blocks and local anesthesia used in conventional medicine, such as for tooth extractions or removing small skin lesions, which have been proven to be effective.

USE: Practitioners first locate energy flow disturbances in the body, then inject anesthetics, such as lidocaine and procaine, at key points that may be far from the pain source. These injections are intended to eliminate the "interference patterns" and restore the body's natural energy flow. The injections may be given into nerves, acupuncture points, glands, scars, and trigger points (see Acupuncture and Myotherapy). A course of treatment may involve one or more injections. A few practitioners use electrical current and lasers instead of injected drugs.

EFFECTS: Most articles on neural therapy have been published in Germany (where neural therapy is widespread), and most of the literature focuses on pain relief. Many of the promoters have claimed positive results, but no clinical studies have been conducted in the United States. There is no scientific evidence that neural therapy is effective in treating cancer or any other disease.

Since there are few studies done on the use of neural therapy, information about side effects is limited. There are methods other than neural therapy that have proven to be effective for relieving acute and chronic pain. In fact, anesthetic drugs are sometimes used to treat some types of chronic pain, such as neuropathic pain. These drugs do not treat the cancer but rather the pain.

■ OHASHIATSU®

OTHER COMMON NAME(S): Shiatsu

Using touch, exercise, meditations, and Eastern healing techniques, Ohashiatsu practitioners claim that one can achieve balance and harmony by altering the flow of vital energy or life force called qi *(or* chi*), through the body rather than focusing on any one area. Ohashiatsu practitioners say this therapy, based on the traditional Japanese practice of shiatsu, offers physical, psychological, and spiritual healing benefits. Promoters say Ohashiatsu is a "step up" from shiatsu because it offers a more complete experience of healing and personal growth. According to its followers, successful Ohashiatsu sessions depend not only on the technical skill of the practitioner but also on the feelings of compassion and empathy the practitioner is able to convey. A connection between the giver and receiver of Ohashiatsu therapy is said to be important to the effectiveness of this practice. There is no scientific evidence to support the claims of physical healing (see Bodywork).*

■ OSTEOPATHY

OTHER COMMON NAME(S): Osteopathic Medicine

There is little scientific evidence that osteopathy is effective in treating cancer or any other condition, except musculoskeletal problems. Research funded by the National Institutes of Health (NIH) will soon be underway.

DESCRIPTION: Osteopathy is a form of physical manipulation that is used to restore the structural balance of the musculoskeletal system (ie, bone and muscles). Doctors of osteopathy (called DOs) use their hands to diagnose and correct muscle, tendon, and joint abnormalities, which they claim are the cause of many diseases. Osteopathy is based on the belief that all systems in the human body work together. Osteopaths claim that if bones and muscles are in balance and functioning properly, the body can heal itself. Practitioners most often recommend osteopathy for head, neck, and back pain, headaches, joint pain, muscle strain, repetitive strain injuries, and sports-related problems. There is some evidence that osteopathy may help relieve musculoskeletal problems.

Osteopathy is promoted as an alternative method to ease pain, improve the quality of a patient's life, minimize the side effects of treatment, enhance other types of treatments, and extend the life of some cancer patients. Some proponents claim that people with cancer, emphysema, heart disorders, high blood pressure, menstrual problems, stomach disorders, and a variety of other conditions can benefit from osteopathy. When used as a complementary method to conventional medicine, they claim osteopathy can reduce the pain from arthritis and the symptoms of asthma, chronic fatigue, and some gynecological problems. There is no scientific evidence to support these claims.

Use: In treating people with various conditions, DOs use several different forms of physical manipulation. *Articulation* involves moving the patient's joints through the normal range of motion. *Counterstrain techniques* involve placing a joint or muscle in a relaxed position and then stretching tightly. *Cranial techniques* involve the manipulation of bones in the skull to relieve pain (especially in the jaw) and treat other conditions (see Craniosacral Therapy). *Functional techniques* involve gently moving the patient's joints until restrictions to movement are found. *Muscle energy techniques* involve stretching the patient's muscles and then forcing the muscles to move against resistance. Hands-on massage may also be used in osteopathy (see Massage). These techniques are sometimes used in combination with conventional medical treatment or after conventional treatments have failed.

Some DOs limit their practice to conventional medicine only, while others may practice manipulative therapy almost exclusively. In recent years, the distinctions between osteopaths and doctors of conventional medical practice have begun to blur.

Effects: There is little scientific evidence that osteopathy alone has a beneficial effect on most diseases, although some studies have indicated that the therapy may help alleviate musculoskeletal problems.

The NIH, through its National Center for Complementary and Alternative Medicine, is making research money available to fund scientific studies on the effectiveness of osteopathy in the management and treatment of musculoskeletal injuries and diseases, especially in children and physically disabled adults.

As with any medical treatment, osteopathic treatments may carry risks of failure or may have serious effects. Some say that it is not recommended for anyone with bone cancer. People with cancer and chronic conditions, such as arthritis and heart disease, should consult their doctor before undergoing any type of therapy that involves manipulation of joints and muscles.

▌ POLARITY THERAPY

OTHER COMMON NAME(S): Polarity Balancing, Polarity Energy Balancing

There is no scientific evidence that shows polarity therapy is effective in treating cancer or any other disease; however, doctors sometimes recommend it as a tool for relaxation when conducted by a trained professional.

DESCRIPTION: Polarity therapy is a system of touch and movement based on the idea that a person's health and well-being are determined by the natural flow of energy through the body. Polarity refers to the positive and negative charges of the body's electromagnetic energy field. It is based on the theory that a smooth flow of energy maintains health, while disruptions in the flow caused by trauma, stress, poor nutrition, and other factors lead to energy imbalances, fatigue, and disease (see Electromagnetic Therapy). The top and right side of the body are believed to have a positive charge, while the feet and left side of the body have a negative charge. The stomach is considered neutral.

Practitioners of polarity therapy claim they can identify the sources of energy blockages and disruptions by observing symptoms such as headaches, tight shoulders and back muscles, muscle spasms, pain, abdominal discomfort, and even tumors. They also claim it can be used to promote relaxation and range of motion, relieve tension, increase energy, and reduce pain, inflammation, and swelling. They further claim polarity therapy enhances the body's ability to fight off serious disease, including cancer. There is no scientific evidence to support this claim.

USE: While the patient lies on a massage table, the polarity therapist applies a variety of hands-on techniques to balance and clear the energy field paths. Some of these include twisting the torso, spinal realignment, curling toes, rocking motions, and moving crystals along the body's natural energy pathways (see Crystals). Some techniques are similar to those used by chiropractors (see Chiropractic). Other aspects of polarity therapy include deep-breathing exercises, dietary management, hydrotherapy (such as whirlpool baths), stretching, and yoga (see

Hydrotherapy and Yoga). During a successful session of polarity therapy, the patient is said to reach a state of deep relaxation. A polarity therapy session lasts about 1 hour or more.

EFFECTS: Claims that polarity therapy is an effective treatment for cancer and other serious diseases have not been proven. The existence of energy field paths in the human body has also not been proven. No clinical research on polarity therapy has been published in peer-reviewed medical journals.

Some patients have reported feeling relaxed and less tense after a polarity therapy session. Some doctors encourage patients to undergo movement therapies because they make people feel better, if only for a short time. Others believe the prolonged physical contact involved in hands-on techniques is beneficial and relaxing to some people.

Polarity therapy, when conducted by a trained professional, is considered safe for relaxation purposes. Improperly applied techniques may cause injury. People with cancer and chronic conditions, such as arthritis and heart disease, should consult their doctor before undergoing any type of therapy that involves manipulation of joints and muscles.

PSYCHIC SURGERY

OTHER COMMON NAME(S): None

There is no scientific evidence that psychic surgery offers any value to people with cancer or any other disease. Psychic surgeons create the illusion that they can remove tumors, unhealthy tissue, and organs by making an invisible incision using only their fingers and hands.

DESCRIPTION: Psychic surgery is used to remove "spirits" or physical manifestations of spiritual problems from a patient by the use of bare fingers and hands without any actual surgery. Some psychic surgeons claim they can cure cancer and other serious diseases by removing tumors or other unhealthy tissue from a patient's body without leaving an incision or wound. There is no scientific evidence to support these claims.

USE: During the procedure, practitioners appear to press their fingers and hands into the patient's abdomen to remove tissue, tumors, or other material believed to be making the patient sick. The practitioners often show their hands that appear bloody to patients as proof of their ability to enter the body without surgical instruments. Critics believe the material they remove is actually dyed cotton pads or other props soaked in animal blood that they hold in a false finger or thumb.

Some psychic surgeons hold up objects such as palm leaves, glass, plastic bags, and corncobs they supposedly removed from the patient. Practitioners will then "close" the wound using their fingers and hands, and then wipe the blood away. No anesthesia is used and the patient feels no pain during the procedure. The patient is asked to stand and walk immediately after the procedure has ended. The skin displays no scars or wounds where the "incision" has been made.

EFFECTS: There is no scientific evidence that psychic surgery has any medical value. It has never been known to remove tumors or cure cancer or any other disease. Consumers should be aware that the claims made by practitioners of psychic surgery have not been proven. There is also a very slight chance of infection from HIV or hepatitis if human blood, instead of animal blood, is used by a psychic surgeon. There has been at least one report of a psychic surgeon in the Philippines who uses human blood for this procedure. Relying on this type of treatment alone, and avoiding traditional medical care, may have serious health consequences.

▧ REFLEXOLOGY

OTHER COMMON NAME(S): Zone Therapy

There is some evidence that reflexology may be useful for relaxation and for reducing some types of pain, although most of the claims for reflexology are unproven. There is no scientific evidence that reflexology cures cancer or any other disease.

DESCRIPTION: Reflexology is a treatment that applies pressure by hand to specific areas of the feet, called *reflex points*, to heal a variety of problems and balance the flow of vital energy or life force called *qi* (or *chi*) throughout the body. Practitioners claim that reflex points on the feet are directly linked to various parts of the body and organs, and when manipulated, they can affect the connected organ or body part. By stimulating these reflex points, a wide variety of health problems can supposedly be treated without medication or special equipment. Reflexology is similar to other forms of body manipulation such as acupuncture and acupressure (see Acupuncture).

Proponents claim reflexology can help conditions such as respiratory infections, headaches, asthma, diabetes, back pain, premenstrual distress, and problems with the skin and gastrointestinal tract. They also say reflexology can stimulate internal organs, boost circulation, and restore bodily functions to normal. They believe that energy travels from the foot to the spine, where it is released to the rest of the body. The practice of reflexology releases endorphins (natural pain killers) and detoxifies the body by dissolving uric acid crystals in the feet. There is no scientific evidence to support these claims.

USE: A reflexologist first gently massages the feet while the person is lying on a massage table. Then the reflexologist applies pressure to selected reflex points on the feet. A person may experience tingling sensations in areas of the body that correspond to the reflex points being manipulated; however, no pain is felt. The whole process can take from 30 minutes to 1 hour.

EFFECTS: There is no scientific evidence that reflexology cures cancer or any other disease. Most evidence regarding reflexology is anecdotal; however, it has been shown to have some effectiveness in promoting relaxation and reducing some types of pain. Because reflexology resembles massage, it can be relaxing and feel good. Further study is needed to determine if reflexology can have any benefits beyond that of massage therapy.

There are no known harmful effects of reflexology. People with cancer and chronic conditions, such as arthritis and heart disease, should consult their doctor before undergoing any type of therapy that involves manipulation of joints and muscles.

■ REIKI

OTHER COMMON NAME(S): Reiki System, Reiki Healing, Usui System of Reiki

There are no scientific studies that show the effectiveness of reiki for treating cancer or any other disease; however, some conventional medical practitioners note it may be useful as a complementary therapy to help reduce stress and improve quality of life.

DESCRIPTION: Reiki (pronounced ray-key) is a form of hands-on treatment used to manipulate energy fields within and around the body (believed to influence a person's physical and spiritual health) to liberate the body's natural healing powers. Reiki is a Japanese word, meaning *universal life energy.* Proponents claim when the energy paths of the body are blocked or disturbed, the result can be disease, weakness, and pain (see also Electromagnetic Therapy). They claim reiki can realign and strengthen the flow of energy, decrease pain, ease muscle tension, speed the healing of injuries and burns, improve sleep, and generally enhance the body's natural ability to heal itself. Reiki is also said to promote relaxation, decrease stress and anxiety, and increase a person's general sense of well-being.

Most practitioners explain that reiki is not used to diagnose or treat specific diseases but to correct any and all underlying physical and emotional problems or imbalances. They also claim it is helpful for people with cancer who suffer pain and discomfort caused by the disease or by the side effects of conventional treatments such as chemotherapy and radiation. There is no scientific evidence to support these claims.

USE: *First-degree reiki* may be compared to the "laying on of hands" practiced in some religious or cultural healing traditions (see Faith Healing, Qigong, Therapeutic Touch). During a reiki session, the practitioner places his or her hands on various parts of the patient's clothed body to channel (redirect) and balance energy within and around the body. The practitioner then attempts to eliminate disturbances or blockages in the patient's energy patterns in order to promote physical healing and spiritual rejuvenation.

A reiki session usually lasts about 1 hour. Many practitioners say that they achieve the best results when patients undergo 3 reiki sessions within a relatively short time, then take a break, and repeat the process. *Second-degree reiki* practitioners claim to be able to send healing over a distance, similar to claims by qigong masters who practice traditional Chinese healing concepts (see Qigong).

EFFECTS: There are many anecdotal reports and case studies about reiki's power to refresh the spirit, speed healing, and increase well-being. Some patients undergoing chemotherapy have reported reduced intensity and frequency of nausea and vomiting after reiki sessions. Some conventional medicine practitioners believe reiki may be useful as a complementary method for relaxation and managing some types of pain; however, there is no scientific evidence that reiki is effective.

A small pilot study found that reiki treatment effectively relieved pain in 20 volunteers, some of whom had cancer. The investigators noted the results were difficult to interpret because there was no comparison group of similar patients who did not receive reiki. More clinical research is needed to determine the benefits of reiki.

Reiki is considered safe. People with cancer and chronic conditions, such as arthritis and heart disease, should consult their doctor before undergoing any type of therapy that involves manipulation of joints and muscles.

▌ ROSEN METHOD

OTHER COMMON NAME(S): None

The Rosen Method, a kind of bodywork, combines full-body massage (to relieve muscle tension) and "talk therapy" (to release unconscious thoughts and painful emotions). A physical therapist named Marion Rosen developed this treatment method in the 1970s based on the belief that repressed emotions cause muscular tension. One of the beliefs of the Rosen philosophy is that people protect themselves from a painful past by separating from their "true selves." Proponents of this therapy claim that the "true self" must be reclaimed through touching, verbal interaction, and breathwork in order to heal. There is no scientific evidence to support the claims of physical healing (see Bioenergetics, Bodywork, and Massage).

▌ RUBENFELD SYNERGY® METHOD

OTHER COMMON NAME(S): None

Practitioners of the Rubenfeld Synergy Method identify and massage tense body parts while encouraging their clients to talk through emotional problems they are experiencing. The Rubenfeld Synergy Method combines the Alexander Technique®, the Feldenkrais Method, Gestalt therapy, and hypnotherapy practices. Developed in the 1960s by Ilana Rubenfeld, the aim of the Rubenfeld Method is personal growth and awareness. This therapy also includes aura analysis and dreamwork. There is no scientific evidence to support the claims of physical healing (see Bodywork and Hypnosis).

▌ SONOPUNCTURE

OTHER COMMON NAME(S): None

Sonopuncture is similar to acupuncture, but an ultrasound device that transmits sound waves is applied, rather than a needle, to the body's acupoints during this treatment method. Sonopuncture is also sometimes combined with tuning forks and other vibration devices. Proponents claim this approach is useful to treat many of the same disorders as acupuncture (see Acupuncture). There is no scientific evidence to support these claims.

◼ THERAPEUTIC TOUCH

OTHER COMMON NAME(S): Energy Field Therapy, Biofield Therapy, TT

There is no evidence to support many of the claims made for Therapeutic Touch or that energy is balanced or transferred by the use of this therapy. It may be useful in reducing anxiety and increasing a sense of well-being in some people.

DESCRIPTION: Therapeutic Touch (TT) is a technique in which the hands are used to direct human energy for healing purposes; however, there is usually no actual physical contact. The practice of TT is based on the belief that the patient's energy field can be identified and rebalanced by a healer. Harmful energy is believed to cause blockages in the patient's normal energy flow. Proponents claim TT removes blockages and other problems in the patient's energy field that cause disease and pain.

TT is promoted to improve or cure conditions such as pain, fever, swelling, infections, wounds, ulcers, thyroid problems, colic, burns, nausea, PMS, diarrhea, and headaches. They also say that TT is useful in treating diseases such as measles, Alzheimer's, AIDS, asthma, autism, multiple sclerosis, stroke, comas, and cancer. There is no scientific evidence to support these claims.

USE: There are 4 parts required to complete an average 20- to 30-minute TT session. The first is called *centering*. During centering, the therapist makes an effort to clear his or her mind in order to "communicate" with the patient's energy field and "locate" areas of energy blockage that are believed to cause pain or disease.

The second part of TT involves an assessment in which the therapist's hands are held about 2 to 6 inches above the patient's body. The therapist then passes both hands, with palms down, head to toe across the patient's body to locate irregularities or blockages in the patient's energy field that signal a health problem.

In the third step, the therapist conducts several passes of the body with his or her hands. At the end of each pass, the therapist releases the harmful energy by flicking his or her hands into the air past the toes of the patient, throwing off the bad energy. Finally, the therapist transfers his or her own excess and healthy energy to the patient. This brings the patient's energy field back into balance and removes the blockages.

EFFECTS: There have been very few well-designed studies of TT. A recent article published in the *Journal of the American Medical*

Association reported that only 1 study of 83 confirmed positive results for TT. Many researchers believe the positive results claimed for TT are due to the placebo effect. That is, the patient wants it to work and believes it will work, so the procedure may create a beneficial result. They believe the simple presence of a person who is interested in helping can promote relaxation and increase a sense of well-being. There is no scientific evidence that TT can cure cancer or any other disease.

Therapeutic touch is generally considered safe. Some of the reported side effects include nausea, dizziness, restlessness, and irritability.

■ TRANSCUTANEOUS ELECTRICAL NERVE STIMULATION

OTHER COMMON NAME(S): TENS

There is some evidence that transcutaneous electrical nerve stimulation (TENS) may help reduce certain types of pain, especially mild pain, for a short time; however, it does not appear to reduce chronic pain.

DESCRIPTION: TENS is a method of pain relief in which a special device transmits electrical impulses through electrodes to an area of the body that is in pain (see Electromagnetic Therapy). Supporters claim that TENS is effective for relieving acute and chronic pain caused by surgery, childbirth, migraines, tension headaches, injuries, arthritis, tendonitis, bursitis, chronic wounds, cancer, and other sources. Some practitioners claim that TENS stimulates the production of the body's natural painkillers. Most TENS practitioners do not claim the therapy cures the underlying causes of pain. There is some evidence that it may offer short-term pain relief for some people, but the long-term benefits have not been proven.

USE: A TENS system consists of an electrical generator connected by wires to a pair of electrodes. The electrodes are attached to the patient's skin near the source of pain. When the generator is switched on, a mild electrical current travels through the electrodes into the body. Patients may feel tingling or warmth during treatment. A session typically lasts from 5 to 15 minutes, and treatments may be applied as often as necessary, depending on the severity of pain. Some practitioners refer to TENS as a sort of "electrical massage."

TENS is used widely by physical therapists and other medical practitioners but can also be performed at home by patients using a portable TENS system. There are more than 100 types of TENS units approved for use by the Food and Drug Administration. A prescription is needed to obtain a system. In a variation of TENS called percutaneous electrical nerve stimulation, the electrical impulses are sent through acupuncture needles (see Acupuncture).

EFFECTS: Research on the effectiveness of TENS therapy for cancer-related pain is limited to small clinical studies and case reports and is somewhat conflicting. Some cancer patients, particularly those with mild pain related to nerve tissue damage, may benefit from TENS for brief periods of time. TENS may also be more effective when used with pain medicines.

There is limited evidence to show TENS effectively decreases chronic pain. More clinical studies are needed to determine what benefit TENS may have for people with cancer in the management of cancer-related pain.

TENS is generally considered safe; however, electrical current that is too intense can burn the skin. The electrodes should not be placed over the eyes, heart, brain, or front of the throat. People with heart problems should not use TENS. The effects of long-term use of TENS on fetuses are unknown, therefore pregnant women should not undergo this therapy.

▨ TUI-NA

OTHER COMMON NAME(S): None

Tui-Na (pronounced twee-nah) uses the principles of looking, listening, smelling, questioning, and palpating (touching) to diagnose areas of the body where energy flow is restricted. Tui-Na has its roots in ancient Chinese culture and actually predates the popular practice of acupuncture. The theory behind Chinese medicine is that to be healthy, a person's vital energy or life force called qi (or chi) must be able to flow freely through the body in a balanced fashion. Tui-Na also attempts to free these energy pathways through 13 basic hand massage techniques that include manual pushing, pressing, pulling, and "wiping" the skin. Practitioners often target and treat the muscles that exist on either side of the spine with this technique. There is no scientific evidence to support the claims of physical healings (see Acupuncture, Bodywork, and Massage).

◼ WATSU®

OTHER COMMON NAME(S): None

Watsu, also known as water shiatsu, is a form of bodywork that is practiced in warm water. A Watsu practitioner stretches, cradles, and massages clients while holding them afloat. The goal of Watsu is to achieve a feeling of peace and simplicity that supposedly is felt in the womb and during early childhood and to release emotional and physical blockages of the body's energy pathways. Practitioners strive to convey a theme of gentleness, acceptance, and unconditional love. Proponents claim that the practice of Watsu can speed both physical and emotional healing processes, although there is no scientific evidence to support the use of this for the treatment of disease (see Bodywork, Hydrotherapy, and Massage).

CHAPTER THREE

HERB, VITAMIN, AND MINERAL METHODS

THIS CATEGORY CONTAINS PLANT-DERIVED preparations that are used for therapeutic purposes, as well as everyday vitamins and minerals. It is noted when there are instances where chemicals extracted from plants are used rather than the plant components.

ACONITE

OTHER COMMON NAME(S): Monkshood, Wolfsbane, Fu-Tzu

Aconite is a Chinese herb used to treat pain related to arthritis, cancer, gout, inflammation, migraine headaches, neuralgia (nerve pain), rheumatism, and sciatica (see Chinese Herbal Medicine). Certain ingredients are extracted from the leaves, flowers, and roots of the plant. It is available as a tincture, tea, or ointment; however, it is not commercially prepared in the United States. Because it is extremely toxic and can cause irregular heartbeats, heart attack, and even death, few sources promote the use of this herb for medicinal purposes. It is dangerous even when used as an ointment. Aconite is on the Commission E (Germany's regulatory agency for herbs) list of unapproved herbs. This means that it is not recommended for use because it has not been proven to be safe or effective. This herb should be avoided, especially by women who are pregnant or breast-feeding.

ALOE

OTHER COMMON NAME(S): Aloe Vera, Aloe Vera Gel, T-UP

The gel inside aloe leaves may be effective in treating minor burns and skin irritations. There are mixed reports about its use as a laxative, and there is no clinical evidence that aloe effectively treats any type of cancer. In fact, used as a cancer treatment, aloe is dangerous and may even be deadly.

DESCRIPTION: The aloe plant, a member of the lily family, is a common household plant originally from Africa. The most common and widely known species of aloe plant is aloe vera. Aloe vera plants have dark green leaves that look like small cacti but are soft and supple. The gel from aloe vera is a thin, clear, jelly-like substance found in the inner portion of aloe leaves.

Aloe is used conventionally for constipation and skin conditions; however, proponents of alternative treatments claim aloe also boosts the immune system and acts directly on abnormal cells, thus preventing or treating cancer. The main aloe product promoted as a cancer cure is a new, unapproved drug called T-UP, which comes in an oral form or can be injected. Aloe proponents claim it is effective against all types of cancer, including liver and prostate cancer, although there is no scientific evidence to support these claims.

USE: Aloe vera is a common ingredient in many skin creams and lotions, cosmetics, and burn and wound ointments. For topical applications to minor burns or skin irritations, aloe gel is applied to the affected area 3 to 5 times a day. Aloe gel may be either purchased as a commercial gel or cream or applied directly from a cut aloe leaf. Since some compounds in aloe gel break down quickly, fresh aloe gel (from the plant) is the best source for beneficial results.

Commission E (Germany's regulatory agency for herbs) has approved aloe for treating constipation. A common dosage is 50 to 200 mg of aloe latex (the residue left behind after the liquid from the gel has evaporated), taken either in liquid or capsule form, which can be used once a day for up to 10 days.

T-UP (concentrated aloe) has been promoted, in liquid form, to be taken either orally or injected directly into the tumor or bloodstream. Practitioners give T-UP injections to people with advanced cases of cancer. Aloe injections are illegal in the United States but are available at clinics in other countries.

EFFECTS: Aloe contains many chemicals, including carbohydrate polymers that soothe and moisturize the skin and anthranoids that give aloe its laxative properties. Mannans are another class of compounds found in aloe that are thought to stimulate wound healing.

There is no evidence that aloe is effective in treating people with cancer. Several people with cancer have died as a direct result of receiving aloe injections. Animal and laboratory studies have found mixed results. One study reported that aloe reduced the growth of liver cancer cells in rats, but another found that it promoted the growth of human liver cancer cells in tissue culture.

The external use of aloe for the relief of minor cuts and burns appears to be safe and effective. There are mixed reports about the safety of taking aloe internally. One report suggested that aloe taken orally might increase cancer risk to humans. Side effects of the internal use of aloe may include abdominal pain, nausea and vomiting, diarrhea, and electrolyte (chemical) imbalance, especially at high doses. It should not be used as a laxative for more than 2 weeks. Women who are pregnant or breast-feeding should not use aloe internally. Aloe injections are dangerous and have caused the deaths of several people.

ALSIHUM

OTHER COMMON NAME(S): Alzium™

Alsihum is an herbal formula manufactured by a company in Israel that is marketed as an alternative therapy for cancer. According to the manufacturer, the compound is a liquid that consists of extracts of 11 herbs in a base of water and alcohol. The herbs include cone flower (Echinacea), cayenne, burdock, myrrh, saffron, and skullcap (see Echinacea and Capsicum.) The manufacturer claims that alsihum may be used by itself or along with conventional cancer treatment to help boost a patient's immune system and kill cancer cells. The company also claims alsihum may destroy cancer cells that are resistant to conventional drugs. In addition, they claim people have used alsihum successfully to treat breast infections, gout, and chronic fatigue syndrome. There is no scientific evidence to support any of these claims. The reported side effects include diarrhea, dizziness, mood swings, and dry mouth. Women who are pregnant or breast-feeding should not use this product. Relying on this type of treatment alone, and avoiding conventional medical care, may have serious health consequences.

ARNICA

OTHER COMMON NAME(S): Arnica Root, Common Arnica, Arnica Flowers, Mountain Arnica, Mountain Tobacco, Leopardsbane, Wolfsbane

This herbal remedy is used for skin wounds, infections, and inflammation. It has not been scientifically proven to be effective. If taken by mouth, it can be poisonous and has been known to cause a number of serious reactions.

DESCRIPTION: Arnica is a perennial plant native to Europe, the northern United States, and Canada. Its daisy-like flower and root (called a rhizome) are often used in herbal medicines. It is promoted for external use to help soothe and heal wounds, sunburn, bruises, sprains, irritation from injuries and burns, arthritis, ulcers, acne, eczema, chapped lips, and irritated nostrils. Arnica contains organic substances that are claimed to reduce inflammation (swelling, redness, and pain) and help heal bacterial infections. The herb is not usually recommended for internal use because it can irritate the stomach and may result in vomiting, diarrhea, and nosebleeds. Some homeopathic practitioners claim it can be used orally to treat fevers, colds, bronchitis (wheezing and a persistent cough), seasickness, inflammation of the mouth and throat, and epilepsy (see Homeopathy). There is no scientific evidence to support these claims.

Commission E (Germany's regulatory agency for herbs) has approved arnica only for external use in treating minor injuries, inflammation of the mouth and throat area, and insect bites. It is considered unsafe for internal use and can cause poisoning in people who are sensitive to the plant.

USE: Arnica is used as a whole or cut herb, powder, tea, liquid, or salve (ointment). The herb is diluted with water and made into a poultice, a soft, moist mass of herbs, which is applied directly to the skin. Arnica ointments usually contain up to 15% of arnica oil or 25% of a tincture of arnica (the herb mixed with alcohol). Blistering and inflammation may occur unless very dilute solutions are used.

EFFECTS: Controlled studies in humans have found that arnica was no more effective than a placebo (inactive substance) in treating injuries. One controlled clinical study actually found that arnica appeared to increase pain and cause more swelling than the placebo in patients who had their wisdom teeth removed.

Small, single doses of the herb are considered safe if applied externally; however, repeated applications can cause skin reactions, severe inflammation, itching, blisters, skin ulcers, and other allergy-related skin problems. Internal use is not recommended because arnica may cause vomiting, diarrhea, internal bleeding, rapid heartbeat, muscle weakness, nervousness, and nosebleeds in some cases. Arnica may reduce the effectiveness of high blood pressure medications and increase the risk of bleeding in people who take blood-thinning medications. Women who are pregnant or breast-feeding should not use this herb.

▨ ASTRAGALUS

OTHER COMMON NAME(S): Milk Vetch, Huang Qi, Huang Ch'i

Animal studies suggest that astragalus may enhance the effect of conventional immune therapy of some cancers. There is no scientific evidence that astragalus can prevent or cure cancer in humans.

DESCRIPTION: Astragalus is a traditional Chinese herbal medicine taken from a plant known as *Astragalus membranaceus*, which is a type of bean or legume (see Chinese Herbal Medicine). The sweet root is used in herbal remedies. It is promoted to kill cancer cells, reduce the toxic effects of chemotherapy, help the body heal burns, protect against heart disease, and fight the common cold and overall weakness. Proponents also claim astragalus can stimulate the spleen, liver, lungs, and circulatory and urinary system, and help treat arthritis, asthma, and nervous conditions. They further claim it can lower blood sugar levels and blood pressure. Many Chinese medicine practitioners say the use of astragalus can help build the flow of vital energy or life force in the body called *qi* (or *chi*), which is essential to good health and well-being. There is no evidence to support any of these claims.

USE: The dried root of the astragalus plant is used in teas, tinctures, and capsules. It is also available as a root slice and a powder. In China, healers sometimes use the dried root in soups or roast the root in honey for use as a medicinal tonic. Astragalus is often combined with other Chinese herbal remedies to enhance the effects of the herbs.

EFFECTS: The scientific evidence for the ability of astragalus to enhance the immune system and fight diseases, including cancer and heart disease, comes only from laboratory and animal studies. Further studies are necessary to determine if these study results apply to humans. There is no scientific evidence that astragalus can prevent or cure cancer in humans or decrease the toxic effects of chemotherapy. Large-scale human studies are needed to verify the benefits, if any, of astragalus in people with cancer.

Astragalus is generally considered safe. Side effects that have been reported include abdominal bloating, loose stools, low blood pressure, and dehydration. People with autoimmune diseases (such as rheumatoid arthritis or lupus) or people taking immune-suppressing medications (such as corticosteroids or cyclosporin) should consult their doctor before taking this herb.

▪ AVELOZ

OTHER COMMON NAME(S): Killwart, Milkbush, Pencil Tree

Aveloz sap is promoted for use as an anticancer agent when placed on the skin or swallowed in liquid form. Preliminary laboratory and animal studies have shown that aveloz sap may actually promote tumor growth, suppress the immune system, and lead to the development of certain cancers. It can also cause burning of the mouth and throat and other serious complications.

DESCRIPTION: Aveloz is a large succulent shrub native to the tropical forests of Brazil, Madagascar, and South Africa. The sap, leaves, and root of various species of the shrub have been used in folk medicine for centuries. The sap of the aveloz shrub has been promoted as a tumor-killing agent for people with cancer. It is also said to burn off warts, cysts, and skin cancers, especially in the face. In various parts of the world, the plant is also used to treat leprosy, earaches, abscesses, toothaches, asthma, colic, cough, rheumatism, and fractures. There is no scientific evidence to support these claims.

USE: Aveloz is sold in the United States in some health food stores and by herbal practitioners in liquid form. To treat cancer, benign tumors, warts, and cysts, practitioners recommend drinking 5 drops of the liquid dissolved in half a glass of water or tea. Aveloz is also sold as an ointment for application directly to the skin to treat warts and tumors.

EFFECTS: The effects of aveloz have only been studied in laboratory and animal research, but the results indicate that aveloz may actually promote tumor growth. Preliminary laboratory and animal studies have suggested that the sap and the aveloz plant itself may suppress the body's immune system, making it less resistant to infections and some cancers. This may lead to an activation of the Epstein-Barr virus and the development of a type of cancer known as Burkitt's lymphoma, which causes tumors in the jaw and abdomen.

Aveloz sap is caustic and harmful to skin and mucous membranes, the skin-like layer of cells that lines the mouth, throat, and other cavities in the body. It can cause burning of the mouth and throat, skin inflammation, conjunctivitis (inflammation of the eyes), diarrhea, nausea, vomiting, and stomach cramps.

▪ BETA CAROTENE

OTHER COMMON NAME(S): Provitamin A, β-carotene

Beta carotene, which occurs naturally in fruits and vegetables, is believed to be an effective cancer-preventing nutrient. As a supplement, however, there is not enough evidence to show that it prevents cancer. It may actually increase the risk of lung cancer among people already at high risk, such as smokers. Research is currently being done to examine the role of carotenoids in cancer treatment.

DESCRIPTION: Beta carotene is the major pigment in many fruits and vegetables that gives them their color. It is a carotenoid that the body converts into vitamin A. Carotenoids are a group of pigments naturally found in fruits and vegetables that also include alpha carotene, lycopene, lutein, and other compounds (see Lycopene).

Beta carotene is an antioxidant, a compound that blocks the action of activated oxygen molecules known as free radicals, which can damage cells. Beta carotene, found in foods, is believed to enhance the activities of natural killer cells (a type of white blood cell) and other cells in the immune system that protect the body against cancer. It is thought to work in the epithelial cells that make up the outer layers of skin and line most of the hollow structures in the body, including the mouth, throat, lungs, stomach, intestines, cervix, bladder, and glands in the breasts. Beta carotene and, sometimes, other carotenoids are also promoted for use as dietary supplements.

USE: Fruits and vegetables are excellent sources of beta carotene and carotenoids, which are believed to play a role in preventing cancer. Beta carotene is found in carrots, squash, sweet potatoes, dark green leafy vegetables such as spinach, and many fruits. A diet rich in green, orange, red, and yellow vegetables and fruits—at least 5 servings a day—is said to significantly decrease the risk of developing stomach, lung, prostate, breast, head, and neck cancer and may slow progression of some cancers. These foods contain many other substances, however, and it is not known if this decrease in risk is due to beta carotene.

Beta carotene supplements are sold in some health food stores, in supermarkets, and over the Internet. The potency and dosages vary by manufacturer. Some supplements include beta carotene with other carotenoids and are sold in pill, powder, and oil form.

EFFECTS: Studies have found that eating foods rich in beta carotene reduces the risk of developing certain cancers; however, it is not known if this is due to beta carotene alone. Well-controlled human studies have not shown that beta carotene supplements reduce the risk of cancer. There is not enough evidence at this time to recommend beta carotene supplements for cancer prevention in the general public. The combination of antioxidants in fruits and vegetables, rather than individual supplements, is most likely to be beneficial to health. More research is needed to understand the benefits of supplemental nutrients and cancer prevention.

Although not harmful, high doses of beta carotene supplements can result in a skin condition known as carotenosis in which the skin turns a yellow-orange color. In cigarette smokers and people exposed to carcinogens (cancer-causing substances), beta carotene supplements can increase the risk of developing lung cancer.

▮ BETULINIC ACID

OTHER COMMON NAME(S): Butalin, Bet A

Betulinic acid may hold promise as an anticancer agent. Some studies have reported antitumor activity for betulinic acid; however, these studies were done with animals and cell cultures. Additional studies are underway to determine its potential role in treating melanoma and certain brain cancers. Well-controlled human studies are needed to determine what effect, if any, betulinic acid may have in treating cancer in humans.

DESCRIPTION: Betulinic acid is a chemical that has a number of plant sources but can also be made chemically from betulin. Betulin is found in the bark of white birch trees, which grow from the Arctic Circle down to Florida and Texas. Some researchers believe that betulinic acid causes some types of tumor cells to start a process of self-destruction called apoptosis. They also believe that betulinic acid slows the progression of melanoma and other types of tumor cells and the human immunodeficiency virus (HIV) and that it has antibacterial properties. Clinical studies are now being conducted to test these claims.

Proponents claim that white birch bark can be used as a remedy for eczema and other skin conditions when applied externally. Other claims for betulinic acid obtained from birch bark include the treatment of diarrhea, dysentery, and cholera.

USE: Betulinic acid is used internally or externally. Tea can be made by infusing a teaspoon of the birch bark in a cup of boiling water for 15 minutes. Proponents recommend from 2 to 5 cups of tea per day. Birch bark containing betulinic acid in natural form can be applied to the skin as well. Pure betulinic acid is not directly available for public use, but raw birch bark is sold in herbal medicine shops.

EFFECTS: Betulinic acid has not been studied in humans, but it is being evaluated in laboratory studies in cultured cancer cell lines and in cancer cells taken from patients. These laboratory studies, using the pure chemical and not the birch bark, suggest that betulinic acid holds some promise for patients with melanoma (a form of skin cancer) and certain nervous system tumors. Three German studies concluded that betulinic acid showed antitumor activity against cells from certain types of nervous system cancers in children. Two laboratory studies conducted at the University of Illinois indicated that betulinic acid might prove useful as an antitumor drug. Further studies are necessary to determine if these laboratory study results apply to humans.

It is not clear if betulinic acid is safe for humans, and more research is underway. Birch bark, available commercially, has not been scientifically studied, and its side effects are not known.

▌ BLACK COHOSH

OTHER COMMON NAME(S): Black Snakeroot, Bugbane, Bugwort, Remifemin®

There is mixed evidence about whether black cohosh is effective in relieving menopausal symptoms. It appears to have some estrogen-like effects, but the mechanism of action is not understood. There is no evidence that it is effective in treating cancer and should not be used for more than 6 consecutive months. The long-term effects are not known.

DESCRIPTION: Black cohosh is a woodland plant of the eastern United States and Canada that grows from 4 to 8 feet tall and has feathery white flowers. The root is used in herbal remedies. It is often referred to as a "woman's remedy" because it is used primarily to relieve premenstrual discomfort, menstrual cramps, and symptoms associated with menopause such as hot flashes. Commission E (Germany's regulatory agency for herbs) has approved black cohosh for these symptoms. Black cohosh is also a source of vitamin A and pantothenic acid.

The beneficial effects of black cohosh are attributed to chemicals in the plant that resemble and mimic the effects of the female hormone estrogen; however, the strength of these effects has been disputed, and it is not clear how it functions in the body. Because some cancers, such as breast and endometrial cancer, are stimulated by estrogen, some herbalists state that black cohosh may be dangerous for people who have cancer. But a contrary opinion holds that since the herb does not actually contain estrogen, it is safe for cancer patients. Some defenders of black cohosh state that the herb reduces the risk of breast and prostate cancer, although there is no evidence to support these claims.

Other conditions that black cohosh has been used to treat include pain relief before, during, and after childbirth; breast pain; ovarian pain; and uterine pain. Other reported uses of black cohosh include arthritis pain relief, lowering blood pressure, sedation, treatment of bronchial infections, spasms associated with whooping cough, and diarrhea.

USE: Black cohosh is the primary ingredient in an over-the-counter German menopausal remedy named Remifemin. Black cohosh can be found in several different forms, including capsules, solutions, tablets, and tinctures. There is no standardized treatment plan for the use of the herb. The typical dosage suggested is 2 tablets of Remifemin twice daily or 40 drops of Remifemin liquid twice daily.

EFFECTS: There have been no published peer-reviewed scientific studies of black cohosh use in people or animals with cancer or even in the laboratory. Previous clinical studies have found black cohosh to be effective in relieving menopausal symptoms such as hot flashes. However, a more recent study on women with breast cancer found that it was no more effective than a placebo for relieving most menopausal symptoms. Larger controlled clinical studies are needed to determine its effects in women with and without cancer. Long-term studies are also needed to determine how safe the herb is when taken over a long time. Not enough scientific information is available about black cohosh to determine whether it is safe. No serious reactions to moderate doses of black cohosh have been reported; however, common side effects include upset stomach, nausea, and vomiting. An excessive dose may cause reduced heart rate, uterine contractions, headache, dizziness, tremors, joint pain, and light-headedness.

The Commission E recommends the herb not be taken for more than 6 consecutive months. It should be used with caution in individuals with high blood pressure and those taking high blood pressure medications. Women who are considering any form of hormone-replacement therapy should consult their doctor before taking black cohosh. Women who are pregnant or breast-feeding should not use this herb.

◼ BLACK WALNUT

OTHER COMMON NAME(S): Black Walnut Hulls, English Walnut, Butternut, Oilnut

There is no scientific evidence that hulls from black walnuts remove parasites from the intestinal tract or that they are effective in treating cancer or any other disease.

DESCRIPTION: The black walnut is a hardwood tree that grows widely in the United States, Canada, and parts of Europe. It can reach a height of more than 100 feet. The nut hulls, inner bark, leaves, and fruit are used in herbal remedies. A few herbal medicine practitioners claim that a tincture made from black walnut hulls combined with wormwood and cloves will kill "cancer-causing parasites," preventing or curing the disease without causing significant side effects. They believe black walnut effectively kills more than 100 types of parasites. There is no scientific evidence to support these claims.

Black walnut is also promoted as a natural remedy for such wide-ranging conditions as acne, thyroid disease, colitis, eczema, hemorrhoids, ringworm, sore throats, tonsillitis, skin irritations, and wounds. Supporters claim black walnut hulls can be used as a mild laxative that eases general digestive problems. A few proponents claim that black walnuts reduce the risk of heart attacks. Because of its claimed antiparasite properties in the stomach and intestines, proponents recommend black walnut for people who travel to areas with contaminated water supplies.

USE: The part of the black walnut tree used as a remedy is the hull of the fruit. Black walnut hull is available in tablets, capsules, and tinctures; however, some claim that only a tincture preparation (with alcohol) is effective.

EFFECTS: There is no scientific evidence that black walnut hulls can cure any diseases, including cancer. The notion that parasites cause cancer or that they can be killed using herbal remedies is unproven. No studies have been done in humans to support any of the claims made for black walnut. Due to the lack of research, little is known about the potential side effects of black walnut hulls.

◼ BROMELAIN

OTHER COMMON NAME(S): None

A small clinical study conducted in Germany recently found that bromelain may have some effect on immune function. No scientific studies have evaluated whether bromelain shrinks tumors or extends the survival of people with cancer. Laboratory studies on the bromelain enzyme have shown it to be effective in treating diarrhea in some animals, but the health benefits to humans have not been proven. More research is needed before any conclusions can be made about the effectiveness of bromelain.

DESCRIPTION: Bromelain is a natural enzyme found in pineapples. The pineapple is a tropical fruit native to Central and South America. Bromelain supplements are promoted as an alternative remedy for various health problems, including joint inflammation and cancer. Proponents claim it reduces swelling and inflammation associated with soft-tissue injuries. Some people also believe that the enzyme is an effective treatment for a number of digestive disorders because it stimulates the contraction of intestinal muscles. Some practitioners claim that bromelain relieves the pain and inflammation caused by joint disorders, such as arthritis and carpal tunnel syndrome, and that it inhibits cancer cell growth when combined with chemotherapy. Supporters also state that bromelain fights bacterial and viral infections and reduces the risk of heart attacks by thinning the blood. There is no scientific evidence to support these claims.

USE: Although bromelain can be obtained naturally by eating pineapples, some people also use supplements. They are available in capsules and ointments in most health food stores. It is also often an ingredient (along with other herbs) in supplements sold for joint health. Recommended dosages vary by manufacturer.

EFFECTS: A recent clinical study found that a bromelain drug taken orally may stimulate one aspect of immune function. This might partially explain its proposed antitumor activity. Other studies suggest that bromelain increases the quantity of immune system hormones produced by white blood cells. No scientific data are available on bromelain's impact on survival or quality of life in people with cancer. More well-controlled research is needed to understand its role, if any, in cancer treatment.

A number of laboratory and animal studies suggest that bromelain is effective in treating diarrhea related to *Escherichia coli* infections and helps prevent platelets from sticking together, thus preventing blood clot formation. Further studies are necessary to determine if these animal study results apply to humans.

Bromelain is generally considered safe. Some people may be allergic to bromelain, and it may cause bleeding when taken with anticoagulant (blood-thinning) medications. Some practitioners advise caution when administering bromelain to people with high blood pressure.

▧ CALCIUM

OTHER COMMON NAME(S): Calcium Carbonate

Many people, especially women, can benefit from monitoring calcium intake to prevent bone problems such as osteoporosis. Calcium supplements will not slow the growth of most cancers, although they are being studied for the treatment or prevention of precancerous changes such as adenomatous polyps of the colon. Calcium supplements may be important for some people with cancer, depending on their specific medical situation (eg, cancer type and stage, type of treatments received). Anyone considering using supplements should consult their doctor to discuss the benefits for their specific situation.

DESCRIPTION: Calcium is a mineral that is found naturally in many foods. Foods and beverages high in calcium include milk and other dairy products (low-fat products are more healthy), leafy green vegetables such as broccoli and greens, nuts, seeds, beans, tofu prepared with calcium, cheese, dried figs, kelp, oysters, and canned fish that still has bones, such as sardines and salmon. Because humans cannot manufacture calcium, it must be obtained from diet or supplements.

Calcium is the building block of bones. It helps the growth and maintenance of bones and teeth, and it assists the heart and other muscle contractions. There is strong evidence that low calcium intake can lead to bone fragility, high blood pressure, and certain cancers. Recent studies have shown that calcium may reduce the risk of developing colon cancer and perhaps some other cancers. When combined with vitamin D, calcium may have the potential to help prevent cancers of the breast and pancreas. Calcium has also been found to be of significant benefit in reducing certain symptoms of premenstrual syndrome. There is some preliminary evidence that calcium may play a role in helping to prevent heart disease and reducing insulin resistance in diabetic patients.

The greatest benefit of calcium to people with cancer may be to reduce the risk of osteopenia (reduced bone mass) and osteoporosis (bone fragility and a severe decrease of bone mass and strength). Both conditions are associated primarily with aging, and osteoporosis is a common problem for postmenopausal women. Osteopenia and osteoporosis can also result from poor nutrition, prolonged drug therapy, disease, and decreased mobility, all of which may apply to people with cancer.

USE: Calcium metabolism is complex and affected by many hormones and factors other than dietary intake. The best source of calcium comes from eating a good balanced diet, which will help to avoid and treat bone problems and calcium balance problems, as well as decrease the risk of some cancers.

Calcium supplements are available in drug stores, grocery stores, and many health food stores. The recommended daily allowance for calcium is 1000 mg per day for men and women aged 19 to 50 years, and 1200 mg per day for people older than 50 years. Some nutritionists recommend that calcium supplements be accompanied with supplements of vitamin D and other important minerals, such as magnesium and potassium.

EFFECTS: A number of important studies to measure calcium's impact on cancer suggest that a diet rich in calcium may decrease the risk of colorectal cancer. While further research is needed to clarify the role of calcium in preventing or reversing cancer growth, there is little doubt that adequate calcium intake is essential for preventing osteopenia and osteoporosis.

For people with cancer, calcium intake may be very important for maintaining bone strength. Some chemotherapy medications can reduce appetite, create swallowing difficulties, or cause nausea and vomiting and result in osteopenia. The chemotherapy drugs methotrexate and doxorubicin may directly damage bones. Radiation therapy can cause osteopenia within the area being treated, and the combination of both radiation and chemotherapy can cause even greater damage to bone structure. Some cancers also can harm bones.

In rare cases, ingesting very high levels of calcium (eg, more than 2400 mg per day) can lead to hypercalcemia (excessive ingestion of calcium), which can cause kidney stones, muscle pain, and mental confusion and is considered a serious medical condition. One study found indirect evidence that excessive levels of dietary or supplemental calcium should be avoided to reduce the risk of advanced prostate cancer. People who are undergoing treatment for cancer should consult their doctor before taking vitamins, minerals, or other supplements that might interact with the cancer drugs prescribed.

▌ CAPSICUM

OTHER COMMON NAME(S): Capsaicin, Chili Pepper, Hot Pepper, Red Pepper, Paprika

Although no research has been reported using the Capsicum annum *plant for people with cancer, capsaicin (the active ingredient) has been studied in oral and topical (applied to the skin) forms. Several studies have shown that capsaicin may be somewhat useful for managing pain related to surgery and mouth sores due to chemotherapy and radiation; however, more research is needed to determine other uses of capsaicin.*

DESCRIPTION: *Capsicum annum* is an annual plant native to Mexico and Central America and cultivated in many warmer regions of the world. Capsicum varieties include cayenne pepper, jalapeños, other hot peppers, and paprika. *Capsaicin*, the active ingredient in capsicum, has been approved by the Food and Drug Administration and is used primarily as a topical cream for pain caused by conditions such as arthritis and general muscle soreness. There is some evidence that capsaicin may be useful in managing postsurgical pain from mastectomy, thoracotomy, amputation, and other surgery related to conventional cancer treatment. Researchers have found that capsaicin may provide temporary relief for mouth sore pain caused by chemotherapy and radiation.

Some proponents claim that capsaicin has antioxidant properties that help to fight the carcinogen nitrosamine (a cancer-causing agent). An antioxidant is a compound that blocks the action of activated oxygen molecules known as free radicals, which can damage cells. Still others claim that it may prevent DNA damage and cancer of the lungs from cigarette smoke; however, these claims have not been proven.

Over the years, the *Capsicum annum* herb has been used by alternative medicine practitioners as a remedy for a variety of conditions, such as upset stomach, menstrual cramps, and headaches, just to name a few. Some practitioners also claim it can prevent colds, heart disease, and stroke; increase sexual potency; and strengthen the heart, although there is no scientific evidence to support these claims.

USE: Capsaicin cream is rubbed directly onto the skin over painful areas. Depending on the concentration of the cream, applications to the skin are recommended for as little as 2 days or as long as 2 months. It is available by prescription or over the counter.

The capsicum herb is available in health food stores as a tonic, in capsules, or in tea. There are some recipes available over the Internet that advocate making a candy with cayenne pepper to relieve the pain of mouth sores from chemotherapy and radiation.

EFFECTS: Although there has been no research done on the use of the *Capsicum annum* herb for people with cancer, capsaicin has been studied for external use. Some clinical research found the topical form of capsaicin to have pain-relieving effects in women who had mastectomies, as well as in people who had pain after surgery. Although it is not a satisfactory treatment by itself, topical capsaicin may be used with other medications to help ease pain.

In a pilot study, oral capsaicin (mixed with taffy) produced substantial pain reduction in patients with mouth sores caused by chemotherapy or radiation therapy. For most of the patients, pain relief was temporary.

The consumption of cayenne, and other peppers, is considered safe in moderate amounts; however, it can cause stomach upset or diarrhea in some cases. Women who are pregnant or breast-feeding should avoid using this remedy internally. Capsaicin cream typically causes temporary stinging, burning, or itching when applied directly to the skin or taken orally. In severe cases, blisters may result. Contact with eyes and mucous membranes should be avoided.

◾ CAT'S CLAW

OTHER COMMON NAME(S): Una de Gato

Cat's claw has been promoted as a remedy to boost the body's immune system, but there is no scientific evidence in humans of its immune-stimulating effects. No data exist showing that cat's claw is effective in preventing or treating cancer or any other disease. There are some serious side effects associated with cat's claw, although the extent of these effects is not known.

DESCRIPTION: Cat's claw is a woody vine that winds its way up trees at higher elevations in the Peruvian rain forests. The plant's name comes from the claw-like thorns that grow on the stem, which can reach up to 100 feet. The root (which can grow to the size of a watermelon) and the inside of the bark are the parts of the plant used in herbal remedies.

The most common claims for cat's claw are that it boosts the immune system and increases the body's ability to fight off infections. The herb also is promoted as a remedy for arthritis, allergies, yeast infections, herpes and other viral infections, parasitic infections, inflammatory bowel disorders, cancer, cardiovascular disease, diabetes, asthma, urinary tract infections, and menstrual disorders. South American folk medicine holds that cat's claw is a contraceptive, and some practitioners claim that it can significantly decrease AIDS-related symptoms. There is no scientific evidence to support these claims.

USE: Cat's claw is taken orally and is available in capsules, tablets, tinctures, elixirs, and tea. Sometimes it can be found as a cream. Practitioner recommendations for how much to take vary widely. Some suggest a dosage of 3000 to 6000 mg per day in pill form, or 4 strong cups of tea. Herbalists may prescribe up to 20 g per day for seriously ill patients. Because herbs are not regulated in the United States, different brands of cat's claw may contain different amounts of active ingredients.

EFFECTS: There has been no rigorous scientific study of cat's claw in humans. All of the reported positive effects of the herb are either anecdotal or the result of laboratory and animal experiments. Some laboratory studies that focused on the alkaloids, or organic compounds, present in cat's claw have found that they may reduce inflammation and heart rate, slow the growth of tumors, and lower blood pressure. One study concluded that some of the alkaloids may provide a strong "immunostimulant action" in rats. Also found were antioxidants—compounds that block the action of activated oxygen molecules known as free radicals, which can damage cells. Further studies are necessary to determine if these animal study results apply to humans.

Research is currently underway to study the effects of cat's claw as a treatment for breast cancer. Until clinical trials are completed, however, the true value and safety of cat's claw remain questionable. Herbalists warn people who are taking anti-ulcer, high blood pressure, anticoagulant, hormonal, or insulin medications not to take cat's claw. Other people who should not take the herb include those who receive injections of foreign proteins, have low blood pressure or an autoimmune disease (eg, multiple sclerosis or tuberculosis), or have had an organ or bone marrow transplant. Studies have also shown that cat's claw contains tannins, which, in high concentrations, may cause gastrointestinal disturbances or even kidney damage. Women who are pregnant or breast-feeding should not use this herb.

▮ CELANDINE

OTHER COMMON NAME(S): Greater Celandine, Ukrain®, Common Celandine, Tetterwort, Celandine Poppy

There is no scientific evidence that celandine, or any synthetic compound derived from the plant, is effective in treating cancer in humans. Animal studies conducted in other countries found that Ukrain had some positive effects; however, there have been no clinical trials to determine if the results apply to humans. Celandine might cause hepatitis when used as an herbal preparation.

DESCRIPTION: The celandine plant, a member of the poppy family, grows in Europe and the temperate and subarctic regions of Asia. The root and aerial parts of the plant are used in herbal remedies.

Celandine is promoted for use in the prevention of gallstones and the treatment of gastrointestinal problems, liver disease, digestive disorders, and eye irritation. Externally, practitioners have used it to remove warts. Supporters have also used celandine as part of antiviral agents to treat herpes, HIV, and the Epstein-Barr virus. There is no scientific evidence to support these claims.

Ukrain is a compound formed from substances derived from celandine, called alkaloids, and other man-made products. It is promoted as a cancer drug. Proponents claim Ukrain improves the overall health of people with several types of cancer, including lung, colon, kidney, ovarian, breast, brain, and skin cancer. They further claim that it helps people with cancer live longer by boosting the immune system and inhibiting tumor growth without any of the major side effects of conventional cancer treatment. Ukrain supposedly keeps cancer cells from getting air and nutrients, causing them to die, and leaves healthy cells undamaged. Proponents also claim that it protects cells from radiation damage; however, there is no scientific evidence for these claims.

USE: Celandine is on the Commission E (Germany's regulatory agency for herbs) list of approved herbs, and it is sold as a whole plant, the top, or just the root and as an extract, tincture, or tea. It is also sold in health food stores and over the Internet. The average dosage is 2 to 5 g per day. It can be taken internally or used externally.

Ukrain is administered through injection at a dosage of 5 to 20 mg approximately 3 times a week for 15 to 20 days. Ukrain is available in Europe, at alternative therapy clinics in the United States, or through mail order.

EFFECTS: There is no scientific evidence to support any of the claims about the benefits of celandine.

There have been some case reports suggesting that treatment with Ukrain may decrease tumor size and provide an improvement in overall health (increased appetite, reduced pain in joints, reduced fever, and so on) for people with cancer. The size and methodology of these studies are not considered by most cancer researchers to be sufficient for supporting the promoters' claims. Controlled clinical trials are needed to determine the safety and antitumor effects of Ukrain, if any, in humans.

Researchers recently found that celandine is often prescribed as an herbal medicine for stomach problems and may be responsible for many unexplained cases of hepatitis. There are also reports that Ukrain has produced pain, nausea, thirst, and swelling in the tumor area. Women who are pregnant or breast-feeding should not use this herb. Relying on this type of treatment alone, and avoiding conventional medical care, may have serious health consequences.

CENTELLA

OTHER COMMON NAME(S): Gotu Kola, Pennywort, Hydrocotyle, Talepetrako

Centella is used in Ayurvedic and Chinese medicine to treat skin wounds (see Ayurveda and Chinese Herbal Medicine). There is no scientific evidence that centella is effective in treating cancer or any other disease.

DESCRIPTION: Centella is a swamp plant that grows naturally in Madagascar, India, Sri Lanka, Indonesia, and many parts of South Africa. Its dried leaves and stems are used in herbal remedies. Also known as *gotu kola*, centella is not related to the kola nut. Proponents claim that centella possesses numerous curative qualities. It has been said that the herb accelerates the healing of open wounds, burns, bedsores, and ulcers. There are claims that it can be used to relieve conditions caused by poor circulation, such as leg cramps, swelling, and phlebitis (inflammation in a vein). Some practitioners maintain that centella reduces fever and relieves congestion caused by colds and upper respiratory infections. Some women use centella for birth control, and some herbalists claim that centella is an antidote for poison mushrooms and arsenic poisoning and, when applied externally, an effective treatment for snakebites, herpes sores, fractures, and sprains.

In some folk medicine traditions, centella is used to treat syphilis, rheumatism, leprosy, mental illness, and epilepsy. It is also used to stimulate urination and to relieve physical and mental exhaustion, diarrhea, eye diseases, inflammation, asthma, high blood pressure, liver disease, dysentery, urinary tract infections, eczema, and psoriasis. Some manufacturers of the herbal supplement claim centella can be used to treat cancer as well. There is no scientific evidence to support any of these claims.

Use: Centella is available in capsules, eye drops, extracts, powder, and ointments from health food stores and over the Internet. Dried centella can be made into a tea. Recommended dosage depends on the condition being treated.

Effects: There is no clinical evidence to support the claims made for centella. A few laboratory studies conducted in India and Europe suggest that an ointment made from centella may speed up wound healing. One study in India reported that centella extract slowed the development of tumors in mice and increased their life span. Further studies are necessary to determine if these animal study results apply to humans. Also, extracted chemicals are not the same as the raw plant. Study results of extracts will not necessarily be consistent with studies using the raw plant.

Centella is generally considered safe; however, there are no clinical studies in humans to fully document side effects. When used directly on the skin, some possible side effects may include a burning sensation, itching, and drowsiness. Women who are pregnant or breast-feeding should not use this herb.

█ CESIUM CHLORIDE

Other common name(s): High pH Therapy

Radioactive cesium (cesium-137) is used in certain types of radiation therapy for cancer patients. However, there is no scientific evidence that nonradioactive cesium chloride supplements have any effect on tumors, and there have been some side effects reported.

Description: Cesium is a rare, naturally occurring element of alkali metal similar in chemical structure to lithium, sodium, and potassium. Cesium chloride is a salt form of this element. Proponents claim that cesium chloride supplements increase the pH level of tumor cells back to a "normal" level, which may be detrimental to the cancer's growth. Since cesium chloride is claimed to work by raising the pH of the tumor cells, its use in therapy has been called *high pH therapy*. There is no scientific evidence to support this theory.

USE: Cesium chloride supplements are available in pill form. Proponents suggest a dosage of 1 to 6 g per day. In a single case report describing the effect of short-term oral administration of cesium chloride in a healthy individual, 3 g of cesium chloride, dissolved in fluid, was taken after the morning and evening meals.

EFFECTS: There is no evidence that the intracellular pH of a cancer cell is any different than a normal cell or that raising the pH of a malignant cell will lead to its death. Because of this, the underlying principle behind high pH therapy has not been proven. Although it was observed that certain areas with low rates of cancers had a high concentration of alkali metals in the soil, a direct benefit of dietary cesium in the protection from cancer has not been demonstrated. More research is needed to determine the benefit of cesium, if any, for people with cancer.

Cesium chloride is not considered toxic; however, the acute and chronic toxicity of this substance is not fully known. Consuming large amounts of cesium could result in nausea and diarrhea. Based on results of animal studies, women who are pregnant or breast-feeding should avoid taking cesium chloride supplements. Relying on this type of treatment alone, and avoiding conventional medical care, may have serious health consequences.

CHAMOMILE

OTHER COMMON NAME(S): German Chamomile, Hungarian Chamomile

Chamomile has not been found to be useful in reducing the side effects of cancer treatment. The effectiveness of chamomile for sedation, inflammation, and intestinal cramps has not been proven in human studies, and its use has resulted in many allergic reactions.

DESCRIPTION: Chamomile is a daisy-like flower. The active compounds in German and Hungarian chamomile are extracted and used in herbal remedies. Other varieties of the plant, such as Roman or English chamomile, which contain similar compounds, are not used as often for herbal remedies. In traditional folk medicine, chamomile has been promoted as a treatment for a long list of ailments. Today, it is most commonly promoted as a sedative to induce sleep and to soothe gastrointestinal discomfort caused by spasms and inflammation. Some proponents also claim that chamomile calms the mind, eases stress, reduces pain from swollen joints and rheumatoid arthritis, speeds the healing of wounds, and can be used to reduce skin inflammation caused by sunburn, rashes, eczema, and dermatitis. The herb is also used to treat menstrual disorders, migraine headaches, eye irritation, and hemorrhoids. There is no scientific evidence to support these claims.

Use: Commission E (Germany's regulatory agency for herbs) has approved the use of German chamomile for gastrointestinal spasms and skin and mucous membrane inflammation. They recommend using it as a tea steeped for 5 to 10 minutes in hot water 3 or 4 times a day. It is also available in capsules and liquid extracts. Bandages containing chamomile are sometimes placed over wounds.

Effects: Well-controlled human studies found that chamomile was not effective in managing some of the side effects of cancer treatment. Animal studies have suggested that chamomile is effective in inducing sleep and reducing inflammation and intestinal cramps; however, these effects have not been clearly demonstrated in humans. In a small clinical study, chamomile extract was found to be effective in inducing deep sleep, but according to Commission E, there is no clinical evidence to support the use of German chamomile as a sedative.

Some researchers report that allergic reactions to chamomile are relatively common and can result in abdominal cramps, airway obstruction, itching, and other symptoms. People who have severe allergies to ragweed should use it with caution. Chamomile may interact with blood-thinning medications, such as warfarin. People taking these medications should consult their doctor before using chamomile. It should also not be taken with alcohol or other sedatives. Women who are pregnant or breast-feeding should not use this herb.

▨ CHAPARRAL

Other common name(s): Greasewood, Creosote Bush

Chaparral is considered a dangerous herb that can cause irreversible, life-threatening liver damage. The Food and Drug Administration (FDA) has cautioned against the internal use of chaparral. Research has not found it to be an effective treatment for cancer or any other disease. A study of nordihy-droguaiaretic acid (NDGA), one of the chemicals in chaparral, concluded that it was not useful in treating people with cancer. Researchers continue to study NDGA in laboratory experiments.

DESCRIPTION: Chaparral is an herb that comes from the leaves of the creosote bush, an evergreen desert shrub. The term *chaparral* refers to a plant community dominated by evergreen shrubs that have small, stiff leaves and grow in dense clusters to heights of 4 to 8 feet in the American West and Southwest.

Proponents claim that it can help relieve pain, reduce inflammation, aid congestion, increase urine elimination, and slow the aging process. It is also promoted as an anticancer agent and an antioxidant (a compound that blocks the action of activated oxygen molecules, known as free radicals, which can damage cells). There is no scientific evidence to support these claims.

Some researchers think NDGA might make other anticancer drugs more effective, but this theory still needs to be tested in animal studies and in clinical trials of people with cancer.

USE: Chaparral is distributed in capsule or tablet form. Chaparral is also made into a tea, which is bitter and has an unpleasant taste. Chaparral is also sometimes found in combination with other herbs in a variety of teas.

EFFECTS: Chaparral does not prevent or inhibit the growth of cancer in humans. It has not been found to be an effective treatment for any other medical condition, although most research has focused on the relationship between chaparral and cancer. One clinical study found that chaparral tea was not an effective anticancer agent. Some laboratory studies have indicated that one of the chemicals in chaparral, NDGA, may possess anticancer properties and may make other anticancer drugs more effective; however, evidence from human studies has not confirmed these findings. Further studies are necessary to determine if these animal study results apply to humans.

Chaparral is highly toxic and can cause severe and permanent liver disease that is sometimes fatal. In 1968, the FDA recommended that the herb not be taken internally. Other side effects of chaparral use can include fatigue, stomach pain, diarrhea, weight loss, fever, and itching. This herb should be avoided, especially by women who are pregnant or breast-feeding.

◼ CHINESE HERBAL MEDICINE

OTHER COMMON NAME(S): Traditional Chinese Medicine, Chinese Herbs

Because of the large number of Chinese herbs used and the different uses recommended by practitioners, it is difficult to comment on Chinese herbal medicine as a whole. There may be some individual herbs or extracts that play a role in the prevention and treatment of cancer and other diseases when combined with conventional treatment. More research is needed to determine the effectiveness of these individual substances.

DESCRIPTION: Chinese herbal medicine is a major aspect of traditional Chinese medicine, which focuses on restoring a balance of energy, body, and spirit to maintain health rather than treating a particular disease or medical condition. Chinese herbal medicine is not based on Western conventional concepts of medical diagnosis and treatment, which treats patients' main complaints, or the patterns of their symptoms, rather than the underlying causes. Practitioners attempt to prevent and treat imbalances, such as those caused by cancer and other diseases, with complex combinations of herbs, minerals, and plant extracts.

Chinese herbal medicine uses a variety of herbs, in different combinations, to restore balance to the body (see Astragalus, Ginkgo, Ginseng, Green Tea, and Siberian Ginseng). Herbal preparations are said to prevent and treat hormone disturbances, infections, breathing disorders, and many other ailments and diseases. Some practitioners claim herbs have the power to prevent and treat a variety of cancers. There is no scientific evidence to support these claims.

Most Chinese herbalists do not claim to cure cancer. They use herbal medicine along with conventional treatment prescribed by oncologists, such as radiation therapy and chemotherapy. They claim that herbal remedies can help ease the side effects of conventional cancer therapies, control pain, improve quality of life, strengthen the immune system, and, in some cases, stop tumor growth and spread.

USE: In China, there are more than 3200 herbs, 300 mineral and animal extracts, and more than 400 formulas used. Herbal formulations may consist of 4 to 12 different ingredients, to be taken in the form of teas, powders, pills, tinctures, or syrups. Chinese herbal remedies are made up of 1 or 2 herbs that are said to have the greatest effect on major aspects of the problem being treated. The other herbs in the formula treat minor aspects of the problem, direct the formula to specific parts of the body, and help the other herbs work more efficiently. Many Chinese herbs are sold individually and in formulas in the United States as well. They may be purchased in health food stores, in some pharmacies, and from herbal medicine practitioners.

EFFECTS: Some herbs and herbal formulations have been evaluated in animal, laboratory, and human studies in both the East and the West. Research results vary widely depending on the specific herb. There is some evidence from controlled studies that some Chinese herbs may contribute to longer survival rates, reduction of side effects, and lower recurrence for some cancers, especially when combined with conventional treatment. Many of these studies, however, are published in Chinese, and some of them do not list the specific herbs that were tested. More controlled research is needed to determine the role of Chinese herbal medicine in cancer treatment and prevention.

Because of the variety of herbs used in Chinese herbal medicine, there is a potential for negative interactions with prescribed drugs. Some herbal preparations contain other ingredients that are not always identified. The Food and Drug Administration has issued a statement warning diabetic patients to avoid several specific brands of Chinese herbal products because they illegally contain certain prescription diabetes drugs. In the last 5 years, Chinese herbal medicines have become the leading cause of liver damage.

A few Chinese herbs are potentially toxic to the human body. Toxic herbs may mistakenly be harvested and shipped for herbal medicines and cause harmful reactions. In addition, the herbal formulas used are often complex and difficult for manufacturers and practitioners to formulate correctly. Women who are pregnant or breast-feeding should consult their doctor before using any of the herbs.

▨ CHLORELLA

OTHER COMMON NAME(S): Sun Chlorella, Green Algae

Chlorella is widely used in Japan for a variety of health conditions; however, there have been no studies that prove its effectiveness for preventing or treating cancer or any other disease.

DESCRIPTION: Chlorella is a single-celled freshwater alga. It reportedly contains a very high amount of chlorophyll, the chemical that gives plants their green color, and is an essential component in photosynthesis, the process by which plants convert light into chemical energy. It is promoted for a wide range of herbal remedy uses. Proponents claim it kills several types of cancers, fights bacterial and viral infections, enhances the immune system, increases the growth of "friendly" organisms in the digestive tract, lowers blood pressure and cholesterol levels, and promotes healing of intestinal ulcers, diverticulosis, and Crohn's disease.

Supporters state that chlorella supplements increase the level of albumin in the bloodstream. Albumin is a protein that promoters claim is protective against diseases such as cancer, diabetes, arthritis, AIDS, pancreatitis, cirrhosis, hepatitis, anemia, and multiple sclerosis. Chlorella is said to prevent cancer through its ability to cleanse the body of toxins. There is no scientific evidence to support these claims.

Chlorella contains vitamin C and carotenoids, both of which are antioxidants (see Beta Carotene and Vitamin C). Antioxidants are compounds that block the action of activated oxygen molecules known as free radicals, which can damage cells. According to proponents, chlorella also contains high concentrations of B-complex vitamins that may help to relieve stress (see Vitamin B Complex). Some herbalists claim that chlorella stimulates macrophages, the immune system cells that attack and consume invading organisms; however, this has not been proven.

USE: Chlorella is available in tablets, liquid extracts, and powder. Some herbalists recommend up to 3 g a day (15 tablets). Although it may be taken on its own, many supporters suggest mixing the powder form of chlorella into foods made with flour, such as bread or cookies.

EFFECTS: There is no scientific evidence showing that chlorella is effective against cancer or any other disease. Limited laboratory and animal research suggests that the algae may have some anticancer properties. One investigation concluded that a protein extract from one type of chlorella prevented the spread of cancer cells in mice. Another study in mice suggested that the extract reduced the side effects of chemotherapy treatment without affecting the potency of anticancer medications. Extracted chemicals are not the same as the raw plant, so study results of extracts will not necessarily be consistent with studies using the raw plant. Further studies are necessary to determine if these animal study results apply to humans.

Although chlorella appears to be safe, no research has been done in humans to determine if the supplement causes any negative side effects or what can be expected from long-term use.

▨ CLOVES

OTHER COMMON NAME(S): Clove Oil, Oil of Cloves

There is no scientific evidence that cloves or clove oil is effective in treating or preventing cancer. Some dentists and patients report that clove oil may relieve gum and tooth pain and may be useful as a topical antiseptic in mouthwash; however, there is limited scientific evidence for this.

DESCRIPTION: The clove is an aromatic spice that grows as an evergreen tree in the tropical regions of Asia and South America. The oil extracted from the plant, leaves, flower buds, and fruit itself is used in herbal remedies. Cloves are said to have antiseptic (germ-killing) and anesthetic (pain-relieving) properties. Undiluted clove oil is often applied topically to relieve pain from toothaches and insect bites. Some proponents also claim that, taken internally, cloves and clove oil combat fungal infections, relieve nausea and vomiting, improve digestion, fight intestinal parasites, stimulate uterine contractions, ease arthritis inflammation, stop migraine headaches, and ease symptoms of colds and allergies. Practitioners of traditional Chinese medicine sometimes treat hiccups and impotence with cloves (see Chinese Herbal Medicine).

One herbalist claims that a mixture of cloves, black walnut hulls, and wormwood cures cancer (see Black Walnut and Wormwood). Others claim that cloves contain antioxidants, compounds that block the action of activated oxygen molecules known as free radicals, which can damage cells. There is no scientific evidence to support these claims.

USE: Cloves are available in capsules, powder, or as a whole herb. Pure and diluted clove oil can also be purchased.

EFFECTS: Commission E (Germany's regulatory agency for herbs) approved clove oil for use as an antiseptic and topical anesthetic. However, no well-controlled clinical studies have been done to evaluate the potential antibacterial, anticarcinogenic, and pain-relieving properties of cloves or clove oil in humans.

A few laboratory studies suggest that clove oil may fight bacteria and prevent convulsions and that compounds taken from cloves show promise as potential anticarcinogenic agents; however, extracted chemicals are not the same as the raw plant. Study results of extracts will not necessarily be consistent with studies using the raw plant. Further studies are necessary to determine if these laboratory study results apply to humans.

Cloves are generally considered safe, although a few people may be allergic to eugenol, the main active ingredient. Excessive application of undiluted clove oil on or near the teeth may cause damage to dental pulp and other soft tissue surrounding teeth. It should be used for tooth and gum conditions only under the supervision of a dentist.

▧ COMFREY

OTHER COMMON NAME(S): Blackwort, Bruisewort, Knitbone, Slippery Root

Although comfrey has been used in folk medicine for many years to help heal wounds, sprains, and fractures, there have been no studies in humans to prove that it is useful. There is also no evidence that comfrey is effective in treating cancer. It is not safe for internal use and should not be consumed.

DESCRIPTION: Comfrey is a fast-growing herb native to Europe and temperate parts of Asia. It now grows in North America as well. The roots and leaves are used in herbal remedies. It has been promoted mainly to speed the healing of wounds, sprains, bruises, and bone fractures and to reduce inflammation and swelling related to these injuries. Comfrey has also been used to treat a number of other ailments, including gastrointestinal ulcers, gallstones, arthritis, colitis, pleurisy, and insect bites. A mouthwash made from comfrey is sometimes used to heal gum disease, hoarseness, and pharyngitis (inflammation of the pharynx). Some proponents also claim comfrey has anticancer properties; however, there is no scientific evidence to support these claims.

USE: Commission E (Germany's regulatory agency for herbs) has approved comfrey for external use only to treat bruises and sprains. Ointments, compresses, and poultices are made from the crushed roots and leaves of comfrey or from liquid extracts pressed from the plant. They are placed directly on bruises, wounds, or sprains; are covered with a dressing; and replaced daily until healing occurs. For internal use, dried comfrey is sometimes prepared as a tea but is also available in tinctures and capsules; however, since it has the potential to cause liver damage, comfrey should not be taken internally.

EFFECTS: There is no evidence showing that comfrey is useful in treating cancer or any other disease. The herb's influence on the healing of wounds, fractures, and other injuries in humans is not known.

Several studies have shown that comfrey contains chemicals called pyrrolizidine alkaloids, which cause severe liver damage when taken internally. Animal studies have also shown that these chemicals lead to the development of liver tumors.

The internal use of comfrey is not considered safe. Experts strongly warn consumers not to eat or drink any preparations that contain comfrey. This herb should be avoided, especially by women who are pregnant or breast-feeding. The US Pharmacopeia reports that the use of comfrey on broken skin should also be avoided because it may be absorbed into the body's system. In July 2001, the Food and Drug Administration advised dietary supplement manufacturers to remove comfrey products from the market and alert customers to stop using the product immediately because the pyrrolizidine alkaloids present a serious health hazard when ingested. The Federal Trade Commission has also taken action against unsafe products containing comfrey.

COPPER

OTHER COMMON NAME(S): None

Some laboratory and animal studies have found that copper has antioxidant properties and may have some anticancer effects. Other animal studies suggest that high copper levels may promote cancer formation and growth. Human studies are needed to determine what role, if any, copper may play in the prevention or treatment of cancer.

DESCRIPTION: Copper is a trace element found naturally in foods such as seafood, organ meats, green vegetables, and nuts. It assists in the regulation of blood pressure and heart rate and the absorption of iron in the body. Some proponents claim copper helps cells in the immune system work properly. There are claims that copper aids the body in other functions such as the healing process, expelling toxins from the body, maintaining connective tissues, forming red blood cells, and preventing heart problems. A lack of copper in the body, some practitioners say, can lead to lowered resistance to infections and a shortened life span after infection. Copper is also used in some preparations of *Iscador*, a species of European mistletoe, for primary tumors of the liver, gallbladder, stomach, and kidneys.

There are also claims that copper actually promotes cancer growth. Proponents of this theory recommend a low copper diet and use of chelating agents that bind to copper and promote its elimination from the body (see Chelation Therapy). There is no scientific evidence to support these claims.

USE: Copper supplements are available in pill form; however, nearly all people are able to get an adequate level of copper in their bodies by maintaining a balanced diet. Fruits and vegetables can contribute up to 30% of a person's total copper intake. The estimated minimum daily requirement is 2 mg.

EFFECTS: There have been no studies in humans to determine whether copper supplements are effective in preventing or treating cancer. Animal studies have shown that copper is useful in maintaining antioxidant defenses. Antioxidant compounds block the action of activated oxygen molecules known as free radicals, which can damage cells. While the involvement of copper in the cancer process via antioxidant effects is still unclear, copper complexes have been shown to have anticancer properties in laboratory studies. Other laboratory and animal studies suggest that high copper levels may promote formation of liver cancer and stimulate growth of brain tumors. Further studies are necessary to determine if these animal and laboratory study results apply to humans.

Copper is a necessary nutrient for absorption of iron into the body. Copper supplements are considered safe; however, most people receive adequate copper intake from a normal balanced diet and do not require supplements. People with Wilson's Disease (a genetic disorder that develops from copper poisoning) should not take copper supplements or multivitamins containing copper. People with diabetes should also avoid these supplements because copper can affect blood sugar levels. Copper toxicity is rare; however, a dosage over 35 mg per day is considered toxic.

◾ ECHINACEA

OTHER COMMON NAME(S): Purple Cone Flower, Kansas Snakeroot, Black Sampson

Although Echinacea has been widely promoted to help fight colds and flu, there is little scientific evidence that it helps boost the immune system. There is also no evidence showing that Echinacea increases resistance to cancer or relieves the side effects of chemotherapy or radiation therapy. Echinacea has some side effects associated with long-term use, as well as the potential to interfere with anesthesia and certain medications.

DESCRIPTION: Echinacea (pronounced ecki-nay-sha) is an herb that grows wild primarily in the Great Plains and eastern regions of North America. It is also cultivated in Europe. There are 3 different species of the plant used in herbal remedies. *Echinacea purpurea* is the most frequently used for research and treatment. Liquid extracts are made from the leaves and roots or from the whole plant.

Echinacea is promoted mainly as a treatment of colds, the flu, and other respiratory infections. In Germany, Echinacea is a common over-the-counter medication, and more than 300 Echinacea products are reportedly sold. Commission E (Germany's regulatory agency for herbs) approved Echinacea for treating respiratory infections, urinary tract infections, and poorly healing wounds. It is also claimed that Echinacea boosts the body's immune system. Some claim that the herb stimulates the anticancer activity of natural killer cells (a type of white blood cell) and therefore could be used as a supplement to chemotherapy or radiation therapy. There is no scientific evidence to support these claims.

USE: Echinacea is available in capsule and liquid form; however, there is controversy over its usefulness in liquid form. Although the dosage may vary, most practitioners recommend 900 mg a day for no longer than 8 weeks to boost the immune system. An injectable form is also available outside the United States.

EFFECTS: Many practitioners and patients are convinced that Echinacea has the ability to fight off infections from colds and the flu. The few reliable studies that have been published have shown mixed results. Studies in Germany concluded that Echinacea did not significantly reduce the number, length, or severity of colds and respiratory infections compared to placebo (an inactive substance or treatment).

In terms of how people with cancer use Echinacea, there is no reliable evidence proving Echinacea increases resistance to cancer or alleviates the immune suppression resulting from chemotherapy. Clearly, more research is needed before scientists can make firm conclusions about Echinacea's effectiveness and how much or what type of preparation to use.

In some cases, Echinacea has been associated with allergic reactions, so people with a history of asthma or allergic rhinitis should use it with caution. Practitioners also caution that Echinacea may cause liver damage or suppress the immune system if used for more than 8 weeks. They urge people taking medications known to cause liver toxicity, such as anabolic steroids, amiodarone (a drug for heart rhythm problems), and the chemotherapy drugs methotrexate and ketoconazole, to avoid Echinacea use. Others who should not take Echinacea include people with autoimmune disorders such as multiple sclerosis or HIV, people with leukemia, people who are undergoing surgery, and women who are pregnant or breast-feeding.

▌ ESSIAC TEA

OTHER COMMON NAME(S): Essiac®, Flor Essence®, Tea of Life®, Herbal Essence®, Vitalitea®

There have been no published human studies showing the effectiveness of Essiac in the treatment of cancer. Some of the specific herbs contained in the mixture have shown some anticancer effects in laboratory experiments. There is no scientific evidence to support its use for the treatment of cancer in humans.

DESCRIPTION: Essiac (pronounced ess-see-ack) is a mixture of herbs that are combined to make a tea. The original formula included burdock root, slippery elm inner bark, sheep sorrel, and Turkish rhubarb. Watercress, blessed thistle, red clover, and kelp were added to later recipes. The different herbs are claimed to relieve inflammation, lubricate bones and joints, stimulate the stomach, and eliminate excess mucus in organs, tissues, lymph glands, and nerve channels.

It was originally claimed that Essiac worked by changing tumors into normal tissue. Proponents claimed a tumor would become larger and harder after a few doses of Essiac, then it would soften, shrink, and be discharged by the body. Promoters claim Essiac strengthens the immune system, improves well-being, relieves pain, increases appetite, reduces tumor size, and extends survival. Some also claim that it cleanses the blood, promotes cell repair, restores energy levels, and detoxifies the body. There is no scientific evidence to support any of these claims.

USE: Essiac is available in dry and liquid formulas, and there are different methods of preparation and dosage according to various manufacturers. Some recommend spring or nonfluoridated water, and most require refrigeration after brewing. A typical dosage is 1 ounce taken 1 to 3 times per day. Practitioners advise that Essiac tea should be taken on an empty stomach, 2 hours before or after meals for at least 1 to 2 years.

Essiac is sold through mail order and is available in the United States in health food stores as a nutritional supplement. In Canada, Essiac cannot be sold or marketed as a drug and is only available directly from the manufacturer or, for people with advanced cancer, through Health Canada. Flor Essence, a leading competitor with a similar formulation, is sold in Canadian stores as an herbal tonic (but is not promoted as a cancer cure).

EFFECTS: Although there have been many testimonials, there have been no clinical trials proving the effectiveness of Essiac. One study found reduced tumor growth after giving oral and intravenous doses of Essiac to mice injected with human cancer cells. Also, some laboratory research found anticancer effects related to the specific herbs studied separately. Further studies are necessary to determine if these animal and laboratory study results apply to humans.

Serious side effects are uncommon. Essiac may have a laxative effect or cause increased urination in some people. If taken with food, it may also cause headache, nausea, diarrhea, and vomiting.

▌ EVENING PRIMROSE

OTHER COMMON NAME(S): Evening Primrose Oil

There is no scientific evidence that evening primrose oil is effective in preventing or treating cancer. While the 2 essential fatty acids found in evening primrose play a role in health and disease, larger clinical studies are needed to determine whether the fatty acids in evening primrose oil are useful in treating cancer or other conditions.

DESCRIPTION: Evening primrose is a flowering plant originally native to North America that now grows throughout much of Europe and parts of Asia. It blooms every other year, and its large, fragrant yellow flowers open at dusk and remain open through the night. In Germany, the plant is called *night candle* for this reason. The oil extracted from the seeds is used in herbal remedies.

Evening primrose is promoted as an herbal remedy for a broad range of conditions, including dermatitis, premenstrual syndrome, eczema, inflammation, hyperactivity in children, high cholesterol, asthmatic cough, upset stomach, psoriasis, rheumatoid arthritis, and diabetic nerve damage. Some proponents also believe the plant has anticancer properties. Claims made for evening primrose are based on the fact that oil from the seeds contains 2 essential fatty acids, which play a key role in many biological processes (see Gamma Linolenic Acid [GLA] and Omega-3 Fatty Acids).

Use: The oil can be purchased in capsules and gelcaps, and the powdered plant can be made into a tea. Daily dosages of evening primrose oil have ranged from 2 to 16 capsules of 500 mg in clinical trials; although in one study, up to 36 capsules per day were used.

Effects: There is little evidence to support claims that evening primrose oil has any effect on cancer or any other disease. Results of studies of evening primrose oil for treating eczema, rheumatoid arthritis, and premenstrual syndrome have been either mixed or not favorable. Most research has been conducted in laboratory settings or involved small numbers of patients. One recent laboratory study concluded that evening primrose oil might help slow the growth of breast cancer in animal tumor models. Other laboratory studies have found that evening primrose oil slowed the growth of skin cancer cells, and a diet enriched with evening primrose oil was thought to enhance the body's ability to fight tumors. Further studies are necessary to determine if these animal and laboratory study results apply to humans. Large-scale human studies are needed to determine the value of evening primrose or its constituent fatty acids in treating any specific condition.

No significant health hazards have been identified with taking evening primrose. Headaches are reported as a possible side effect. One article reported that the acid in primrose oil (GLA) might lower seizure thresholds, so it should not be used with anticonvulsant medication. Women who are pregnant or breast-feeding should not use this herb.

◼ FLAXSEED

Other common name(s): Flaxseed Oil, Linseed, Lint Bells, Linum

Flaxseed and its oil have been promoted since the 1950s as a dietary nutrient with anticancer properties. Most of the evidence for its ability to prevent cancer from occurring or growing has come from a few studies in animals. Only recently has there been some evidence suggesting that flaxseed supplements along with low-fat diets may be useful in men with early-stage prostate cancer. Controlled clinical studies are needed to determine its usefulness in treating cancer in humans.

Description: Flax is an annual plant cultivated for its fiber, which is used in making linen. Flaxseed and its oil are used in herbal remedies. Herbalists promote the use of flaxseed for constipation, abdominal problems, respiratory problems, sore throat, eczema, menstrual problems, and arthritis. The oil extracted from flaxseeds is said to lower cholesterol levels, boost the immune system, and prevent cancer. Flaxseed oil is high in alpha-linolenic acid, an omega-3 fatty acid, which is thought to have beneficial effects against cancer when consumed (see Omega-3 Fatty Acids).

Recently, attention has focused on the flaxseed itself, which is a rich source of lignans, compounds that can act as antiestrogens or weak estrogens and may play a role in preventing estrogen-dependent cancers such as breast cancer. Lignans may also function as antioxidants and may slow cell growth by mechanisms not yet understood. When flaxseeds are consumed, the lignans are chemically converted into active forms by bacteria in the intestine.

USE: Flaxseed is available in flour, meal, and seed form. It may be found in some multigrain breads, cereals, breakfast bars, and muffins. The toasted seeds are sometimes mixed into bread dough or sprinkled over salads, yogurt, or cereal. Flaxseed meal can be used in the same way. Flaxseed oil is available in many health food stores in liquid form and is sometimes mixed into cottage cheese. The oil is also available in soft-gel capsules.

EFFECTS: Most of the evidence for an anticancer effect of flaxseed and flaxseed oil comes from animal research. One small study of men with prostate cancer found that a low-fat diet supplemented with ground flaxseed reduced serum testosterone, slowed the growth rate of cancer cells, and increased the death rate of cancer cells. More research in humans is needed to determine the usefulness of flaxseed in cancer treatment and prevention.

Flaxseeds and flaxseed oil can spoil if they are not kept refrigerated. Some possible side effects include diarrhea, gas, and nausea. Flaxseed oil should not be used with other laxatives or stool softeners. People who have inflammatory disease of the intestine, esophagus, or stomach should avoid flaxseed. The immature pods of flaxseed are poisonous.

▨ FLOWER REMEDIES

OTHER COMMON NAME(S): Bach Remedies

There is no scientific evidence that flower remedies are effective in treating cancer or any other disease. Numerous testimonials state that flower remedies are particularly effective for stabilizing emotions, although no scientific studies have been conducted to determine if they provide any health benefits.

DESCRIPTION: Flower remedies are essences from flowers that have been diluted in water and brandy. Essences are oils in a flower that contain its scent. There are 38 different formulas used that contain various combinations of flowers. Proponents claim that flower remedies ease stress and reduce negative emotions, which in turn stimulates the body's healing processes to help fight disease. They believe that underlying emotional problems or disorders cause physical disease. They do not claim that flower remedies cure diseases, only that they assist the body's natural defenses. Supporters suggest that flower remedies can help improve sleep, reduce stress, calm fears, ease childbirth, reduce alcoholic tremors, and lessen skeletal and muscular pain. There is no scientific evidence to support these claims.

Particular flowers are believed to be associated with 7 categories of emotional problems that include fear, uncertainty, general disinterest, loneliness, oversensitivity, despondency, and relationship problems.

USE: Drops of flower essence preparations are placed directly under the tongue or in a glass of water or juice. The flowers are collected early in the morning when they are in full bloom and soaked in spring water in bright sunlight for 3 hours. The blossoms are removed from the flowering plant, and the blossom-soaked water is placed in a sterile bottle and mixed with an equal amount of brandy. The liquid is then highly diluted, so very small amounts remain in the final remedy formula (see Homeopathy). Practitioners determine which combination of flower essences to prescribe based on the patient's emotional condition, not on specific diseases that are present.

EFFECTS: Despite numerous anecdotal reports claiming flower remedies improve health, there is no scientific evidence showing that the treatment results in any measurable positive results. They may produce a placebo effect, in which believing that something can or will happen generates a positive result.

There are no known harmful effects reported with the ingestion of flower remedies.

▨ FOLIC ACID

OTHER COMMON NAME(S): Folate, Folacin, Vitamin B Complex

Folic acid may reduce the risk of some cancers, although the amount needed to lower the risk is unknown. Low levels of folic acid have been associated

with higher rates of colorectal cancer and some birth defects. High doses of folic acid can interfere with the effectiveness of the chemotherapy drug methotrexate.

DESCRIPTION: Folic acid is a B-complex vitamin found in many vegetables, beans, fruits, whole grains, and some fortified breakfast cereals (see Vitamin B Complex). It helps in the metabolism of DNA and is especially important for the development of blood cells. Folic acid is promoted primarily as a nutritional requirement for a healthy diet to reduce the risk of some types of cancer, birth defects (eg, spina bifida and anencephaly), and peripheral blood vessel disease.

USE: Folic acid is found in dark green leafy vegetables, citrus fruit, poultry, liver, and fortified grain-based cereals. Folic acid supplements are available in tablet and powder form in drug stores and health food stores. The recommended daily allowance is 400 micrograms (μg) per day. The US Public Health Service recommends that all women who might become pregnant take 400 μg of folic acid every day to prevent birth defects.

EFFECTS: Research from clinical studies has shown a connection between lower intake of folic acid and a greater risk of colorectal cancer. Other investigations have reported a connection between low levels of folic acid and cancer of the breast, lung, esophagus, and stomach. The exact way low levels of folic acid can promote the development of cancer is unknown; however, folic acid is essential for the production of chemicals that form DNA during cell reproduction and cell repair. Scientists believe low levels of folic acid can lead to a change in the chemicals that affect DNA, which can lead to cancer. Other theories suggest low folic acid levels impair the ability to ward off cancer-producing cells.

The amount of folic acid needed to reduce cancer risk has still not been determined. Many scientists believe that few people eat enough green vegetables and fruit to give them adequate protection. That is why some experts favor fortifying grain-based foods with folic acid. Research suggests men and women of all ages should consume approximately 400 μg per day, preferably in the form of a balanced diet that includes large amounts of fruit and vegetables with a multivitamin supplement containing folic acid.

Folic acid is considered a safe and necessary dietary nutrient; however, if taken in extremely large doses, it can be toxic. High doses of folate also interfere with the effectiveness of the chemotherapy drug methotrexate.

FU ZHEN THERAPY

OTHER COMMON NAME(S): None

Fu Zhen therapy is a Chinese herbal remedy promoted to enhance the immune system, improve digestion, and stimulate energy levels (see Chinese Herbal Medicine). The herbs reportedly used most often in Fu Zhen include astragalus, ligustrum, ginseng, codonopsis, atractylodes, and ganoderma (see Astragalus and Ginseng). Proponents claim that Fu Zhen is effective for treating cancer when used as a complementary therapy along with chemotherapy and radiation treatments. There is no scientific evidence to support these claims.

GERMANIUM

OTHER COMMON NAME(S): Germanium Sesquioxide

There is no scientific evidence that germanium supplements are effective in preventing or treating cancer, and there is some information to suggest that they may be harmful. A study conducted by the Food and Drug Administration (FDA) reported that products containing germanium present a potential hazard to humans.

DESCRIPTION: Germanium is a trace mineral. Inorganic germanium is mined and widely used as a semiconductor in the electronics industry. Organic germanium is found in some plants. Both forms of germanium may be included in dietary supplements, though the organic form is more commonly used. Proponents claim it effectively combats leukemia and cancers of the lung, bladder, larynx, breast, and uterus. They also claim it can be used to treat neurosis, asthma, diabetes, hypertension, cardiac insufficiency, sinus inflammation, neuralgia (nerve pain), and cirrhosis of the liver. Supporters contend that germanium stimulates the body's production of interferon (a naturally occurring anticancer agent) and boosts the immune system by enhancing the activity of natural killer cells (a type of white blood cell), which attack invading microorganisms. There is no scientific evidence to support these claims.

USE: Germanium supplements are available in capsules ranging from 250 to 325 mg. There is no standardized dose. These supplements are available in health food stores and over the Internet.

EFFECTS: There is no scientific evidence to show that germanium supplements promote health or increase the body's production of interferon. Germanium is not an essential element in animals or humans and does not play a role in biological processes.

In a study conducted by the FDA, at least 31 cases of kidney failure and death have been linked to products containing inorganic germanium. The FDA study did not conclusively show that organic germanium is toxic; however, because organic germanium could be contaminated with the dangerous inorganic germanium, products containing germanium present a potential hazard to humans. Although it is not clear if germanium supplements pose any danger for humans, adverse effects have included kidney failure, anemia, muscle weakness, peripheral neuropathy (a disturbance in the nervous system), and even death. Women who are pregnant or breast-feeding should not use this mineral.

▨ GINGER

OTHER COMMON NAME(S): Ginger Root

Ginger has a long history as a pungent spice for cooking, and as an herbal remedy for upset stomach, travel sickness, and loss of appetite. Some controlled studies in humans show ginger reduces nausea and vomiting. It may interfere with blood clotting and should only be used with a doctor's approval by cancer patients attempting to control nausea related to chemotherapy.

DESCRIPTION: Ginger is a plant native to southeast Asia that is also grown in the United States, China, India, and various tropical regions. The root is usually the part of the plant used in herbal remedies. Ginger has been used to control or prevent nausea, vomiting, and motion sickness. Proponents also claim it can be used as an anti-inflammatory (a drug that reduces pain and swelling as in arthritis), a cold remedy, an aid to digestion, and a remedy for intestinal gas. Some research findings show that ginger can be taken to relieve nausea in cancer patients who are receiving chemotherapy. Some proponents have claimed ginger is able to prevent tumors from developing; however, this has not been scientifically proven.

USE: Ginger has been approved by Commission E (Germany's regulatory agency for herbs) for indigestion and the prevention of motion sickness. Ginger is available as a tea, in powder form, in tablets, in capsules, and in candied form in Asian food stores.

Ginger root (fresh or dried) is used in cooking and preparing herbal remedies and soft drinks. For nausea, the usual dosage is from 250 mg to 1 g of powdered ginger taken with a liquid several times per day.

EFFECTS: There have been no human studies of ginger's ability to stop tumor growth. Recent preliminary results in animals showing some effect in slowing or preventing tumor growth are not well understood but warrant further investigation. It is too early in the research process to say if ginger will have the same effect in humans.

Ginger reduces nausea, according to some, but not all, controlled studies in humans. Studies also show that ginger reduces motion sickness and severe vomiting in pregnancy. Studies of ginger's ability to reduce nausea and vomiting associated with surgery have had mixed results. At least one study found ginger had no effect after surgery, while other studies have found a significant decrease in nausea and vomiting after surgery when ginger was given before the operation. These inconsistencies may be due to the difficulty in measuring symptoms of nausea.

Experts from the US Pharmacopeial Convention have determined that there is not enough medical and scientific evidence to support recommending ginger for the prevention of nausea and vomiting. People with cancer should consult their doctor before taking ginger because it has the potential to interfere with blood clotting and prolong bleeding time. Published studies are in disagreement about the likelihood of this side effect. The risk of serious bleeding may be increased if the person is also taking medication that can lower platelet (blood cells that help the blood to clot) counts or an anticoagulant (a drug that interferes with blood clotting, such as warfarin). In rare cases, some people have experienced an allergic reaction to ginger and occasional mild upset stomach. People should also consult their doctor about the use of ginger for morning sickness or for gallstone problems.

▚ GINKGO

OTHER COMMON NAME(S): Ginkgo Biloba

Ginkgo has shown some benefit in the treatment of mild to moderate dementia (decline in mental ability). Other studies have shown that it can help improve blood circulation and flow to the brain. Few side effects have been reported with its use; however, it has the potential to interfere with blood clotting, anesthesia, and some medications. There is no scientific evidence that it is effective in preventing or treating cancer.

DESCRIPTION: Ginkgo is an extract of leaves from a ginkgo tree, the world's oldest surviving species of tree from China, Japan, and Korea. It is promoted as an aid to memory and concentration. Widely used in Europe, the extract has recently become popular in the United States. Recent claims include an improvement of memory and vision in older people and a slowing of the progression of Alzheimer's disease or dementia.

Ginkgo is sometimes promoted for tinnitus (ringing in the ears), dizziness, motion sickness, and intermittent cramp-like pain in the lower legs. In addition, it has been used as a treatment for Raynaud's disease, a blood vessel disorder in which the toes or fingers turn pale when exposed to cold because of an insufficient blood supply. European doctors have also used ginkgo in stroke patients to limit tissue damage to the heart.

Although not usually promoted as a cancer treatment, herbalists note that ginkgo contains a compound called ginkgolide B that may counteract a body chemical thought to promote tumor growth. There is no scientific evidence to support this claim.

USE: Ginkgo leaf extract is on the Commission E (Germany's regulatory agency for herbs) list of approved herbs and can be taken in pill or liquid form by mouth. The average dosage of ginkgo extract is 120 to 240 mg per day for up to 3 months. Proponents do not recommend the crude, dried leaf preparations because they claim that these do not contain an adequate amount of the active ingredients.

EFFECTS: Some studies have found positive results with ginkgo extract. A 1996 laboratory study of aging mice found that ginkgo extracts improved short term memory, fluidity within cell membranes of neurons, and passive avoidance learning. One controlled human study found evidence that ginkgo extract could improve cognitive and social function in some patients with mild to moderate forms of dementia resulting from Alzheimer's disease or multiple heart attacks. Other clinical trials have shown improved blood circulation and flow to the brain and other parts of the body with use of the extract. There have been no scientific studies on ginkgo related to cancer or tumor growth.

Ginkgo is generally considered safe. Some possible side effects include headache and mild stomach upset. Because of its potential to inhibit the chemical thought to promote tumor growth, ginkgo is not recommended for people who are undergoing surgery or who are using aspirin, nonsteroidal anti-inflammatory drugs (eg, ibuprofen), or anticoagulants (drugs that inhibit abnormal blood clotting). People with seizure disorders are advised to avoid using ginkgo because it may reduce the effects of seizure medication. Women who are pregnant or breast-feeding should not use this herb.

▌ GINSENG

OTHER COMMON NAME(S): None

There is no scientific evidence that ginseng is effective in preventing or treating cancer. Although some population studies suggest it may have a protective effect, clinical trials are needed to determine if it is useful. Ginseng has been known to produce undesirable side effects and may even be dangerous when taken with certain medications, as well as when undergoing surgery.

DESCRIPTION: Ginseng is a perennial plant that grows in China, Korea, Japan, Russia, and the United States. The part of the plant used in herbal remedies is the dried root. It is promoted as an ancient herb that, due to its complex physical nature, can help the body prevent and fight diseases, including cancer. Promoters claim ginseng helps provide energy to people who are fatigued, and it is sometimes used during recovery from illness. There are also claims that ginseng relieves anxiety, protects the heart, strengthens stomach functions, prevents arteriosclerosis, stabilizes blood pressure and insulin levels, and even delays the effects of aging. There is no scientific evidence to support these claims.

USE: Ginseng is available as a powder, capsule, and tea or is sometimes mixed with foods. There is no standard dosage; however, Commission E (Germany's regulatory agency for herbs) suggests 1 to 2 g per day of ginseng root for up to 3 months. There is a lot of variation among ginseng products. Since it is expensive, some packagers dilute it or substitute less expensive ingredients to make it affordable to the consumer. Some ginseng products from areas of the world such as Siberia, Alaska, and Brazil are mislabeled. True ginseng has the word *Panax* as part of its Latin (scientific) name.

EFFECTS: Ginseng has been known for 3000 years, but despite research, scientists still are not certain whether the herb has cancer-prevention properties. Most of the studies with ginseng have been done in China and Korea, and only recently in the United States. Some investigations have suggested that ginseng can inhibit cancer formation by enhancing DNA repair at the cellular level or by bolstering the immune system. But many studies of this herb have suffered from design problems, and results have been contradictory. Some scientists have found that it raises blood pressure, while others have reported that it lowers blood pressure. In some studies, certain chemicals in the root seem to act as stimulants, but in others, they seem to work like sedatives. The only conclusions that can be reached with any certainty at this time are that ginseng is a complex herb and its medicinal effects are not clearly defined. It is clear that more research is needed to determine the benefit of ginseng, if any, for people with cancer.

There are several known side effects associated with the use of ginseng. Ginseng has been known to cause hypertension, headaches, insomnia, restlessness, and, in women, swollen breasts and vaginal bleeding. Because of its estrogen-like effects, women who are pregnant or breast-feeding should not use ginseng. In fact, some doctors believe it can cause breast cancer to recur in women who have had the disease previously. Ginseng can alter bleeding times, so it should not be used when undergoing surgery or with drugs that interfere with blood clotting, such as warfarin. If used with phenelzine sulfate, an antidepressant, ginseng can cause headaches, tremors, and manic episodes. People with cancer should consult their doctor before taking this herb.

▩ GOLDENSEAL

OTHER COMMON NAME(S): Eye Balm, Eye Root, Goldsiegel, Ground Raspberry, Indian Dye, Indian Turmeric, Jaundice Root, Yellow Paint, Yellow Puccoon, Yellow Root

There is no evidence that goldenseal is effective in treating cancer or any other disease. Some components of the herb (berberine and hydrastine) have been studied for potential pharmacological uses. Goldenseal can have toxic side effects, and high doses can be lethal.

DESCRIPTION: Goldenseal is an herb native to the United States and cultivated elsewhere. It takes its name from the golden-yellow scars that appear at the top of the root when the stem is broken off and that resemble an old-fashioned wax letter seal. The roots of the plant are used in herbal remedies.

Practitioners promote the use of goldenseal for a wide variety of conditions, including digestive problems (eg, peptic ulcers, colitis), urinary tract inflammation, constipation, hemorrhage after childbirth, painful menstruation, and cancer, to name a few. Some claim that goldenseal stimulates the immune system. Externally, goldenseal has been used to treat skin conditions, wounds, and herpes sores.

Berberine, a chemical contained in goldenseal, is said to have the ability to fight off infection caused by some bacteria, fungi, and yeast and can act as a mild sedative. Some claim that berberine stimulates the heart and is more effective than aspirin for reducing fevers. Another chemical in goldenseal, hydrastine, is said to reduce blood pressure. There is no scientific evidence to support these claims.

USE: Goldenseal can be taken internally in the form of capsules, extracts, tinctures, and teas. The ground root powder can also be purchased. The amount of goldenseal used varies depending on the way it is ingested (eg, tincture versus dried root).

Proponents use tooth powder and gargle made from goldenseal to treat tooth and gum infections and also apply the powder to herpes lesions and skin wounds. They also use solutions made from goldenseal in eyedrops for conjunctivitis (inflammation of the eye) and also as eardrops and douches.

EFFECTS: There is no clinical evidence to support the use of the herb for cancer or any other medical condition. In one recent animal study, goldenseal appeared to stimulate the immune system. Berberine, a chemical component of goldenseal, has been studied for its blood-thinning and cardiac stimulant properties in animals. Hydrastine, another component of goldenseal, has been found to produce severe changes in blood pressure. Further studies are necessary to determine if these animal and laboratory study results apply to humans.

Goldenseal may produce toxic effects, including digestive complaints, nervousness, depression, constipation, rapid heartbeat, diarrhea, gastrointestinal cramps and pain, mouth ulcers, nausea, seizures, and vomiting, and central nervous system depression. High doses may cause respiratory problems, paralysis, and even death. Long-term use may lead to vitamin B deficiency, hallucinations, and deliria. Women who are pregnant or breast-feeding should not use this herb in any form. Due to the potential harmful effects of goldenseal, a doctor should be consulted before taking the herb for any condition, including cancer.

▨ GREEN TEA

OTHER COMMON NAME(S): Black Tea, Chinese Tea

Some researchers believe green tea may have a protective effect against some cancers because it contains antioxidants. Results from human studies have been mixed. More research is needed to determine its role in cancer prevention.

DESCRIPTION: Green tea is a drink made from the steamed and dried leaves of the *Camellia sinesis* plant, a shrub native to Asia. Black tea is also made from this plant, but unlike green tea, it is made from leaves that have been dried and fermented.

Green tea is widely consumed in Japan, China, and other Asian nations and is becoming more popular in Western countries. Some reports indicate green tea may have the ability to help prevent certain cancers from developing, including prostate, stomach, and esophageal cancers. Green tea contains chemicals known as polyphenols, which have antioxidant properties. An antioxidant is a compound that blocks the action of activated oxygen molecules known as free radicals, which can damage cells. One major element in green tea is *epigallocatechin-3-gallate* (EGCG), a compound that is believed to block production of an enzyme required for cancer cell growth. EGCG may work by suppressing the formation of blood vessels, a process called angiogenesis, thereby cutting off the supply of blood to cancer cells.

Herbalists use green tea and extracts of its leaves for stomach problems, vomiting, and diarrhea and to reduce tooth decay, blood pressure, cholesterol levels, and blockages of the blood vessels in the heart that can lead to heart attacks. Green tea is also promoted as an herb that can prevent certain bacterial infections. In the past 5 years, some researchers have suggested that black tea may also be effective in cancer prevention. These claims are currently under investigation.

USE: Three cups a day or more is the amount typically taken in Asian countries. Green tea is usually brewed using 1 to 2 teaspoons of the dried tea in a cup of boiling water or is steeped for 3 to 15 minutes. Green tea extracts are also available in capsule form. Proponents recommend 3 capsules of green tea extract a day, but this dosage and its effects remain uncertain.

EFFECTS: Although animal and laboratory studies have shown a positive benefit of green tea consumption in protecting against cancer, studies in humans have been mixed. Researchers from the Shanghai Cancer Institute and the National Cancer Institute conducted a large population study in 1994 comparing green tea drinkers to nongreen tea drinkers. They found that green tea drinking was associated with 60% fewer cancers of the esophagus for people who did not smoke. Well-controlled human studies are needed to determine the effectiveness of green tea in protecting against cancer.

Green tea is generally considered safe. Asians have consumed this tea for thousands of years with few dangerous side effects. Some people may develop allergic reactions and should stop drinking it. Drinking large amounts of tea may cause nutritional and other problems because of the caffeine content and the strong binding activities of the polyphenols. Because caffeine acts as a stimulant, people with irregular heartbeats or who have anxiety attacks should not drink more than 2 cups a day. Women who are pregnant or breast-feeding should not drink green tea in large amounts.

◼ HANSI™

OTHER COMMON NAME(S): None

HANSI is an herbal preparation consisting of very small dilutions from plants of the desert and rain forests such as cactus, aloe, arnica, lachesis, and licopodium in a 2% to 8% alcohol base (see Homeopathy). Proponents claim that HANSI enhances the immune system, prevents and stops the progression of some cancers, increases tolerance of side effects from chemotherapy and radiation therapy, and effectively treats chronic fatigue syndrome, AIDS, and asthma. HANSI is taken orally or delivered by injection for up to 2 years. The basic formula includes about 10 components whose proportions are adjusted according to the condition being treated and whether the drug will be delivered orally or by injection. The Food and Drug Administration has not approved HANSI injections.

There is no scientific evidence that HANSI is effective in treating cancer or any other disease. Not enough is known about HANSI to determine if it is safe or if it poses any dangers to humans. Relying on this type of treatment alone, and avoiding conventional medical care, may have serious health consequences.

◼ HOXSEY HERBAL TREATMENT

OTHER COMMON NAME(S): Hoxsey Method, Hoxsey Treatment, Hoxsey Herbs, Hoxsey Formula

There is no scientific evidence that the Hoxsey herbal treatment is effective in treating cancer, and there have been no clinical trials of the treatment. In some animal studies, a few of the herbs contained in the Hoxsey formula were studied separately and showed some anticancer activity. It is not known if the combination of the herbs taken together has harmful effects. The paste made for external application can severely burn, disfigure, and scar the skin.

DESCRIPTION: The Hoxsey herbal treatment is an herbal mixture taken internally or applied externally. The pastes or salves that are applied externally contain antimony trisulfide, zinc chloride, bloodroot, and a yellow powder consisting of arsenic sulfide, sulfur, and talc. Both the paste and powder can burn the skin (see Cancer Salves). The Hoxsey herbal treatment is specifically promoted to treat people with cancer. Its proponents claim the internal formula eliminates toxins from the body, strengthens the immune system, and enhances its ability to slowly absorb and excrete tumors. The external treatment is used to treat skin cancer. It allegedly keeps cancer from spreading and helps destroy cancer cells. The goal of treatment is to restore the body's chemistry to a normal state. There is no scientific evidence to support these claims.

USE: The herbal mixture used internally is a liquid that contains a combination of numerous herbs, including pokeweed, burdock root, licorice, barberry, buckthorn bark, stillingia root, red clover, prickly ash bark, potassium iodide, and cascara, and sometimes other ingredients (see Pokeweed, Licorice, and Red Clover). The external preparation, usually a paste or salve, is rubbed directly onto cancerous tumors. Internal and external dosages vary depending on the patient and whether the tumor is inside the body or on the skin. The Hoxsey herbal treatment is currently illegal in the United States, although it can be obtained through clinics in Mexico.

The Hoxsey treatment now also includes antiseptic douches and washes, laxative tablets, nutritional supplements, and dietary restrictions that prohibit pork, vinegar, tomatoes, pickles, carbonated drinks, alcohol, bleached flour, sugar, and salt.

EFFECTS: There is no evidence that the Hoxsey herbal treatment has any value in the treatment of cancer in humans. Only 2 human studies of the Hoxsey herbal treatment have been published. One was published in a pamphlet provided by the Tijuana clinic and simply contains a description of 9 patients who received the treatment. It concluded that the treatment is effective. The other study involved 39 people with various types of cancer who took the Hoxsey herbal treatment. Ten patients died after an average of 15 months, and 23 never completed the study. Only 6 patients were disease-free after 48 months.

The paste made for external application can severely burn, disfigure, and scar the skin. Some of the ingredients in the internal formula, such as buckthorn, can cause nausea, vomiting, and diarrhea when taken in large quantities. Cascara can also cause diarrhea. Pokeweed is a poisonous plant that can also cause undesirable side effects such as nausea, vomiting, diarrhea, and abdominal cramps. Red clover may increase the risk of bleeding for people who take anticoagulant (blood-thinning) medications. It also has estrogenic activity, which means it should be avoided by women with estrogen-positive breast tumors. Women who are pregnant or breast-feeding should not use this treatment in any form. Relying on this type of treatment alone, and avoiding conventional medical care, may have serious health consequences.

▨ INDIAN SNAKEROOT

OTHER COMMON NAME(S): Snakeroot, Rauwolfia, Serpentwood, Reserpine

The drug reserpine is used in conventional medicine to treat high blood pressure and anxiety; however, there is no scientific evidence that Indian snakeroot is effective in treating cancer, liver disease, or mental illness. It also has many dangerous side effects.

DESCRIPTION: Indian snakeroot is a plant that grows in India, Thailand, and other parts of Asia, South America, and Africa. There are more than 100 species of Indian snakeroot. *Rauwolfia serpentina* is the one most commonly used in herbal remedies. Reserpine, a chemical found in the roots, is responsible for most of the plant's therapeutic effects. According to proponents, Indian snakeroot lowers high blood pressure, eases anxiety and tension, reduces fever, stops diarrhea and dysentery, and can be used to treat some psychiatric illnesses. Some believe that Indian snakeroot inhibits the reproduction of cancer cells; however, there is no scientific evidence to support this claim.

USE: Indian snakeroot is on the Commission E (Germany's regulatory agency for herbs) list of approved herbs for treating mild hypertension. The supplements are available as tablets or in liquid form. Powdered Indian snakeroot can also be brewed as a tea. An average daily dosage is 600 mg. Reserpine, which is a prescription medicine approved by the Food and Drug Administration, is given as pills or injections.

EFFECTS: The drug reserpine, which is extracted from Indian snakeroot, is widely known to be an effective drug for lowering blood pressure and as a tranquilizer. But there is little or no evidence to suggest that reserpine or other chemicals found in Indian snakeroot are effective treatments for mental illness, liver disease, or cancer.

Indian snakeroot is associated with many adverse effects, including depression, decreased heart rate, low blood pressure, decreased sex drive and performance, increased appetite, weight gain, swelling, stomach complaints, diarrhea, nasal congestion, nightmares and hallucinations, gastrointestinal ulcers, decreased motor coordination, and dry mouth. Indian snakeroot can also impair physical abilities and coordination.

People with a history of depression, peptic ulcers, or ulcerative colitis and women with a history of breast cancer should not take Indian snakeroot. Due to the potential for increased blood pressure, increased heart rate, or uncontrollable muscle movements, people taking sleeping pills, appetite suppressants, heart medications, and antipsychotic drugs should also avoid Indian snakeroot. The use of alcohol should also be avoided due to the reduction of physical reflexes. Women who are pregnant or breast-feeding should not use this herb.

▮ KAMPO

OTHER COMMON NAME(S): Kampoyaku, Juzen-taiho-to, Hochu-ekki-to, Sho-Saiko

Despite the popularity of kampo among Japanese doctors and patients, there is no scientific evidence that Japanese herbal preparations are effective in preventing or treating cancer or any other disease.

DESCRIPTION: Kampo is the name for traditional Japanese herbal medicine that involves the use of more than 210 different herbal preparations. Proponents claim that the common kampo preparations Juzen-taiho-to and Hochu-ekki-to boost the anticancer activities of cells called natural killer cells (a type of white blood cell). Another popular kampo preparation, Sho-saiko, is claimed to enhance the function of macrophages, which attack cancer cells. They also say that some kampo remedies are more effective than conventional methods for treating chronic prostatitis (inflammation of the prostate gland). Practitioners of kampo claim that specific herbal formulas can be used to treat other conditions, such as constipation, gastritis, irritable bowel syndrome, allergies, asthma, arthritis, and hypertension. There is no scientific evidence to support these claims.

USE: Kampo practitioners may prescribe one or more herbal mixtures that are prepared by hand. The formula depends on the patient's particular complaint or condition. Unlike Western medicine, kampo does not give names to diseases. Patients are diagnosed based on a concept called *sho*, which involves visual and auditory observations, detailed questioning, and physical examination. Signs and symptoms are then interpreted according to the ancient Chinese theories of yin and yang, which depends a great deal on the intuition of the practitioner.

EFFECTS: Very little research has been conducted on kampo as a cancer therapy, and there is no scientific evidence to show that Japanese herbal preparations cure cancer or slow its growth. In one laboratory animal study conducted in Japan, researchers concluded that the kampo preparations Juzen-taiho-to and Shimotsu-to significantly reduced the spread of colon cancer cells to the liver and of melanoma (skin cancer) cells to the lungs. Several other Japanese studies found that kampo remedies did nothing to stop or slow the spread of cancer. Well-controlled human studies are needed to test the claims that kampo is effective against cancer and other diseases or that it improves general health and well-being.

It is not known whether kampo is safe. No research has been done to determine the possible side effects. Women who are pregnant or breast-feeding should not use these herbs.

◾ KAVA

OTHER COMMON NAME(S): Kava-Kava, Kavalactones

Studies support the use of kava for reducing anxiety, although it is not certain how it works. The safe dosage of kava needed to reduce anxiety has not been determined. Side effects appear to increase with large doses, and it has the potential to interfere with anesthesia as well as some medications.

DESCRIPTION: Kava is a large shrub with broad, heart-shaped leaves and is a member of the pepper family. It is native to many islands of the South Pacific. The roots of the plant are used in herbal remedies. Kava is promoted primarily for anxiety, nervous tension, stress, restlessness, and, at higher doses, insomnia. Many users say the herb enhances mood and brings on a sense of well-being, relaxation, and even euphoria. In South Pacific folk medicine, kava has been used to treat uterine inflammations, headaches, colds, rheumatism, and menopausal symptoms. They also drink it to relieve headaches, restore vigor, promote urination, soothe upset stomachs, ease symptoms of asthma and tuberculosis, and cure fungal infections. Some users believe that kava inhibits gonorrhea. As a cream, kava is used to soothe stings and skin inflammations.

Kava has no direct application to cancer treatment, but its ability to ease anxiety may be of interest to people with cancer. There are other effective medications for treating anxiety that patients should discuss with their doctor.

USE: Kava is on the Commission E (Germany's regulatory agency for herbs) list of approved herbs. It is available in tablets, capsules, cream, and powder, which can be made into tea or mixed with other drinks. Daily dosages range from 100 to 200 mg of kavalactones, the active ingredient in kava. A safe dosage has not been determined, and it should not be taken for more than 3 months.

EFFECTS: Kava has been the focus of dozens of medical studies, many of which support the claims made about the herb's antianxiety properties. Kava does indeed appear to ease symptoms of anxiety and stress. In clinical studies, patients with varying levels of anxiety took kava extract and reported relief within days or weeks. Some researchers have found that kava compares favorably to prescription antianxiety medications, yet causes fewer side effects and is not addictive. For instance, one study showed that kava does not impair reaction time and may even improve concentration. In comparison, common prescription drugs for anxiety slow reaction time.

In rare cases, moderate use of kava can lead to a scaly rash. Commission E reports that kava may reduce motor reflexes and judgment when driving or operating heavy machinery. Some evidence suggests that kava should not be taken with antianxiety medicines or alcohol, which could cause extreme drowsiness. Because of its potential to interact with anesthetics, it should not be used by people who are undergoing surgery. Women who are pregnant or breast-feeding, people taking antidepressants or antipsychotic drugs, and children aged 12 and younger should not use kava.

Heavy or long-term use can sometimes lead to metabolic abnormalities including increased levels of liver enzymes. Regulatory officials in Germany recently reported concerns about cases of liver problems associated with kava, and this information is being scientifically evaluated by the Food and Drug Administration and several trade associations. According to the American Botanical Council, Kava should not be used by anyone with a history of liver problems or who is taking any medications that have negative effects on the liver (such as acetaminophen). They recommend that Kava not be used on a daily basis for more than 4 weeks and should be discontinued if symptoms of jaundice (eg, dark urine, yellowing of the eyes) occur.

Other possible side effects of kava include an increase of symptoms of Parkinson's disease, absence of urination, numbness of the mouth, and painful twisting movements of the trunk.

▌ LARCH

OTHER COMMON NAME(S): American Larch, European Larch, *Larch Arabinogalactan*, Common Larch

There is no scientific evidence that larch is effective in treating cancer or any other disease. Limited laboratory evidence suggests that a polysaccharide found in larch may stimulate the immune system, but clinical trials are needed to determine what effect, if any, it may have in humans.

DESCRIPTION: The larch is a tall, deciduous tree of the *Larix* genus that grows in central Europe, North America, northern Russia, and Siberia. The bark and its resin are used in herbal remedies. Proponents believe that larch can be used to treat bronchitis, colds, and other respiratory conditions. The polysaccharide found in larch, called *larch arabino-galactan*, is said to stimulate the immune system and increase the effectiveness of some drugs (including chemotherapy medications). Some claim that the compound also inhibits the spread of cancer to the liver, although there has been no scientific evidence to support these claims.

USE: Larch is available in the form of ointments, gels, and oils. *Larch arabinogalactan* is available as a fiber supplement in powder form.

EFFECTS: In one laboratory study, researchers at the University of Minnesota concluded that *larch arabinogalactan* is a safe source of dietary fiber and may be effective in boosting the immune system; however, the company that owns the patent to the extract sponsored the research. Another laboratory study conducted in Germany found that *arabino-galactan* from a species of the larch tree stimulated the action of natural killer cells (a type of white blood cell). Further studies are necessary to determine if these laboratory study results apply to humans.

The *Larix* genus is listed in the Food and Drug Administration's Poisonous Plant Database. This is a list of plants that are associated with toxic effects. There have been no definitive conclusions as to its safety or toxicity.

▟ LICORICE

OTHER COMMON NAME(S): Sweet Root, Licorice Root

Licorice appears to have some use in the treatment of peptic ulcers; however, it is associated with side effects that can cause serious problems. Licorice can cause a fluid imbalance in the body involving salt and water metabolism. More research is needed to determine if licorice extract has any role in cancer prevention or treatment.

DESCRIPTION: Licorice is a perennial plant that grows in southern Europe, Asia, and the Mediterranean. The dried roots and underground stems of the plant are used in herbal remedies. It is promoted as an herb that can treat peptic ulcers, eczema, skin infections, cold sores, menopausal symptoms, liver disease, respiratory ailments, inflammatory problems, chronic fatigue syndrome, AIDS, and even cancer. It has also been promoted to relieve symptoms of Addison's disease (a hormone deficiency), lower cholesterol and triglyceride levels, strengthen the immune system, and treat hepatitis.

Many food products are widely available that contain small traces of licorice. Some licorice candy sold in the United States is actually flavored with anise and does not contain licorice. Glycyrrhizin, an active ingredient from the plant, is used as a flavoring in candy, gum, cookies, beverages, and cough syrup.

USE: Licorice is packaged as capsules, tablets, and a liquid extract. It can be purchased at grocery stores, health food stores, or pharmacies. According to Commission E (Germany's regulatory agency for herbs), the recommended dosage is 200 to 600 mg for no more than 4 weeks for peptic ulcers.

EFFECTS: Research suggests that licorice can treat peptic ulcers by increasing the production of prostaglandins (substances present in many tissues that control functions such as blood pressure or smooth muscle control), which is essential to the healing of ulcers.

The value of licorice as a cancer-prevention agent has not been proven. It has been reported to have anticancer properties in mice by increasing the activity of certain enzymes that detoxify cancer-causing chemicals. Further studies are necessary to determine if these animal study results apply to humans.

Regular consumption of licorice has been shown to cause headaches, lethargy, water retention, high blood pressure, and muscle weakness. In extremely large amounts, it can cause heart failure. People with high blood pressure, irregular heartbeat, or cardiovascular, kidney, or liver diseases should avoid its use unless administered under the supervision of a doctor. Women who are pregnant or breast-feeding should not consume licorice.

▨ MARIJUANA

OTHER COMMON NAME(S): Pot, Grass, Cannabis, Weed, Hemp

The cannabinoid drug delta-9-tetrahydrocannabinol (THC) has been approved by the Food and Drug Administration (FDA), for medical use only, in relieving nausea and vomiting, and for helping to increase appetite. Use of the raw marijuana plant, however, is illegal in the United States.

DESCRIPTION: Marijuana, scientifically known as *Cannabis sativa*, is an annual plant that grows wild throughout the world in warm and tropical climates and is cultivated commercially. Parts of the plant (leaves and buds) have been used in herbal remedies for centuries. Scientists have identified 66 biologically active ingredients, called cannabinoids, in marijuana. The most potent of these is thought to be the chemical THC.

There is some evidence that THC has the potential to relieve pain, control nausea and vomiting, prevent or reduce the severity of glaucoma, and stimulate appetite of people with cancer and AIDS. Some supporters claim that marijuana dilates the respiratory tract (which may ease the severity of asthma attacks), has antibacterial actions, and inhibits tumor growth. Others claim that marijuana can be used to effectively control convulsions and muscle spasms in people who have multiple sclerosis, epilepsy, and spinal cord injuries. There is no scientific evidence to support these claims.

USE: THC has been available by prescription (as dronabinol) since 1985 in the form of pills and suppositories. Several pharmaceutical companies are also developing inhalers to deliver therapeutic doses of THC. In raw form, marijuana is most commonly smoked in pipes or homemade cigarettes. It is also eaten directly or mixed with foods. Raw marijuana is illegal in the United States and is not approved by the FDA for medical applications.

EFFECTS: Much of the research into marijuana has been centered on cannabinoids (the active ingredients in marijuana). Research findings about THC are mixed. One comprehensive review concluded that oral THC is as effective or more effective for reducing nausea associated with chemotherapy than commonly used prescription drugs, and that it may be useful at low doses for appetite stimulation in patients with AIDS. Researchers also found that THC reduces eye pressure in people who have glaucoma. Based on potential toxic side effects, the therapeutic benefits of THC should be carefully weighed against its potential risks. It was concluded that current evidence does not support the use of smoked marijuana as a medication, and that additional research is needed.

In the most in-depth investigation into the medical use of marijuana, the Institute of Medicine found that cannabinoids, particularly THC, have some potential to relieve pain, control nausea and vomiting, and stimulate appetite. In addition, cannabinoids probably affect control of movement and memory, but their effects on the immune system are unclear. They found some of the effects of cannabinoids, such as anxiety reduction, sedation, and euphoria, may be beneficial for certain patients and situations, and undesirable for others. They also found that smoking marijuana delivers harmful substances, and may be an important risk factor in the development of respiratory diseases and certain types of cancers.

The National Cancer Institute (NCI) notes that THC may be useful for some people with cancer who have chemotherapy-induced nausea and vomiting that cannot be controlled by other drugs. But THC also causes a high similar to that caused by smoking natural marijuana. The NCI also said that more studies are needed to fully evaluate the potential use of marijuana for people with cancer.

Smoking or eating raw marijuana can cause a number of effects, including feelings of euphoria, short-term memory loss, difficulty in completing complex tasks, alterations in the perception of time and space, sedation, anxiety, confusion, and inability to concentrate. Other side effects include low blood pressure, tachycardia (fast heartbeat), and heart palpitations. Many researchers agree that marijuana contains known carcinogens (substances that can cause cancer). They caution that smoking marijuana may decrease reproductive function, as well as increase the risk of respiratory diseases and cancers of the lungs, mouth, and tongue. It may also suppress the body's immune system, and increase the risk of leukemia in children whose mothers smoked marijuana during pregnancy. Women who are pregnant or breast-feeding should not use marijuana.

The symptoms of a marijuana overdose include nausea, vomiting, hacking cough, disturbances to heart rhythms, and numbness in the limbs. Chronic use can also lead to laryngitis, bronchitis, and general apathy.

■ MILK THISTLE

OTHER COMMON NAME(S): Mary Thistle, Marian Thistle, Holy Thistle, Lady Thistle, Silymarin

Laboratory research has shown that silymarin, an antioxidant found in milk thistle seeds, may be a useful agent for treating various liver diseases. Controlled studies are needed to determine if these findings apply to humans, as well as to determine what role silymarin plays in preventing or treating cancer or reducing the side effects of chemotherapy.

DESCRIPTION: Milk thistle, a plant that belongs to the same family as daisies, grows in Mediterranean regions, Europe, North America, South America, and Australia. The parts used in herbal remedies are the seeds, which contain a compound called silymarin. Proponents claim that silymarin (also called milk thistle fruit) is a potent antioxidant—compounds that block the action of activated oxygen molecules known as free radicals, which can damage cells. Some also claim that milk thistle detoxifies and protects the liver and is an effective treatment for hepatitis C, jaundice, and cirrhosis. They also claim it strengthens the spleen and gallbladder, benefits people with diabetes, and slows the growth of certain types of cancer cells, including skin cancer, breast cancer, and prostate cancer. Some believe that milk thistle is an antidote for certain varieties of poisonous mushrooms.

USE: Milk thistle supplements are available in capsules, tablets, powder, and liquid extract. Powdered milk thistle can be made into a tea. A typical dosage ranges from 200 to 400 mg of silymarin daily.

EFFECTS: Silymarin has been studied extensively in the laboratory for the treatment of acute and chronic liver disease. Commission E (Germany's regulatory agency for herbs) approved the use of milk thistle fruit (ie, silymarin) as a treatment for toxic liver disease, and as a supportive treatment for chronic inflammatory liver disease and cirrhosis of the liver. Research in mice found that silymarin provided protection against skin cancer, and research in the laboratory found that silymarin reduced growth of breast and prostate cancer cells. Further studies are necessary to determine if these animal and laboratory study results apply to humans. There is no scientific evidence that silymarin is effective in preventing or treating cancer in humans.

Milk thistle is generally considered safe; however, one case study reported that a woman suffered sweating, nausea, abdominal pain, diarrhea, vomiting, and weakness whenever she took milk thistle extract. It is not know for certain whether her reaction was caused by the herb or by another ingredient in her supplements. Milk thistle extract may act as a mild laxative. Women who are pregnant or breast-feeding should not use this herb.

▨ MISTLETOE

OTHER COMMON NAME(S): All Heal, Bird Lime, Devil's Fuge, Golden Bough

A number of laboratory experiments suggest mistletoe may have the potential to treat cancer, but these results have not yet been reflected in clinical trials. Studies are needed to determine if there are any anticancer effects in humans.

DESCRIPTION: Mistletoe is a semiparasitic plant that grows on several species of trees native to England, Europe, and western Asia. It differs from the mistletoe found in the United States. The leaves and twigs of mistletoe are used in herbal remedies.

It is claimed that mistletoe stimulates the immune system, helping the body fight more efficiently against cancer and other diseases. Mistletoe extracts are promoted as a remedy for a wide range of cancers, including tumors of the cervix, ovaries, breast, stomach, colon, lung, and also as a treatment for leukemias, sarcomas, and lymphomas. Supporters claim mistletoe extract injected directly into or near a tumor can slow and possibly reverse the growth of cancer cells, even in advanced cases of cancer. They also claim mistletoe can lower blood pressure, decrease heart rate, relax spasms, and relieve symptoms of arthritis and rheumatism. It is further claimed to have sedative effects, and is promoted to relieve the side effects of chemotherapy and radiation. There is no scientific evidence to support these claims.

USE: Commission E (Germany's regulatory agency for herbs) has approved mistletoe as symptom relief for malignant tumors (to help treat symptoms, not cure disease). The herb is prepared as an injectable whole plant extract, and is not used orally. The plant itself is poisonous and not safe to eat.

For people with cancer, mistletoe extracts are injected under the skin near the tumor. Daily injections are often given before and after surgery, chemotherapy, or radiation therapy, and may continue for 10 to 14 days. Mistletoe injections promoted to prevent cancer may involve 3 to 7 injections a week over several months to several years.

EFFECTS: Researchers have completed numerous studies of mistletoe and its effects on cancer. Most of them are not considered scientifically reliable. No controlled human studies have shown mistletoe to have any significant antitumor activity. Other reviews of recent research have also suggested that mistletoe has no measurable effect on cancer growth.

Mistletoe preparations vary widely depending on how they are prepared (eg, fermented or nonfermented), the particular species from which they are obtained, and the season in which the plant was harvested. Researchers are working to identify the most important components, which are thought to be proteins in the plant called lectins. A number of laboratory experiments suggest that mistletoe extracts may have some potential to combat and kill cancer cells, but these results have yet to be reflected in human trials. Laboratory experiments also hint that mistletoe increases the activity of lymphocytes, which are cells that attack invading organisms.

Mistletoe is generally considered safe. Possible side effects include temporary redness at the injection site, headaches, fever, and chills. In rare cases, people allergic to mistletoe can develop a severe reaction and potentially life-threatening condition called *anaphylactic shock*. Some researchers suggest using purified preparations of mistletoe lectins to reduce the occurrence of toxic effects.

Mistletoe should not be eaten because all parts of the plant are poisonous. Consuming mistletoe has been known to cause seizures and death. Other symptoms include blurred vision, nausea and vomiting, stomach pain, diarrhea, irregular heartbeat, confusion, convulsions, disorientation, and drowsiness. Women who are pregnant or breast-feeding should not use this herb.

▌ MOLYBDENUM

OTHER COMMON NAME(S): None

Molybdenum is an essential element in human nutrition, but its precise function and interactions with other chemicals are not well understood. Some evidence suggests that too little molybdenum in the diet may be responsible for some health problems; however, more research is needed to determine its role, if any, in preventing cancer and other diseases.

DESCRIPTION: Molybdenum is a scarce mineral that is present in very small quantities in the human body. The mineral is involved in many important biological processes, possibly including development of the nervous system, waste processing in the kidneys, and energy production in cells.

Proponents claim molybdenum is an antioxidant that prevents cancer by protecting cells from free radicals, the destructive molecules that may damage cells. Some supporters also claim that molybdenum prevents anemia, gout, dental cavities, and sexual impotence; however, there is no scientific evidence to support these claims.

USE: Diet is the major source of molybdenum for most people. Common sources of molybdenum include legumes, cereals, leafy vegetables, liver, and milk. Humans require very small amounts of molybdenum, which a well-balanced diet usually provides.

Molybdenum is also sold as a supplement in some health food stores and over the Internet. It is usually found in capsule form in combination with other nutrients. A typical dosage is 75 micrograms (µg) daily.

EFFECTS: Although researchers believe that molybdenum plays an important role in human health, its precise function and interactions with other chemicals are not well known. Some animal research suggests molybdenum supplements reduce the incidence of tumors in the esophagus and stomach of animals, and breast cancer in rats. Further studies are necessary to determine if these animal study results apply to humans.

Little is known about the effects of too much or too little molybdenum in the body. Overdoses are extremely rare. Some research indicates that high levels of the mineral can irritate the upper respiratory tract, and cause swelling and deformities of the knees, hands, and feet. High levels may also cause gout. Molybdenum deficiencies are very rare in humans; therefore, most practitioners do not recommend supplements. People who eat diets that are very low in molybdenum may be at increased risk for vision problems, rapid heart rate, and rapid breathing; however, the impact on health may be minimal and cause no symptoms at all.

▚ MUGWORT

OTHER COMMON NAME(S): Ai Ye, Felon Herb, St. John's Plant, Wild Wormwood

There is no scientific evidence that mugwort is effective in treating gastrointestinal problems or any other medical condition, including cancer.

DESCRIPTION: Mugwort is a perennial flowering plant that is a member of the daisy family, and should not be confused with wormwood or St. John's Wort. It is native to Asia, Europe, and North America. The dried leaves and roots of the plant are used in herbal remedies. It is promoted to treat gastrointestinal disorders such as colic, persistent vomiting, diarrhea, constipation, flatulence, and cramps. The herb has also been promoted as a treatment for a wide range of other conditions, including headaches, nose bleeds, muscle spasms, epilepsy, circulatory problems, menopausal and menstrual complaints, chills, fever, rheumatism, asthma, dermatitis, dysentery, gout, and infertility. Proponents also claim mugwort oil has antibacterial and antifungal properties, and is used to treat worm infestations and snakebites.

Some proponents also claim mugwort is a sedative and use it to treat neuroses, hysteria, general irritability, restlessness, insomnia, anxiety, mild depression, anorexia, and opium addiction. Dried mugwort is used in moxibustion treatments to treat cancer (see Moxibustion). There is no scientific evidence to support these claims.

USE: Mugwort is available as dried leaves and roots, extracts, tinctures, teas, and pills. It can be used as a poultice as well. Mugwort is on the Commission E (Germany's regulatory agency for herbs) list of unapproved herbs. This means that it is not recommended for use because it has not been proven to be safe or effective.

EFFECTS: Research on mugwort has focused on its properties related to allergic sensitivities. No research or clinical studies have been done on the alternative use of mugwort. There is no scientific evidence to support any of the claims made for mugwort, including its use in moxibustion as a treatment for people with cancer.

Mugwort is generally considered safe; however, it may increase the effects of anticoagulant medications (drugs that slow blood clotting). People with bleeding abnormalities are advised not to take mugwort. Mugwort pollen is known to cause hay fever in some people. The herb may also cause uterine contractions. Women who are pregnant or breast-feeding should not use this herb.

▊ OLEANDER

OTHER COMMON NAME(S): Oleander Leaf, Dogbane, Laurier Rose, Rose Bay, Anvirzel™

There is no scientific evidence that oleander is effective in treating cancer or any other disease. There have been reports of poisoning and death from ingestion of oleander, oleander leaf tea, and some of its extracts. Even a small amount of oleander can cause fatal respiratory paralysis and cardiac effects. One of the substances in oleander that causes the dangerous effects on the heart is called oleandrin. Because of these dangerous effects, oleander should not be used.

DESCRIPTION: Oleander is a poisonous evergreen shrub identified by its fragrant white, rose, or purple flowers, whorled leaves, and long follicles containing seeds. It grows in mild climates or as an indoor plant. The active ingredients are extracted from the leaves. Even though oleander is poisonous, heavily diluted oleander preparations have been promoted to treat a variety of conditions including muscle cramps, asthma, corns, menstrual pain, epilepsy, paralysis, skin diseases, heart problems, and cancer. It has also been used in folk remedies as an insecticide.

USE: There is no established therapeutic dosage of oleander extract. Oleander leaf is on the Commission E (Germany's regulatory agency for herbs) list of unapproved herbs. This means that it is not recommended for use because it has not been proven to be safe or effective. The raw botanical (herb, flower, or other plant part) can be toxic.

An oleander extract with the trade name of Anvirzel is available, but it has not been approved for study or use by the Food and Drug Administration (FDA) as an investigational new drug (IND). In March 2000, the FDA requested the company who manufactures Anvirzel to immediately cease distribution and use of materials that promote the product as an IND, including misleading information on their web site.

EFFECTS: The effectiveness of oleander has not been proven. There have been no controlled studies of oleander or its extract. Although there are claims that Anvirzel improves quality of life, reduces pain, increases energy, and causes cancer regression and remission, there is no scientific evidence to support these claims. Clinical trials on Anvirzel are underway.

The oleander plant is poisonous, and people have died from eating parts of the plant. Death has resulted from heart failure or respiratory paralysis. Some of the symptoms and signs of oleander toxicity are nausea, vomiting, colic, appetite loss, dizziness, drowsiness, hyperkalemia (high potassium levels), rapid heart rate, heart block, dilated pupils, bloody diarrhea, seizures, loss of consciousness, and slow irregular pulse. There have been reports of death occurring after oral and/or rectal administration of the extract from the plant. The FDA has received reports of at least 2 deaths associated with the use of Anvirzel prior to the filing of the IND. This herb should be avoided, especially by women who are pregnant or breast-feeding.

◼ ORTHOMOLECULAR MEDICINE

OTHER COMMON NAME(S): None

Orthomolecular medicine is the use of very high doses of vitamins, minerals, or hormones to prevent and treat a wide variety of conditions. The dosages are well above the recommended daily allowance (RDA) and are sometimes used along with special diets and conventional treatment. Proponents believe that taking megadoses of these nutrients may correct "biochemical abnormalities," and thereby reverse a wide variety of conditions, such as alcoholism, arthritis, asthma, allergies, cancer, depression, epilepsy, heart disease, high blood pressure, hyperactivity, migraine headaches, mental retardation, and schizophrenia. There is no scientific evidence to support these claims. While a balanced diet may be sufficient for people who are healthy, proponents of orthomolecular medicine claim that sick people need far more nutrients than the RDA provides. Consuming large amounts of supplements, however, can be dangerous.

◼ PAU D'ARCO

OTHER COMMON NAME(S): Lapachol, Lapacho, Lapacho Morado, Lapacho Colorado, Ipe Roxo, Ipes, Taheebo, Tahuari, Trumpet Bush, Trumpet Tree

Although some laboratory and animal studies suggest that lapachol, an ingredient in pau d'arco, may have some effects against certain diseases, no well-designed, controlled studies have shown that this substance is effective against cancer in humans. Pau d'arco also has potentially dangerous side effects.

DESCRIPTION: Pau d'arco is a large tree that grows in the rainforests of Central and South America. There are about 100 species of the tree, which produces large, purple flowers, and can grow to 150 feet tall and 6 feet in diameter. The inner bark of the tree is used in herbal remedies. It is promoted as a cure for dozens of diseases and medical conditions, including arthritis, ulcers, diabetes, and cancer. Proponents also claim that when taken internally, it relieves infections, reduces inflammation, promotes digestion, strengthens the immune system, flushes toxins from the body, and protects against cardiovascular disease and high blood pressure. There is no scientific evidence to support these claims. They also use it to treat lupus, osteomyelitis, Parkinson's disease, psoriasis, and to relieve pain. Applied externally, practitioners have used it to treat skin inflammation, fungal infections, hemorrhoids, eczema, and wounds.

USE: Pau d'arco is available in capsules, tablets, salves, extracts, powder, and teas from health food stores and over the Internet. Recommended dosages vary by manufacturer. When making tea, practitioners say the bark must be boiled for at least 8 minutes to release the active ingredients.

EFFECTS: Pau d'arco contains at least 20 active compounds, including quercetin and other flavonoids, whose effects are not yet known. One of the active ingredients that has been studied is called lapachol. In laboratory animals, lapachol was found to be effective against malaria and certain kinds of animal tumor cells, such as sarcoma, but did not affect other kinds of cancer, including leukemia and adenocarcinoma. Further studies are necessary to determine if these animal and laboratory study results apply to humans.

There have only been a few studies on lapachol in humans. An uncontrolled study in the early 1970s found no toxic effects on liver or kidney tissue. Doses high enough to affect tumors posed a serious risk of side effects, such as prevention of blood clotting. Based on these results, approval was not sought for lapachol as a new anticancer drug, research in the area was discontinued, and in Canada, a ban on the substance was recently imposed.

Pau d'arco has some potentially serious side effects. Some of the chemicals in pau d'arco, such as hydroquinone, are known to be toxic. High doses may cause liver and kidney damage. Even low doses of the pau d'arco can cause vomiting and diarrhea and interfere with blood clotting. This herb should be avoided, especially by women who are pregnant or breast-feeding.

PC-SPES

OTHER COMMON NAME(S): None

Recent studies have found that PC-SPES shows promise with patients whose cancer did not respond to conventional hormone therapy. Common side effects include breast enlargement and tenderness, hot flashes, and decreased libido. More research is needed to determine whether PC-SPES is an effective and safe treatment for prostate cancer. It was recently recalled from the market due to contamination with other prescription drugs.

DESCRIPTION: PC-SPES is a combination of 8 herbs that contain a range of plant chemicals including flavonoids, alkanoids, polysaccharides, amino acids, and trace minerals such as selenium, calcium, magnesium, zinc, and copper (see Calcium, Copper, Selenium, and Zinc). The herbs include chrysanthemum, isatis, licorice, *Ganoderma lucidum, Panax pseudo-ginseng,* Rabdosia rubescens, saw palmetto, and skullcap (see Licorice, Ginseng, Rabdosia Rubescens, and Saw Palmetto). *PC* stands for prostate cancer; *SPES* is the Latin word for hope.

PC-SPES is promoted primarily as a treatment for prostate cancer. Proponents claim that the herbal preparation may prevent or delay the recurrence of prostate cancer, inhibit the growth of prostate tumors, lengthen the survival time of prostate cancer patients, improve the effectiveness of conventional treatments, and delay the use of chemotherapy. Some also state that PC-SPES stimulates the immune system, prevents benign prostatic hyperplasia (enlargement of the prostate gland), neutralizes blood toxins, suppresses cancer-causing genes, reduces inflammation, and has antioxidant qualities.

USE: PC-SPES comes in capsules and is taken daily, in varying dosages. It is available in health food stores, from some nutritionists, and directly from the manufacturer. One study found that the potency of PC-SPES varies widely from batch to batch, so it can be difficult to know if the formula contains the correct amount of active ingredients.

EFFECTS: PC-SPES shows some promise as a treatment for prostate cancer, but more research, which is currently underway, is needed before firm conclusions can be reached. Some recent clinical trials have found that PC-SPES may be useful in treating prostate cancer when the disease does not respond to conventional hormone therapy. For patients who do respond to conventional hormone therapy, PC-SPES does not currently appear to offer any advantages. For example, it is not an appropriate treatment for men with early-stage prostate cancer who can be treated with surgery or radiation therapy.

Side effects associated with the use of PC-SPES can be troubling. Recent studies have found that PC-SPES contains compounds that act like estrogen in the body. Such estrogen compounds can cause hot flashes, increased breast size, and nipple tenderness in men taking PC-SPES. The estrogenic activity of PC-SPES appears to interfere with male hormones by lowering testosterone levels, which can reduce sex drive. There is also an increased risk of developing blood clots and thromboembolism, in which a piece of a blood clot breaks free and clogs a blood vessel. This potentially life-threatening condition is rare (occurring in about 4% to 10% of patients), and may be prevented by combining PC-SPES with clot-preventing drugs.

In February 2002, PC-SPES was recalled from the market after the product was found to contain other prescription drugs that could cause serious health problems. The manufacturer has planned to apply a new quality control process to protect against such contamination in the future.

◥ PEPPERMINT

OTHER COMMON NAME(S): Peppermint Oil, Mint, Balm Mint, Brandy Mint, Green Mint

There is no scientific evidence that peppermint oil is effective in treating side effects related to chemotherapy and radiation, although there is some evidence that it may be effective in controlling nausea after surgery. There is mixed evidence about its effectiveness in treating symptoms of irritable bowel syndrome, such as stomach cramps.

DESCRIPTION: Peppermint is a plant native to Europe, and is now cultivated widely in the United States and Canada. The oil from the leaves and flowering tops of the plant is used in herbal remedies. Proponents claim peppermint oil improves digestion and relieves many gastrointestinal ailments, including gas, indigestion, cramps, diarrhea, and symptoms of irritable bowel syndrome and food poisoning. Some state it has a soothing effect and reduces anxiety.

Sprays and inhalants containing peppermint oil are promoted to relieve sore throats, toothaches, colds, coughs, laryngitis, bronchitis and nasal congestion, and inflammation of the mouth and throat. Some claim salves made from menthol (one of the major active ingredients in peppermint) ease muscle pain and soreness associated with injuries, arthritis, rheumatism, and neuralgia (nerve pain). Menthol vapors are also believed to relieve respiratory and sinus congestion.

Aromatherapists claim peppermint scent alone increases concentration, stimulates the mind and body, decreases inflammation, improves digestion, and relieves stomach pain (see Aromatherapy).

Use: Peppermint oil is the most frequently used form of the plant. The pure oil, or a liquid extract containing the oil, can be taken as is or swallowed in capsules. Peppermint oil is on the Commission E (Germany's regulatory agency for herbs) list of approved herbs. Common dosages are 1 to 2 capsules 3 times a day for irritable bowel syndrome; 1 tablespoon of leaves in a cup of boiling water for tea, 2 or 3 times a day; 3 to 4 drops in hot water for inhalation; 1% to 5% essential oil for nasal ointments; and 5% to 20% essential oil for other ointments applied to the skin.

Effects: There are many anecdotal reports that support the use of peppermint as a treatment for various digestive and respiratory complaints. There is not enough scientific evidence to conclude that peppermint lives up to all the claims made by proponents, including its use as a treatment for stomach cancer or any other type of cancer.

Although there is no scientific evidence that peppermint oil is effective in treating side effects related to chemotherapy and radiation, one controlled study found it to be useful in controlling nausea after surgery. There is debate about whether peppermint oil is effective in treating irritable bowel syndrome. Some preliminary evidence suggests that instilling peppermint oil into the colon during a barium enema (and perhaps colonoscopy) may reduce spasms and decrease the need for intravenous antispasm medications; however, more well-controlled human studies are needed to make definite conclusions.

Peppermint is considered safe, but may cause irritation when applied to the skin. Because peppermint may increase symptoms associated with esophageal reflux disease and hiatal hernia, people with these conditions are advised to avoid the herb. People with gallstones or liver damage should also use caution when using peppermint. Products containing peppermint oil should not be applied to faces of infants or small children.

▌ PHYTOCHEMICALS

Other common name(s): Antioxidants, Flavonoids, Carotenoids, Sulfides, Polyphenols

Some phytochemicals have either antioxidant or hormone-like actions. Eating fruits, vegetables, and grains reduces cancer risk, and researchers are looking for specific compounds in these foods that may account for the beneficial effects in humans. There is no evidence that taking phytochemical supplements is as beneficial as consuming the fruits, vegetables, beans, and grains from which they are taken.

DESCRIPTION: The term phytochemicals refers to a wide variety of compounds produced by plants. Phytochemicals are found in fruits, vegetables, beans, grains, and other plants. Scientists have identified thousands of phytochemicals, although only a small fraction has been studied closely. Some of the more commonly known phytochemicals include beta carotene, ascorbic acid (vitamin C), folic acid, and vitamin E (see Beta Carotene, Folic Acid, Vitamin C, and Vitamin E). There are several major groups of phytochemicals: polyphenols (which includes flavonoids and phytoestrogens), antioxidants, carotenoids (which includes lycopene), and sulfides.

Phytochemicals are promoted for the prevention and treatment of numerous health conditions, including cancer, heart disease, diabetes, and high blood pressure. There is some evidence that phytochemicals may help prevent the formation of carcinogens (potential cancer-causing substances), block the action of carcinogens on their target organs or tissues or act on cells to suppress cancer development. Some scientists estimate that people can reduce their risk of cancer by 30% to 40% simply by eating more fruits, vegetables, and other plant sources that contain phytochemicals.

USE: Phytochemicals are present in virtually all fruits, vegetables, legumes (beans and peas), and grains , so it is quite easy for most people to include them in their diet. For instance, a carrot contains more than 100 phytochemicals. According to one estimate, more than 4000 phytochemicals are catalogued, but only about 150 have been studied in detail. Some of the better-known phytochemicals, such as vitamin A, vitamin E, beta carotene, and lycopene, are also available as supplements. Most nutrition researchers believe that single supplements are not as beneficial as the foods from which they are derived.

EFFECTS: It has become widely accepted that a diet rich in fruits, vegetables, legumes, and grains reduces the risk of cancer, heart disease, and other diseases. But only recently have researchers begun to try to determine the effects of specific phytochemicals contained in those foods.

Much of the evidence so far has come from observations of cultures whose diets consist mainly of plant sources and that appear to experience noticeably lower rates of certain types of cancer and heart disease. Researchers have conducted many laboratory and clinical studies examining the relationship between cancer risk and eating fruits and vegetables, legumes, and grains. Much of the evidence indicates that a higher consumption of these foods is associated with a reduced risk of some cancers and other diseases.

Researchers have also shown much interest in phytochemical supplements. Studies so far indicate that the value of most phytochemicals decreases when they are obtained through supplements and not through diet. Until conclusive research findings emerge, health care professionals advise a balanced diet with emphasis on fruits, vegetables, legumes, and whole grains. According to the American Cancer Society dietary guidelines, at least 5 servings of fruits and vegetables per day are recommended. Experts also stress that diet, regardless of how healthy, may reduce the risk of cancer and other diseases, but other crucial factors such as genetics and the environment clearly play a role as well.

Because of the number of phytochemicals and the complexity of the chemical processes they are involved in, researchers face the challenging task of trying to determine which phytochemicals in foods are truly beneficial to health, which may fight cancer and other diseases, and which may even be harmful. It is known, however, that phytochemical supplements should not be taken with benzodiazepine-type drugs, such as Valium or other sedatives. Some phytochemical supplements may actually be toxic when taken in large doses.

▩ POKEWEED

OTHER COMMON NAME(S): Common Pokeweed, Pokeroot, Poke Salad, Pokeberry, Poke, Virginia Poke, Inkberry, Cancer Root, Crowberry, Bear's Grape, American Nightshade, Pigeon Berry

Some research has shown that a protein contained in pokeweed, called pokeweed antiviral protein, has antitumor effects in mice and laboratory studies. Clinical trials have not yet been done to determine if these effects apply to humans. All parts of the mature plant contain chemically active substances such as phytolaccine, formic acid, tannin, and resin acid, and all parts are at least mildly poisonous when eaten.

DESCRIPTION: Pokeweed is a shrub that is native to eastern North America and cultivated throughout the world. It can grow to a height of more than 10 feet. The berries and dried roots, which are the most potent sections of the plant, are used in herbal remedies. Proponents claim that pokeweed can be used internally to treat a number of conditions, including rheumatoid arthritis, tonsillitis, mumps, swollen glands, chronic excess mucus, bronchitis, mastitis, and constipation. They also say that the herb is an effective treatment for fungal infections, joint inflammation, hemorrhoids, breast abscesses, ulcers, and bad breath. Herbalists also claim that external application of a preparation made from the plant relieves itching, inflammation, and skin diseases. There is no scientific evidence to support these claims.

Some supporters also believe that the plant has anticancer and antiviral properties, protects cells against HIV, and may prevent the virus from replicating. Current studies are investigating the possible benefits of pokeweed as an anticancer agent in osteosarcomas (bone cancers) and certain kinds of leukemia.

USE: Pokeweed supplements are available as liquid extracts, tinctures, powders, and poultices. There is no standard dosage for pokeweed. Pokeweed berries are one of the ingredients in the Hoxsey formula (see Hoxsey Herbal Treatment). For research purposes, scientists have learned to chemically manufacture pokeweed antiviral protein because it is difficult to remove from the plant.

EFFECTS: Research has shown that pokeweed contains a compound that appears to enhance the immune system and has some anticancer effects in animals. Further studies are necessary to determine if these animal study results apply to humans.

All parts of the pokeweed are poisonous, particularly the berries, roots, and seeds. Cooking the plant reduces its toxicity. The effects of eating the uncooked plant can include nausea, vomiting, diarrhea, abdominal cramps, headaches, blurred vision, confusion, dermatitis, dizziness, and weakness. Pokeweed may be fatal in children.

Pokeweed should not be used by people who are taking antidepressants, Antabuse®, oral contraceptives, or fertility drugs. The plant may cause menstrual cycle irregularities and may also stimulate contractions of the uterus. Women who are pregnant or breast-feeding should not use pokeweed.

■ POTASSIUM

OTHER COMMON NAME(S): None

Potassium is a mineral that is essential to normal body functioning. Most people get all the potassium they need in their diet. There is no scientific evidence that potassium supplements can prevent or treat cancer in humans. Excess potassium in the body can be toxic.

DESCRIPTION: Potassium is an essential mineral found in most foods. Along with sodium and calcium, potassium helps regulate major body functions, including normal heart rhythm, blood pressure, water and pH balance (acidity and alkalinity), digestion, nerve impulses, and muscle contractions. The body cannot manufacture potassium on its own and must obtain it from a variety of foods.

Some alternative medical practitioners maintain that low levels of potassium in the body may be linked to cancer, heart disease, high blood pressure, osteoporosis, depression, and schizophrenia. Some proponents claim that a diet high in sodium and low in potassium promotes tumor growth by changing the normal pH and water balance in human cells.

USE: There is no recommended daily allowance for potassium, but the Estimated Minimum Daily Requirement is 2 g. Because most foods contain potassium, people usually get plenty of potassium from their normal food intake. The kidneys control blood levels of potassium and eliminate excess in the urine.

Supplements may be needed only by those who have low levels of potassium in their bloodstream, a condition known as hypokalemia. The causes of hypokalemia can include digestive disorders that result in diarrhea and vomiting, some types of diuretics (drugs that remove water from the body through urine), overuse of laxatives, diabetes, certain kidney diseases, and excessive sweating.

EFFECTS: Some animal and human studies have indicated that a diet high in potassium and low in sodium might help prevent high blood pressure in some people. Similar studies of the effects of a high-potassium diet on cancer have not shown a positive link between potassium intake and the prevention or development of cancer.

Some population studies have found that in a number of countries where there are high-potassium diets, there are lower cancer rates, and in areas where there are low-potassium diets, there are higher cancer rates. These types of studies do not prove a direct connection because there may be many other factors involved.

One researcher has suggested a link between an increased risk of cancer and low-potassium and high-sodium levels in cells; however, there is no scientific evidence that shows that changes in dietary potassium have any impact on potassium concentrations inside cancer cells. Potassium concentration in the body is actually regulated by the kidneys. Further studies are needed to determine the effects of a high-potassium/low-sodium diet on the prevention or formation of cancer.

People with symptoms of hypokalemia should consult their doctor before taking potassium supplements. These symptoms include tiredness, sleepiness, dizziness, muscle fatigue, and, in more serious cases, abnormal heartbeat or muscle paralysis. Taking excessive potassium supplements can cause potassium to build up in the blood, resulting in a condition known as hyperkalemia. The symptoms of hyperkalemia include muscle numbness and tingling, abnormalities in heart rhythm, muscle paralysis, and possibly even heart failure. Severe kidney failure and Addison's disease (a hormone deficiency) may also cause hyperkalemia.

▧ PSYLLIUM

OTHER COMMON NAME(S): Psyllium Seed Husk, Isphagula, Isapgol

Although psyllium and other fiber supplements are useful in treating constipation and may reduce cholesterol, fruits and vegetables are considered to be more effective in lowering cancer risk. Psyllium should be taken with an adequate amount of water to avoid choking or obstruction of the esophagus, throat, and intestines.

DESCRIPTION: Psyllium (pronounced silly-um) comes from the crushed seeds of the *Plantago ovata* plant, an herb native to parts of Asia, Mediterranean regions of Europe, and North Africa. It is now cultivated extensively in India and Pakistan, as well as in the southwestern United States.

The psyllium seed husk is the part used in herbal remedies, primarily as a fiber supplement to promote bowel movements and ease constipation. Fiber is the indigestible material in plant foods, also known as roughage. High-fiber diets help the digestive tract function properly. Psyllium absorbs water and expands as it travels through the digestive tract, which is why it is referred to as a bulk-forming laxative. Psyllium is sometimes used to treat side effects of conventional cancer treatment, such as diarrhea and constipation.

USE: Psyllium seed husk is approved by Commission E (Germany's regulatory agency for herbs) for chronic constipation. It is also supported by the Food and Drug Administration, which has issued a food-specific positive health claim for oats that includes psyllium fiber.

Psyllium is available as a powder, tablet, or capsule. In any form, it must be taken with adequate amounts of water (1 or 2 glasses per 3.5 g). Commission E recommends 4 to 20 g per day of the drug as needed. Psyllium is also available as the most common ingredient contained in laxatives that are used by over 4 million Americans a day. These laxatives are available over the counter and by prescription.

EFFECTS: Psyllium has been found to be effective in treating constipation, and research suggests that it may also help reduce cholesterol. It is well known that a diet high in fiber helps the digestive tract perform most efficiently. An inadequate amount of fiber in the diet can lead to constipation, hemorrhoids, and diverticulitis. Most nutritionists agree that the best source of fiber is from the diet in the form of beans, vegetables, whole grains, and fruits.

Some nutritionists believe that dietary fiber may help reduce the risk of colorectal cancer, although it is not yet known whether the protective factor is fiber itself or other components of the plant. Conflicting results from studies of dietary fiber and colorectal cancer risk have caused some confusion among the general public and some health professionals. Studies clearly show that a diet high in fruits and vegetables can lower colorectal cancer risk, as well as the risk of several other diseases.

The use of psyllium is generally safe; however, excessive amounts can cause abdominal distention, diarrhea, gas, and gastrointestinal obstruction. Not drinking enough water with psyllium can cause choking or obstruction of the esophagus, throat, and intestines. Some people are allergic to the plant, as well as to the psyllium powder.

Psyllium may delay the absorption of some medications taken at the same time. Diabetic patients who are insulin-dependent may need to reduce insulin doses while taking psyllium products. Patients with a history of intestinal obstruction, fecal impaction, and narrowing of the gastrointestinal tract and those who have difficulty controlling diabetes should avoid psyllium.

▉ PYCNOGENOL

OTHER COMMON NAME(S): Pinebark Extract, Pycnogenol™

Although interest in pycnogenol as a potent antioxidant is growing among medical researchers, there is little data from clinical trials to support the health claims made for any form of pycnogenol.

DESCRIPTION: The name pycnogenol (pronounced pick-naw-gin-all) is used in several ways. Pycnogenol often refers to a trademarked compound extracted from the bark of the European coastal pine tree (*Pinus maritima*) that contains naturally occurring chemicals called proanthocyanidins. Pycnogenol is also the name of a variety of compounds that contain proanthocyanidins taken from a variety of natural sources, such as grape seeds (see Grapes) and other plants.

Proponents claim that pycnogenol is one of the most powerful antioxidants. Antioxidants are compounds that block the action of activated oxygen molecules known as free radicals, which can damage cells. Supporters believe that pycnogenol protects against arthritis, complications from diabetes, cancer, heart disease, and circulatory problems, such as swelling and varicose veins. Other reported benefits include helping to improve memory, reducing the effects of stress, improving flexibility in joints, and reducing inflammation. Some claim that Pycnogenol supplements are much more effective in eliminating free radicals than vitamins E and C (see Vitamin C and Vitamin E). There is no scientific evidence to support these claims.

USE: Pycnogenol is available as tablets and capsules. Practitioners use 25 to 300 mg per day for up to 3 weeks. They suggest a maintenance dosage of 40 to 800 mg per day.

EFFECTS: There is not enough data from clinical trials to support the health claims made for any form of pycnogenol, although interest in proanthocyanidins among medical researchers is growing. There are anecdotal reports that pycnogenol is effective in treating circulatory disorders. The results of one animal study suggest that pycnogenol from a pine tree bark extract may protect against lung cancer. More research is needed to determine if pycnogenol may have any benefit for people with cancer or any other disease.

Pycnogenol has been reported to be safe; however, not enough information is known about any possible drug interaction effects.

RABDOSIA RUBESCENS

OTHER COMMON NAME(S): None

Rabdosia rubescens is a Chinese herb promoted as a treatment for cancer of the esophagus. It is also one of the 8 herbs used in PC-SPES, an herbal formula promoted as a treatment for prostate cancer (see PC-SPES). There is no scientific evidence to support the claims for Rabdosia rubescens.

RED CLOVER

OTHER COMMON NAME(S): Purple Clover, Trefoil, Wild Clover

There is no scientific evidence that red clover is effective in treating or preventing cancer, menopausal symptoms, or any other medical conditions. It may also increase the risk of excessive bleeding in some people.

DESCRIPTION: Red clover is a native plant of Europe, central Asia, and northern Africa. It now grows in many other parts of the world. The flower head is the part of the plant used in herbal remedies. Proponents claim that it is useful for relieving menopausal symptoms because it contains chemicals that are similar to the hormone estrogen. They also claim that the herb suppresses coughs (particularly whooping cough), speeds wound healing, eases chronic skin conditions such as psoriasis, and is an anticoagulant (a compound that slows blood clotting). People who take prescription anticoagulant medication may be able to reduce their dosage by taking red clover supplements, according to some practitioners.

Other supporters claim that red clover is effective for treating cancers of the breast, ovaries, and lymphatic system. A few claim that the herb acts as an antibiotic, an appetite suppressant, and a relaxant; however, there is no scientific evidence to support these claims.

USE: Red clover supplements are available as tablets, as capsules, or in liquid extract form. Dried red clover can be brewed into a tea. Practitioners generally use a daily dosage of about 4 g of dried red clover, or 1.5 to 3 ml of liquid extract. The liquid extract can be rubbed directly on skin or applied with a compress.

EFFECTS: Scientists have identified estrogen-like substances called isoflavonoids and anticoagulant chemicals called coumarins in red clover. The therapeutic claims made for the herb have not been verified in humans through controlled clinical studies.

One laboratory study found that red clover contains substances similar to the hormones estrogen and progesterone. Most studies suggest that long-term use (10 years or more) of estrogen replacement therapy after menopause may increase the risk of breast and endometrial cancers. Scientists have been seeking alternatives to estrogen that do not increase the risk of cancer.

In a small clinical study, researchers concluded that a diet supplemented with red clover sprouts and other plants that contain estrogen-like substances may reduce the severity of menopause. This conclusion needs to be confirmed in other studies before red clover can be routinely recommended.

Not enough is known about the herb to determine its safety. Patients with bleeding problems or who take anticoagulant medications should avoid red clover because it may increase the risk of serious bleeding. Women with a history of estrogen receptor-positive cancers or who are pregnant or breast-feeding should not use this herb.

■ SAW PALMETTO

OTHER COMMON NAME(S): None

There is some scientific evidence that saw palmetto relieves symptoms associated with benign prostatic hyperplasia (BPH—an enlarged prostate gland), such as difficult and frequent urination; however, saw palmetto is not an effective treatment for prostate cancer.

DESCRIPTION: Saw palmetto is a low-growing palm tree found in the West Indies and in coastal regions of the southeastern United States. The tree grows 6 to 10 feet in height and has a crown of large leaves. The berries are used in herbal remedies. Saw palmetto is promoted as a treatment for prostatitis (inflamed prostate gland) and the symptoms of benign prostatic hyperplasia (BPH). Chemicals in saw palmetto berries are believed to interfere with the action of prostate hormones that stimulate cell growth. Some proponents claim it also increases sex drive and fertility and can be used to treat low thyroid function, although there is no scientific evidence to support these claims.

USE: Saw palmetto supplements are available as capsules, tablets, extracts, and tea. There is no standard dosage. In some clinical studies for the treatment of BPH, patients received 320 mg per day, divided into 2 doses.

EFFECTS: Saw palmetto is not effective as a treatment for prostate cancer, but it may aid in relieving some of the symptoms of BPH (a noncancerous condition), which include difficult and frequent urination. A recent review concluded that the extract improved urinary symptoms, such as frequent nighttime urination and problems with urine flow. The improvements from using palmetto extract were similar to those seen in men who took the prescription drug finasteride for BPH. Saw palmetto also caused fewer and milder side effects than finasteride. Finasteride appears to reduce the size of the prostate, but it is still not clear whether saw palmetto causes the prostate to shrink. More research is needed to determine saw palmetto's long-term effectiveness and ability to prevent complications from BPH. There is no published scientific evidence that saw palmetto has any value in the treatment of prostate cancer.

The long-term effects and safety of saw palmetto are unknown. Side effects are not common but may include headache, nausea, vomiting, upset stomach, dizziness, constipation or diarrhea, difficulty sleeping, fatigue, and, in rare instances, heart pain. Men who have difficult, frequent, or urgent urination should see a doctor as soon as possible, rather than treating themselves with saw palmetto. Similar symptoms can also result from prostate cancer, and self-treatment with saw palmetto may delay diagnosis and treatment of cancer.

It is not known if saw palmetto interferes with the measurement of prostate-specific antigen (PSA), a protein made by prostate cells, which is used to determine the presence and extent of prostate cancer. The effects of saw palmetto on blood PSA levels have not yet been determined. Since saw palmetto affects testosterone metabolism in the same way as finasteride, some doctors recommend that men also have a baseline PSA test and digital rectal examination before starting treatment with saw palmetto.

◤ SELENIUM

OTHER COMMON NAME(S): None

Selenium shows promise as a nutrient that may prevent the development and progression of cancer; however, more research is needed. A small amount of selenium is all the human body needs. Large amounts in supplement form can be toxic.

DESCRIPTION: Selenium is an essential mineral nutrient for both humans and animals. It is found in soil all over the world in varying amounts. It is said to help preserve elasticity in body tissues, slow the aging process, improve the flow of oxygen to the heart, and help prevent abnormal blood clotting. Researchers think selenium is an antioxidant, a compound that blocks the action of activated oxygen molecules known as free radicals, which can damage cells. Selenium may stimulate the formation of antibodies (proteins that help fight invading microorganisms) in response to vaccines. Selenium may also play a role in normal growth, development, and fertility.

Selenium is claimed to protect the body against cancer by causing cancer cells to die before they have a chance to grow and spread; however, this has not yet been proven.

USE: The best nutritional sources of selenium are seafood, liver, kidney, whole grains, cereals, and Brazil nuts. Selenium is also present in drinking water in very low levels. Selenium in food and water is easily absorbed by the human body and used where needed. A very small amount of selenium is good for the body, but too much can be toxic and have a negative effect on the immune system. The recommended intake of selenium is 5.5 micrograms (µg) a day for adults.

Since a normal diet provides about 50 to 150 µg per day, supplements are usually not needed. Some research suggests that supplements may help prevent certain types of cancer, but the amount of the supplements should not exceed 400 µg per day taken on a regular basis. Supplements are available in drug and health food stores.

EFFECTS: Both animal and human studies suggest that selenium may play a role in lowering a person's risk of developing cancer, as well as reducing death rates of those with cancer. Epidemiological studies indicate that in areas of the world where selenium levels in the soil are high, mortality rates from cancer are significantly lower. Although animal studies have also shown a protective effect from selenium against the development of various cancers, observational studies in humans have had mixed results. More long-term controlled human studies are needed. A comprehensive report by the National Academy of Sciences concluded that there is not enough evidence that taking high doses of antioxidants can prevent chronic diseases.

Taking selenium supplements can be toxic to the human body if the supplements raise selenium levels beyond what the body can tolerate. No one knows for sure what that level is, however. The signs of selenium poisoning include deformed nails, vomiting, fatigue, numbness and loss of control in the arms and legs, as well as loss of hair, teeth, and nails. Massive overdoses can result in death. In rare cases, eating vegetables grown in areas where selenium levels in the soil are high, such as the western United States, may also cause selenium poisoning.

On the other hand, a deficiency of selenium resulting from eating a poor diet over a long time or eating vegetables grown in selenium-poor soil can cause heart disease, muscle pain, and premature aging.

▨ SIBERIAN GINSENG

OTHER COMMON NAME(S): None

There is no scientific evidence that Siberian ginseng is effective in treating cancer or reducing the side effects of chemotherapy or radiation therapy. There have been no studies of its safety or long-term effects.

DESCRIPTION: Siberian ginseng is an herb that grows in Siberia, China, Korea, and Japan. Siberian ginseng should not be confused with Asian ginseng or American ginseng, which belong to a different family of herbs. The dried root and other underground parts of the plant are used in herbal remedies. Proponents of Siberian ginseng claim that it stimulates the immune system, increases energy, improves concentration and memory, quickens recovery from disease, and heightens mental acuity and physical prowess. Some practitioners claim that the herb regulates blood pressure, reduces inflammation, has a restorative effect on many organs, lowers blood sugar levels, and enables chemotherapy drugs to penetrate cancer cells more easily. There is no scientific evidence to support these claims.

USE: Siberian ginseng is on the Commission E (Germany's regulatory agency for herbs) list of approved herbs, and the supplements are available in tablets and liquid extracts. The powdered or cut root can be brewed as a tea. An average dosage is 2 to 3 g per day. Typically, Siberian ginseng is taken regularly for 6 to 8 weeks, followed by a 1- or 2-week break before resuming.

EFFECTS: Few animal studies of Siberian ginseng have been published in peer-reviewed medical journals. There is no evidence that demonstrates the herb's effectiveness against cancer, and there is little evidence that supplements enhance athletic ability. One clinical study in the United States concluded that Siberian ginseng did not improve performance during aerobic exercise.

Health risks associated with Siberian ginseng have not been established, although side effects seem to be rare. A few cases of diarrhea and insomnia have been reported. People with high blood pressure should avoid the supplements. There have been no studies of Siberian ginseng's long-term effects.

▌ SIX FLAVOR TEA

OTHER COMMON NAME(S): Liu Wei Di Huang, Gold Book Tea, Jin Gui Shen Qi

Six Flavor Tea is a Chinese herbal tonic that is promoted to enhance conventional treatment of small-cell lung cancer (see Chinese Herbal Medicine). It is primarily sold as a treatment for kidney deficiencies, which practitioners claim can cause a buildup of disease-causing toxins. They contend Six Flavor Tea can also treat weakness or pain in the lower back, insomnia, night sweats, dizziness, ringing in the ears, impotence, and high blood pressure. There is no scientific evidence to support any of these claims.

▌ ST. JOHN'S WORT

OTHER COMMON NAME(S): Goatweed, Amber, Klamath Weed, Tipton Weed, Kira®, Tension Tamer®, Hypercalm®

St. John's wort has been shown to be effective in treating mild to moderate depression with fewer side effects than standard antidepressants (ie, tricyclics), although recent research has found that it is not useful in treating severe depression. More research is needed to compare it with newer antidepressants. St. John's wort also has the potential to interfere with anesthesia as well as a number of prescription drugs.

DESCRIPTION: St. John's wort is a shrub-like perennial plant with bright yellow flowers that is native to Europe, western Asia, and northern Africa. It is also cultivated in the United States and other parts of the world. The parts of the plant used in herbal remedies are taken from the flowering tops. St. John's wort is widely used in Europe to treat depression, anxiety, and sleep disorders. In Germany, doctors prescribe it more often than Prozac®, a popular antidepressant drug. Hypericin is the most commonly studied active ingredient in St. John's wort.

The herb is also promoted to treat bronchial inflammation, burns, wounds, bed-wetting, stomach problems, hemorrhoids, hypothyroidism, insect bites and stings, skin diseases, insomnia, migraines, kidney disorders, and scabies. There is no scientific evidence to support these further claims.

USE: Commission E (Germany's regulatory agency for herbs) has approved St. John's wort for the treatment of depression and anxiety, as well as for burns and skin lesions. It is available by prescription only in Germany; however, it can be purchased in drug and health food stores in the

United States. An average daily dosage is 300 mg (0.3% hypericin, the standardized amount) of standardized extract preparation 3 times per day for 4 to 6 weeks. There is a wide range of potency and purity of the different extracts that are available. Researchers have found that most brands of St. John's wort contain lower potency than is listed on the label.

EFFECTS: Clinical trials have shown that hypericin is effective in treating mild to moderate depression with fewer side effects than standard antidepressants (ie, tricyclics); however, St. John's wort may not work with all types of depression. A recent multicenter study found that it is not effective in treating severe cases of depression. Its long-term effectiveness is also unknown, and there is no data about how it compares to newer antidepressants such as Prozac (ie, selective serotonin reuptake inhibitors). It is unclear how the hypericin in St. John's wort works to relieve depression. Some think that the active ingredient may even be another compound in the herb.

Information on the long-term effects or usage of St. John's wort is not currently known. Side effects are not common but include gastrointestinal discomfort, fatigue, dry mouth, dizziness, rash, and hypersensitivity to sunlight. St. John's wort should not be used with alcohol, narcotics, amphetamines, anticoagulants, antibiotics, or cold and flu medicines such as pseudoephedrine. It should not be used with other antidepressants because it could cause serotonin syndrome—a potentially fatal complication involving changes in thoughts, behavior, and autonomic and central nervous system functioning caused by an increase in serotonin activity. People with severe depression or manic depression and women who are pregnant or breast-feeding should not use St. John's wort.

In response to a report in the medical journal *Lancet*, the Food and Drug Administration issued a public health alert on St. John's wort on February 10, 2000. The herb may interfere with a number of prescription drugs such as warfarin, indinavir, cyclosporine, digoxin, oral contraceptives, and antiretroviral medications (used for HIV). People taking any prescription medications or other herbal preparations should consult their doctors before taking St. John's wort. Because of its potential to interact with anesthetics, it should not be used by people who are undergoing surgery.

▪ STRYCHNOS NUX-VOMICA

OTHER COMMON NAME(S): Poison Nut, Strychnos Seed, Quaker Buttons

There is no scientific evidence that Strychnos nux-vomica *is effective in*

treating the side effects of conventional cancer treatment or any other conditions. The chemicals in the seeds are poisonous and may cause convulsions and death.

DESCRIPTION: *Strychnos nux-vomica* is the name of an evergreen tree native to southeast Asia, especially India and Myanmar. Its dried seeds and bark (called *nux vomica*) are used in herbal remedies. The seeds contain organic substances, strychnine and brucine, that act as stimulants in the human body. In herbal medicine, *Strychnos nux-vomica* is recommended for upset stomach, vomiting, abdominal pain, constipation, intestinal irritation, hangovers, heartburn, insomnia, certain heart diseases, circulatory problems, eye diseases, depression, migraine headaches, nervous conditions, problems related to menopause, and respiratory diseases in older people. In folk medicine, it is used as a healing tonic and appetite stimulant. There is no evidence to support these claims.

USE: The seeds of the *Strychnos nux-vomica* tree are removed from the ripened berries of the tree and dried in the sun. Various herbal preparations are made from the dried seeds, including tablets, liquid extracts, and tinctures. Some practitioners use single doses that range from 0.02 g to 1 g. The maximum daily dosage should not exceed 2 g.

EFFECTS: *Strychnos nux-vomica* has not been proven to be effective for the treatment of any disease. Since the herb contains strychnine, which is poisonous to humans, conventional medical practitioners do not recommend it as a medicine. Some research has shown that the level of toxicity of *nux vomica* preparations may depend greatly on how the seeds are processed. The herbal remedy is on the Commission E (Germany's regulatory agency for herbs) list of unapproved herbs. This means that it is not recommended for use because it has not been proven to be safe or effective.

The strychnine in *nux vomica* is a poison that, in doses of 5 mg or more (equal to 30 to 50 mg of the herb formulation), may cause anxiety, restlessness, painful convulsions of the body, breathing difficulties, and even death resulting from suffocation or exhaustion. In addition, long-term intake of strychnine can cause liver damage. This herb should be avoided, especially by women who are pregnant or breast-feeding.

▌ TEA TREE OIL

OTHER COMMON NAME(S): Australian Tea Tree Oil, Melaleuca Oil

Tea tree oil has been used in Australia for many years to treat skin infections.

It holds promise today as an alternative to antibiotics that are resistant to certain bacteria; however, there is no evidence that it boosts the immune system. Tea tree oil is toxic when swallowed, and it should never be taken internally.

DESCRIPTION: Tea tree oil is concentrated plant oil that is distilled through a steam process from the leaves of a large myrtle tree native to Australian coastal areas known as *Melaleuca alternifolia* (or tea tree). The oil is used as an herbal remedy. Some proponents believe tea tree oil may be an antibiotic and antiseptic that is effective in combating germs. It has been used to treat cuts, minor burns, athlete's foot, and insect bites. Some claim it can treat bacterial and fungal skin infections, wound infections, gum infections, acne, head lice, eczema, yeast infections, colds, pneumonia, and other respiratory illnesses.

While no one claims tea tree oil can prevent or treat cancer, some proponents claim the oil can boost the immune system. In addition, household cleaners that contain tea tree oil have been promoted as alternatives to products that contain possible cancer-causing chemicals, such as formaldehyde. One herbalist claims that tea tree oil can be used as a "lymphatic recharge" for a "sluggish" lymphatic system. There is no scientific evidence to support these claims.

USE: Tea tree oil can be dissolved in water or used in full strength. It is available as an ointment, cream, lotion, and soap. Tea tree oil is often sold in dark glass bottles with a dropper on the cap to prevent light from affecting its potency. When used to treat infections and skin conditions, the oil can be applied directly to the skin in full strength or in diluted form using cotton swabs. The oil can also be found in deodorants, shampoos, soaps, antiseptic first-aid creams, and household cleaning products.

Tea tree oil should never be taken internally. For colds and other respiratory illnesses, the oil is added to a vaporizer so that the fumes can be inhaled to kill germs in the nose and throat. Drops of the oil can be added to bath water to treat skin diseases. The oil is sometimes mixed in water as a mouthwash to prevent gum infections.

EFFECTS: Recent laboratory experiments suggest that tea tree oil holds promise as an antibiotic when spread on top of the skin to treat the bacteria *Staphylococcus* (staph) and other infectious agents that are resistant to certain antibiotics. Further studies are necessary to determine if laboratory results apply to humans. There is also no clinical evidence for the effectiveness of tea tree oil for treating skin problems and infections.

Tea tree oil is toxic when swallowed. As a result, it can cause drowsiness, poor muscle coordination, vomiting, diarrhea, and stomach upset. In rare cases, some people develop allergic reactions, such as inflammation of the skin. There is some evidence that the oil should not be used on burns. The oil is not recommended for children. Women who are pregnant or breast-feeding should not use this oil.

█ THUJA

OTHER COMMON NAME(S): Eastern White Cedar, Yellow Cedar, Tree of Life, Arborvitae, Hackmatack, Swamp Cedar

There is no scientific evidence that thuja or its extract is safe or effective. Taken internally, this herb can cause serious side effects and may be toxic in large doses.

DESCRIPTION: Thuja is an eastern white cedar tree. It is an evergreen in the cypress family that is native to eastern North America. The tree is also grown in Europe as an ornamental plant. The parts used in herbal remedies are the leaves, branches, and needles, which contain the oil thujone (see Wormwood).

Thuja is promoted as a treatment for many medical conditions, including cancer. Some proponents claim that thuja decreases the toxic effects of chemotherapy and radiation therapy.

Herbalists prescribe thuja to treat coughs and other respiratory ailments (including strep throat and respiratory distress related to congestive heart failure) and viral and bacterial infections. They also use it as a diuretic (to increase urination) and an astringent (to purify the blood, reduce inflammation, and cleanse the body of toxins). Thuja is sometimes used together with antibiotics to treat bacterial skin infections and herpes sores. It has even been used by practitioners to stimulate abortions. Thuja ointment is applied to the skin for ailments such as psoriasis, eczema, vaginal infections, warts, muscular aches, and rheumatism. There is no scientific evidence to support any of these claims.

USE: Liquid extracts, tinctures, and tea made from thuja are taken internally. There is no standardized dosage. Thuja ointment is applied directly to the skin. Thuja oil and capsules are available in health food stores and on the Internet.

EFFECTS: There is no scientific evidence that thuja is effective in treating cancer or any other disease. The medical literature contains no studies on the effects of thuja in humans, and there is very little scientific data to verify that the herb has any therapeutic value. Many supporters base their claims on limited laboratory experiments or anecdotal reports.

Taken internally in large doses, thuja is potentially toxic, although the amount that constitutes a high dose has not been determined. Some people who have consumed thuja reportedly experienced asthma attacks, gastrointestinal irritation, excess stimulation of the nervous system, and spontaneous abortion. People with seizure disorders or gastrointestinal problems (such as ulcers or gastritis) should avoid thuja. Women who are pregnant or breast-feeding should not use this herbal treatment. In fact, because so little is known about thuja, it is not recommended for any use.

▨ TURMERIC

OTHER COMMON NAME(S): Indian Saffron, Indian Valerian, Jiang Huang, Radix, Red Valerian

Turmeric is a common food flavoring and coloring in Asian cuisine. Animal and laboratory studies have found that curcumin, the active ingredient in turmeric, demonstrated some anticancer effects. However, clinical research is needed to determine curcumin's role in cancer prevention and treatment in humans.

DESCRIPTION: Turmeric is a spice grown in India and other tropical regions of Asia. It has a long history of use in herbal remedies, particularly in China, India, and Indonesia. The root of the plant contains the active ingredient, curcumin. Some researchers believe turmeric may prevent and slow the growth of a number of cancers, particularly tumors of the esophagus, mouth, intestines, stomach, breast, and skin, although there is no evidence from human studies to support these claims. Some researchers have speculated that curcumin, after it enters the body, changes into tetrahydrocurcumin, which may be a potent antioxidant. An antioxidant is a compound that blocks the action of activated oxygen molecules known as free radicals, which can damage cells.

Turmeric is promoted primarily as an anti-inflammatory herbal remedy that is said to produce far fewer side effects than conventional pain relievers. Some practitioners prescribe turmeric to relieve inflammation caused by arthritis, muscle sprains, swelling, and pain caused by injuries or surgical incisions. It is also promoted as a treatment for rheumatism and as an antiseptic for cleaning wounds. Some proponents claim turmeric interferes with the actions of some viruses, including hepatitis and HIV.

Supporters also claim that turmeric protects against liver diseases, stimulates the gallbladder and circulatory systems, reduces cholesterol levels, dissolves blood clots, helps stop external and internal bleeding, and relieves painful menstruation and angina (chest pains usually associated with heart disease). It is also used as a remedy for digestive problems such as irritable bowel syndrome, colitis, Crohn's disease, and illnesses caused by the parasite *Giardia* and by the bacteria *Salmonella*. There is no scientific evidence to support any of these claims.

USE: Turmeric root is on the Commission E (Germany's regulatory agency for herbs) list of approved herbs, and it is available in powdered form in most grocery stores. It can also be made into a tea or purchased as a tincture or tablets. An ointment made from turmeric can be applied to the skin. Although there is no standardized dosage for turmeric, some practitioners recommend taking a teaspoon with each meal.

EFFECTS: Researchers have studied turmeric extensively to determine if it is an effective antioxidant and anti-inflammatory agent and whether it holds any promise as a cancer drug. All of the evidence so far comes from laboratory or animal studies. Further studies are necessary to determine if these animal and laboratory study results apply to humans.

When used as a spice in foods, turmeric is considered safe. More research is needed to establish the safety of turmeric when used in herbal remedies. Little is known about the potential risks of taking the larger quantities used to treat disease. An overdose may result in stomach pain. Contact dermatitis (skin allergy) and stomach ulcers have been reported after long-term use.

People taking anticoagulant medications, drugs that suppress the immune system, or nonsteroidal pain relievers (such as ibuprofen) should avoid turmeric. Persons with bleeding disorders, obstructions of the bile duct, or a history of ulcers also should avoid turmeric. Women who are pregnant or breast-feeding should not use this herb.

▓ VALERIAN

OTHER COMMON NAME(S): Valerian Tea, Valerian Root, Valerian Extract

Valerian is an herb used for anxiety and insomnia. Although some research suggests that it is effective, the results have been conflicting and the methods

have been flawed. More research is needed to make definite conclusions about its effectiveness. Valerian has some side effects associated with long-term use, as well as the potential to interfere with anesthesia and other medications.

DESCRIPTION: Valerian is a flowering plant native to Europe, Asia, and the Americas. In herbal remedies, the plant's foul-smelling root is chopped up and made into a tea or extract that is used primarily as a sedative. Herbal practitioners claim that valerian root or extract can lessen anxiety and nervous tension, aid sleep, help people quit smoking, ease congestion, and relieve muscle spasms. There are no claims that valerian is useful for treating or preventing cancer.

USE: Valerian root is on the Commission E (Germany's regulatory agency for herbs) list of approved herbs. Supplements are available in tablets, capsules, or tinctures, and it can also be brewed as a tea. To ease sleep and combat insomnia, the usual dose of valerian extract in tablet form is 300 to 900 mg to be taken an hour before bedtime. For stress and anxiety, the recommended dosage is 50 to 100 mg taken 2 to 3 times per day.

EFFECTS: At least 3 controlled human studies have been conducted in the United States comparing valerian with a placebo (an inactive substance). These studies showed that those who took valerian experienced less insomnia and had improved quality of sleep. One well-controlled human study conducted in Germany compared a combination of valerian and St. John's wort to diazepam (an antianxiety drug) in 100 people with anxiety symptoms and found significantly greater symptom improvement in those who took the herbs (see St. John's Wort). While promising, these studies are limited by small sample sizes and short follow-up periods.

On the basis of animal studies and several clinical trials in Europe, German health officials have approved valerian as a sleep aid and mild sedative. Expert advisors to the US Pharmacopeial Convention have concluded that the scientific evidence is insufficient and too conflicting to recommend valerian for the treatment of insomnia. More research is needed to determine the effectiveness of valerian.

Valerian is considered to be relatively safe; however, some people may experience restlessness and heart palpitations, especially with long-term use of valerian as a sedative. Long-term or excessive use is not recommended due to the potential side effects, which include headaches, blurred vision, heart palpitations, excitability, hypersensitivity reactions, insomnia, and nausea. Valerian should not be taken with alcohol, certain antihistamines, muscle relaxants, psychotropic drugs, sedatives, barbiturates, or narcotics. Because of its potential to interact with anesthetics, people who are undergoing surgery should not use valerian. Abrupt discontinuation may cause withdrawal symptoms in some cases, so the dose of valerian should be tapered several weeks before surgery. People with liver or kidney disease should seek their doctor's advice before taking valerian. In very high doses, the herb may weaken the heartbeat and cause paralysis. Women who are pregnant or breast-feeding should not take valerian.

▨ VENUS FLYTRAP

OTHER COMMON NAME(S): Carnivora®, Plumbagin

There is no scientific evidence that the extract from the Venus flytrap plant is effective in treating skin cancer or any other type of cancer. Some side effects have been reported with its use.

DESCRIPTION: The Venus flytrap is a perennial plant that traps and eats insects. It is found in low-lying wetlands of the southeastern United States. Some believe that the primary active ingredient in the Venus flytrap is plumbagin, although this has not been confirmed. Carnivora is a commercially available liquid that is extracted from the plant. Proponents claim that Carnivora has immune stimulant and anticancer properties. Some even claim that Carnivora applied directly to some skin cancer lesions could substitute for radiation therapy and chemotherapy. One practitioner claims that Carnivora can cause the total reversal of skin and other forms of cancer. Supporters also claim that Carnivora is effective for treating colitis, Crohn's disease, rheumatoid arthritis, multiple sclerosis, neurodermatitis, chronic fatigue syndrome, HIV, and certain types of herpes. There is no scientific evidence to support any of these claims.

USE: Proponents suggest that full-strength or diluted Carnivora can be placed under the tongue or mixed with water to make a drink. Carnivora can also be injected into the skin, inhaled through a vaporizer, or applied directly to the skin. There is no standardized dosage for the drug. One practitioner gives patients 30 drops of Carnivora mixed with water or tea 5 times per day or applies the extract directly to skin lesions. Carnivora contains 30% alcohol.

EFFECTS: There is no scientific evidence to support any of the claims made for Carnivora. It is also not clear whether plumbagin is actually the active ingredient in the Venus flytrap plant. Most of the studies that have been done were conducted by the doctor who patented the drug, and who also has a large financial stake in a clinic that administers the drug and in the manufacturing company.

An animal study conducted in India to study the effects of plumbagin from the Indian medicinal plant *Plumbago rosea* combined with radiation therapy was inconclusive. A second animal study in India found that plumbagin demonstrated a small degree of antitumor activity. The results of several other studies from India were positive but inconclusive. A laboratory study in Japan indicated that plumbagin had some effect against intestinal tumors. Further studies are necessary to determine if these animal and laboratory study results apply to humans.

Carnivora does not appear to be toxic, but not enough is known about the active ingredients for scientists to ensure that it is safe. Reported side effects from Carnivora injections include nausea and vomiting. Relying on this treatment alone, and avoiding conventional medical care, may have serious health consequences.

VITAE ELIXXIR

OTHER COMMON NAME(S): None

Vitae Elixxir is an herbal and mineral mixture that is promoted as a treatment for arthritis, multiple sclerosis, lymphomas, leukemias, and multiple myeloma. There is no scientific evidence to support these claims. The ingredients of the formula are not well documented, and people have reported that it has an unpleasant taste. It is taken orally by drops mixed with food and drink. Proponents also recommend mixing Vitae Elixxir with DMSO to make a footbath for people with advanced cancer who cannot tolerate taking the preparation orally; however, it has not been proven to be effective (see DMSO).

VITAMIN A

OTHER COMMON NAME(S): None

Vitamin A has not been proven to be effective in preventing cancer in humans. Clinical studies are currently being done to examine the role of vitamin A and other retinoids (molecules that are similar to vitamin A but different in structure and origin) in cancer prevention and treatment. High doses of vitamin A are toxic, and long-term use of high-dose supplements may increase the risk of lung cancer among people at high risk, such as smokers.

DESCRIPTION: Vitamin A is obtained in the diet from animal sources and is also derived from beta carotene in plant foods (see Beta Carotene). Beta carotene is converted to vitamin A in the small intestine and stored in the liver until needed by the body. Vitamin A and closely related molecules are also known as retinoids. Vitamin A is essential for normal growth, bone development, reproduction, vision, the maintenance of healthy skin and mucous membranes (which line the nose and mouth), and protection against infections in the respiratory, digestive, and urinary tracts. It enters the body directly as vitamin A from animal products and indirectly as beta carotene from many fruits and vegetables.

Some research suggests that vitamin A and some other retinoids have the ability to modify cancer cells and prevent normal cells from becoming cancerous. This is currently under investigation. Some proponents say that vitamin A supplements prevent cancer; however, most scientific studies do not support this claim.

USE: Vitamin A is a fat-soluble vitamin, which means that it is absorbed from dietary fats in the intestine and stored in the liver until needed by the body. It does not need to be consumed every day. The best way to get this vitamin is to eat a well-balanced diet. People who eat a balanced diet of fruits, vegetables, dairy products, and animal fats usually obtain enough vitamin A, although supplements are available. The recommended daily allowance of vitamin A is 4000 IU (2.4 mg) per day for women and 5000 IU (3 mg) per day for men.

EFFECTS: Studies on vitamin A have produced mixed results, and there have been no consistent findings showing a decreased risk of cancer due to vitamin A in the diet. The use of vitamin A supplements has also not been proven to be effective in reducing cancer risk in humans. It appears that the combination of antioxidants in fruits, vegetables, legumes, and grains, rather than individual vitamins, is more likely to be beneficial (see Phytochemicals).

Some laboratory, animal, and human studies have found that certain retinoids may also inhibit cancer development. Retinoids have shown significant activity in the reversal of certain cancers; however, further clinical research is needed. Several large clinical trials involving retinoids are currently being conducted. Retinoids are not currently used as a cancer therapy, except for a rare type of leukemia, promyelocytic leukemia, which often responds to a combination of retinoic acid (a retinoid) and chemotherapy.

High doses of vitamin A supplements can cause nausea, tiredness, headaches, itchiness, scaling of the skin, diarrhea, and loss of appetite. High doses of vitamin A supplements should be avoided because they can cause bone pain, hair loss, irregular menstruation in women, birth defects if taken during pregnancy, as well as temporary or permanent liver damage. In one study, researchers found that supplements did not benefit the patients studied and may have increased the incidence of lung cancer and cardiovascular disease in cigarette smokers and asbestos workers. A deficiency of vitamin A, which is rare in developed countries, can cause a lowered resistance to infection, poor night vision or even blindness, poor growth in children, weak bones and teeth, inflamed eyes, diarrhea, and poor appetite.

▌ VITAMIN B COMPLEX

OTHER COMMON NAME(S): B Vitamins, Vitamin B_1, Vitamin B_2, Vitamin B_3, Vitamin B_5, Vitamin B_6, Vitamin B_7, Vitamin B_9, Vitamin B_{12}

There is not enough scientific evidence to determine what amount of B vitamins are needed to reduce the risk of cancer or other diseases. Vitamin B_9 may have some protective effect against colon cancer, but more studies are needed (see Folic Acid). There is no evidence that B vitamins are an effective treatment for people who already have cancer.

DESCRIPTION: B vitamins are essential nutrients for growth, development, and a variety of other bodily functions. They play a major role in the activities of enzymes (proteins) that regulate chemical reactions in the body. B vitamins are found in a variety of plant and animal food sources. Some alternative medical practitioners claim that deficiencies in B vitamins weaken the immune system and make the body vulnerable to cancer. They recommend high doses of B vitamins as treatments for people with cancer. Current scientific evidence has not found any effect of B vitamin supplements on the growth and spread of cancer. Many scientific studies in progress are studying the relationships between vitamin intake and the risk of developing certain cancers.

USE: Nutritionists maintain that a balanced diet that includes plenty of fresh fruits and vegetables is sufficient to provide the body with all the

B vitamins it needs. Only small amounts of these vitamins are needed to fulfill the recommended daily allowance (RDA). The RDA of vitamin B₉ (folic acid) is 400 micrograms (µg) a day. The National Academy of Science recommends that adults aged 50 and older receive B vitamin supplements, or foods enriched with these vitamins, in order to prevent deficiency, which is common in this age group.

Supplements that contain several of the B vitamins, usually in combination with other nutrients, are sold in grocery stores, in health food stores, and over the Internet in pill form. Doses vary by manufacturer.

EFFECTS: There is some evidence showing that increased intake of vitamin B₉ (folic acid) may lower colorectal cancer risk, but the evidence is not conclusive. The study also reported that vitamin B₆ may reduce elevated levels of homocysteine (an amino acid) in the blood. Decreased levels of homocysteine have been linked with decreased risk of heart disease; however, other studies have not shown a positive benefit from B₆ in relation to vascular and heart disease. Some studies have also shown a possible link between intake of certain B vitamins and cancers of the breast and prostate. While these results are preliminary and not conclusive, they deserve further study. It is still unclear what intake levels are needed to reduce the risk of these diseases or whether an increase in B vitamin intake will produce any positive effect.

Supplements containing B vitamins are generally considered safe but should not be taken in large doses. Some possible side effects include gouty arthritis, hyperglycemia, and skin problems. Overdoses can also lead to heart and liver problems. High doses of folic acid supplements can interfere with at least one chemotherapy drug, methotrexate.

Women who are pregnant and breast-feeding require more folic acid than others. All women of childbearing age may be urged by their doctors to increase their intake of folic acid to help prevent certain birth defects in their children.

B vitamin deficiency can cause anemia, tiredness, loss of appetite, abdominal pain, depression, numbness and tingling in the arms and legs, muscle cramps, respiratory infections, hair loss, eczema, poor growth in children, and birth defects in the fetuses of pregnant women.

▧ VITAMIN C

OTHER COMMON NAME(S): None

Many studies have shown a connection between eating foods rich in vitamin

C, such as fruits and vegetables, and a reduced risk of cancer. Studies of supplement use and cancer have found mixed results that make it difficult to determine the role of supplements and their effect on cancer risk. High doses of vitamin C can cause a number of side effects.

DESCRIPTION: Vitamin C is an essential vitamin the human body needs to function well. It is water-soluble, which means that the body uses what it needs and eliminates the rest, and it must be obtained from the diet. Vitamin C is found in abundance in citrus fruits, such as oranges, grapefruit, and lemons, and in green leafy vegetables, potatoes, strawberries, bell peppers, and cantaloupe.

Vitamin C is an antioxidant, a compound that blocks the action of activated oxygen molecules known as free radicals, which can damage cells. Vitamin C is thought by some to enhance the immune system by stimulating the activities of natural killer cells (a type of white blood cell) and anticancer agents. Some claim that the vitamin can prevent a variety of cancers from developing. It is also said to prevent tumors from spreading, help the body heal after cancer surgery, enhance the effects of certain anticancer drugs, and reduce the toxic effects of other drugs used in chemotherapy. These claims are currently under investigation. It is also unclear whether consuming vitamin C supplements can reduce cancer risk.

Vitamin C may help control high blood pressure according to a recent study. Some practitioners recommend high doses of vitamin C supplements to protect against and treat colds, although this has not been proven.

USE: The recommended daily allowance of vitamin C for women is 75 mg per day and for men is 90 mg per day, although some experts argue that it should be increased to 100 to 200 mg per day. The upper limit from both food and supplements is 2000 mg per day. Vitamin C supplements are available in powder or chewable pill form at grocery stores, health food stores, and drug stores and over the Internet. Recommended dosages vary by manufacturer.

EFFECTS: Many scientific studies of the protective effects of vitamin C have shown that consuming a diet high in fruits and vegetables (containing vitamin C), rather than supplements, significantly reduces the risk of developing certain cancers. More recent research of vitamin C supplements has not shown the same strong protective effects against formation of cancer. Apparently, vitamin C is most beneficial when consumed naturally in fruits and vegetables because of the other active ingredients in the food.

Some scientists believe that taking high doses of antioxidant vitamins may actually interfere with the effectiveness of radiation and some chemotherapy drugs. No studies have yet been done in humans to test this theory. A recent review suggests that a combination of antioxidant vitamin supplements together with diet and lifestyle changes may actually improve the effectiveness of standard and experimental cancer therapies. More research is needed to evaluate the effects.

The vitamin C supplements are generally considered safe unless dosages are higher than 2000 mg per day. Dosages over this amount can cause headaches, diarrhea, nausea, heartburn, stomach cramps, and possibly kidney stones. Many doctors routinely recommend that people with cancer avoid gram-size doses of vitamin C during treatment. People with cancer should consult their doctors before taking vitamin C or other vitamin supplements.

◤ VITAMIN E

OTHER COMMON NAME(S): None

There is some evidence of the protective effects of vitamin E against prostate and colorectal cancer; however, more research is needed to confirm its role. There is no evidence that vitamin E significantly affects the growth of cancers that have already formed. High doses of vitamin E supplements can cause undesirable side effects.

DESCRIPTION: Vitamin E is an essential nutrient that the human body needs to function normally, help build normal cells, and form red blood cells. The main sources of vitamin E in the diet are vegetable oils (especially safflower oil, sunflower oil, and cottonseed oil), green leafy vegetables, nuts, cereals, meats, egg yolks, wheat germ, and whole-wheat products. It is an antioxidant, a compound that blocks the action of activated oxygen molecules known as free radicals, which can damage cells. Some proponents claim vitamin E plays a role in protecting the body against cancer by bolstering the immune system. Some doctors believe the vitamin can also increase the effectiveness of some drugs used in chemotherapy and reduce some of the side effects of radiation therapy. In contrast, others believe high doses of vitamin E might interfere with the effectiveness of radiation therapy and chemotherapy. These claims are currently under investigation.

The claim that vitamin E supplements protect against heart attacks is still being examined. There are also unsupported claims that vitamin

E eases the inflammation associated with arthritis, speeds the healing of wounds in people who have suffered burns or have had surgery, and slows the progress of Parkinson's and Alzheimer's disease.

USE: A balanced diet normally provides adequate amounts of vitamin E for the body's needs, especially a diet low in fat, high in green leafy vegetables, and high in fiber from grains and cereals. The recommended daily allowance (RDA) of vitamin E for adults is 15 mg per day from food. The upper limit of intake from supplements is 1000 mg per day. Supplements are not usually necessary unless the body has a deficiency of vitamin E, which can lead to a destruction of red blood cells and result in anemia, with symptoms such as tiredness and shortness of breath.

EFFECTS: A large, well-controlled human study found no beneficial effect of increased doses of vitamin E supplements on lung cancer incidence and found mixed results for other cancers. The study did find lower rates of prostate and colorectal cancer among those who received vitamin E but higher rates of bladder, stomach, and other cancers. A review of research reported some protective effects of vitamin E against prostate and colon cancer; however, there have been methodological problems in measuring the association of supplement use and cancer risk. For example, one study found people who take supplements are more likely to exercise regularly, eat 4 or more servings of fruits and vegetables per day, and eat a low-fat diet.

There is not enough evidence to support claims that taking high doses of antioxidants can prevent chronic diseases. Some scientists believe that taking high doses of antioxidant vitamins may actually interfere with the effectiveness of radiation and some chemotherapy drugs. No studies have yet been done in humans to test this theory. Vitamin E supplements found in multivitamins are generally considered safe as long as the levels are consistent with the RDA. Excessive doses of vitamin E supplements taken over a long time can cause nausea, vomiting, stomach pain, and diarrhea. High doses of supplements may also slow the way the body absorbs vitamins A, D, and K and result in deficiencies of these vitamins. Megadoses of vitamin E supplements are not advised for people who are taking blood-thinning drugs, such as warfarin, because the supplements might counteract the effects of the drugs. People with cancer should consult their doctor before taking vitamin E or other vitamin supplements.

▚ VITAMIN K

OTHER COMMON NAME(S): Vitamin K$_1$, Vitamin K$_2$, Vitamin K$_3$

Vitamin K is necessary for normal blood clotting. The human body obtains vitamin K from certain foods and bacteria that normally live in the intestines. There is no scientific evidence supporting the use of vitamin K supplements in cancer treatment or prevention.

DESCRIPTION: Vitamin K is an essential nutrient that the liver needs to promote blood clotting and prevent abnormal bleeding. There are 3 forms of vitamin K: vitamin K$_1$ (phylloquinone or phytonadione), vitamin K$_2$ (menaquinone), and vitamin K$_3$ (menadione). Some alternative medical practitioners claim that vitamin K$_3$ is an anticancer agent. Others claim that high doses of both vitamin C and vitamin K$_3$ supplements can inhibit tumor growth when taken together; however, this has not been scientifically proven.

USE: Most people get all the vitamin K they need from natural sources. The recommended daily allowance is 60 micrograms (µg) per day for women and 80 µg per day for men. Dietary sources of vitamin K, such as green leafy vegetables, cereals, and dairy products, provide the body with about half of the normal supply of the vitamin, while intestinal bacteria produce the rest (in the form of vitamin K$_2$).

Only those who have symptoms of a vitamin K deficiency may need to take supplements (in the form of vitamin K$_3$, a potent synthetic form). Newborns are usually given vitamin K supplements, either by injection or by mouth, while in the hospital. Babies who received the supplements in the hospital do not need supplements after they leave.

Vitamin K is also promoted for topical use in some cosmetic or herbal creams to lighten the redness from broken capillaries and to treat skin irritation (burns and sunburns) and scarring. Applications are usually recommended for several weeks.

EFFECTS: There is overwhelming scientific evidence that vitamin K is necessary for blood clotting. Because newborn infants lack the bacteria in their intestines to produce vitamin K and are at risk of uncontrolled bleeding, injections are commonly given at birth. Studies published in the early 1990s suggested a link between childhood cancer (ie, acute lymphoblastic leukemia) and injections of vitamin K supplements in newborn babies; however, most supplement studies have not found any association between vitamin K injections and childhood cancer.

There have been some studies examining whether vitamin K₃ can help overcome resistance to certain types of chemotherapy drugs. Results in animal and cell cultures are mixed, but there is no evidence of any significant effects in humans yet. There is no evidence that vitamin K₃ is an active anticancer agent in human patients when used alone. More research is needed on vitamin K₃ and related compounds to determine if they may have any positive effects for people with cancer.

Natural vitamin K is considered safe as a normal part of a daily diet. Supplements of the vitamin are not usually needed unless recommended by a doctor. Research showing a possible link between the development of leukemia in children who were given injections of vitamin K supplements shortly after birth has led to a recommendation that newborns be given only oral supplements. The effectiveness of this method has not been proven and is not currently licensed.

▨ WILD YAM

OTHER COMMON NAME(S): Wild Mexican Yam, Chinese Yam, Colic Root, Rheumatism Root

Although creams containing wild yam extracts are becoming popular among women as an alternative to hormone replacement therapy (HRT), there is no scientific evidence that they are safe or effective. Neither estrogen nor progesterone are found in wild yams.

DESCRIPTION: Although wild yam is native to North America, the Mexican and the Chinese yam are the 2 types of yams promoted for therapeutic use. The roots and other underground parts of wild yams are used in herbal remedies. These plants are different from yams and sweet potatoes sold as food.

Proponents claim that a cream made from the wild Mexican yam contains natural progesterone (a hormone that plays a vital role in women's health) and is therefore effective in treating premenstrual and menopausal symptoms. They say that using the cream as an alternative to HRT will significantly lower the risk of breast and endometrial cancer, although there is no scientific evidence to support this claim. Cream marketers also claim that their product helps women lose weight, increases energy and stamina, and enhances sex drive.

Supporters claim that the wild Mexican Yam, when taken internally, eases arthritis pain, the symptoms of morning sickness, painful menstruation, bronchitis, asthma, whooping cough, and cramps and relieves gastrointestinal ailments such as Crohn's disease, colitis, and chronic diarrhea.

The Chinese yam is claimed to stimulate appetite and to be a remedy for chronic diarrhea, asthma, uncontrollable or frequent urination, diabetes, and emotional instability. Used externally, proponents claim the Chinese yam can speed the healing of boils and abscesses. Herbalists also use it to treat colic (see Homeopathy).

USE: Wild yam creams are rubbed directly onto the skin and are available from health food stores. In homeopathic medicine, the wild yam from the *Dioscorea villosa* plant is used fresh or dried and put in liquid extracts. The Chinese yam can also be used fresh or baked with flour or clay. Wild yam cream and wild Mexican yam capsules are available in herbal shops and over the Internet. Doses vary by manufacturer.

EFFECTS: Contrary to claims, the wild Mexican yam cannot supply the body with progesterone. The plant contains the chemical diosgenin, which can be converted into progesterone through a lengthy process in the laboratory. The body cannot convert diosgenin into progesterone itself. Some of the chemicals in the plant resemble estrogen, another hormone that is important in female physiology, but their effects on the body are very different from those of progesterone. There are drugs manufactured from diosgenin that are used to treat asthma, arthritis, and eczema and to control fertility.

There is no scientific evidence showing that the wild yam has any effect on the symptoms of menopause or premenstrual syndrome.

Large doses of wild yam may cause nausea, vomiting, and diarrhea. This treatment should not be used as a replacement for HRT. Women who are pregnant or breast-feeding should not use wild yam products.

▌ WORMWOOD

OTHER COMMON NAME(S): Absinthe, Absinthium

There is no scientific evidence that wormwood is effective in treating the side effects of conventional cancer treatment or any other conditions. The plant contains a volatile oil with a high level of thujone, the active component of wormwood oil, which can cause convulsions (see Thuja). In fact, it may be considered harmful when taken internally because there are reports that it can cause serious problems to the liver, as well as neurological symptoms, such as convulsions, numbness of legs and arms, loss of intellect, delirium, and paralysis.

DESCRIPTION: Wormwood is a shrubby perennial plant whose upper shoots and leaves are used in herbal remedies. It is native to Europe, northern Africa, and western Asia. It is promoted as a sedative and anti-inflammatory. There are also claims that it can treat loss of appetite, stomach disorders, and liver and gallbladder complaints. In folk medicine, it is used for a wide range of stomach disorders, fever, and irregular menstruation. It is also used to destroy intestinal worms. Externally, it is applied to poorly healing wounds, ulcers, skin blotches, and insect bites. It is also used in Moxibustion treatments for cancer (see Moxibustion). There is no scientific evidence to support these claims.

USE: Wormwood combinations are taken in small doses for a short time. It is taken in liquid form either in water (tincture) or as a tea preparation, as well as in capsules. Wormwood is also applied externally. Although pure wormwood is not available, "thujone-free" wormwood extract has been approved by the Food and Drug Administration for use in foods and as flavoring in alcoholic beverages such as vermouth.

EFFECTS: No studies have shown any evidence to support the use of wormwood for the treatment of cancer or the side effects of conventional cancer treatment. There is also not enough evidence to support the numerous other indications for which wormwood is recommended. *Artemisia annua*, a related herb known as sweet wormwood, and some of its derivatives have been shown to be effective in the treatment of malaria. In fact, drugs derived from artemisinin, the active ingredient in sweet wormwood, may be registered soon in Europe for the treatment of malaria.

Due to the thujone content, taking large doses of wormwood internally can lead to vomiting, stomach and intestinal cramps, headaches, dizziness, and disturbances of the central nervous system. High doses of wormwood can also lead to liver failure. It may also lower the seizure threshold and offset the beneficial effects from known anticonvulsants such as phenobarbital.

The ingestion of thujone, the active ingredient in oil of wormwood and absinthe, can lead to *absinthism*, a syndrome of hallucinations, sleeplessness, tremors, convulsions, and paralysis associated with long-term use of the liqueur absinthe. This herb should be avoided, especially by women who are pregnant or breast-feeding.

YOHIMBINE

OTHER COMMON NAME(S): Yohimbe, Yohimbe Bark, Yohimbine

Hydrochloride, Actibine®, Aphrodyne®, Yocon®, Yohimex®, Yomax®

Yohimbe bark has been used as an aphrodisiac (sexual stimulant) for many years, and yohimbine has recently been studied as a potential treatment for erectile dysfunction (male impotence). Clinical trials of yohimbine have found contradictory results regarding its effectiveness. Yohimbe bark has been declared an unsafe herb in Germany because of such complications as increased heart rate and blood pressure and even kidney failure.

DESCRIPTION: Yohimbe is an evergreen tree that grows in the jungles of Africa. It can reach a height of 90 feet. The dried bark is used in herbal remedies. Yohimbine hydrochloride is the most important component of yohimbe bark, and it is available as a Food and Drug Administration (FDA)-approved drug for the treatment of impotence. The evidence about its effectiveness is mixed. Yohimbine has also been promoted to treat exhaustion, overdose from clonidine, and a form of low blood pressure that occurs when standing.

USE: Yohimbine is available in tablets, capsules, and liquid extracts. The drug yohimbine hydrochloride is regulated by the FDA for the treatment of impotence and is available only as a prescription. The standard recommended dosage is 5.4 mg taken 3 times per day for not more than 10 weeks.

In contrast, the yohimbe bark extracts and yohimbine sold in health food stores and on the Internet contain varying amounts of yohimbine and other ingredients. The US Department of Agriculture lists the yohimbine bark used in herbal remedies as an unsafe herb. Yohimbe bark is on the Commission E (Germany's regulatory agency for herbs) list of unapproved herbs. This means that it is not recommended for use because it has not been proven to be safe or effective.

EFFECTS: Clinical trials have found contradictory results regarding the effectiveness of yohimbine for treating impotence. A review of clinical research found that yohimbine is a reasonable option for the treatment of certain types of impotence and that the benefits of the drug seem to outweigh its risks. Additionally, the American Urological Association guidelines on treatment of organic erectile dysfunction state that evidence clearly shows that yohimbine is better than a placebo (an inactive substance or treatment). No studies have been done to compare yohimbine to other treatments for impotence. It is apparent that more research needs to be done to clarify the role of yohimbine in the treatment of impotence. Some studies were done using the drug yohimbine hydrochloride, and extracted chemicals are not the same as the raw plant. Study results of extracts will not necessarily be consistent with studies using the raw plant.

Yohimbine and yohimbe bark may increase heart rate and raise blood pressure at dosages from 20 to 30 mg per day. Yohimbine has been associated with psychotic episodes. Other side effects include difficulty breathing, chest pain and palpitations, anxiety, queasiness, insomnia, and vomiting. The less common side effects that do not usually require medical attention include dizziness, headache, flushing, nausea, nervousness, sweating, and tremors.

People with high blood pressure, heart, kidney or liver disease or who take antidepressants should avoid the drug. Yohimbine should not be used by elderly people or women who are pregnant or breast-feeding.

▌ ZINC

OTHER COMMON NAME(S): Zinc Gluconate, Zinc Sulfate

Some studies have found that zinc supplements may help reduce cancer risk in animals, but this has not been proven in humans. Research has found a correlation between increased risk of some cancers and low zinc levels in the diet; however, no controlled clinical trials have been done to show the effectiveness of zinc supplements in cancer prevention or treatment. High doses of zinc can lead to some serious side effects.

DESCRIPTION: Zinc is a trace mineral found in the diet that plays a key role in many bodily processes, including the building of DNA and RNA, energy production, cell metabolism, and regulation of the immune system.

Some people claim zinc protects against certain types of cancer, reduces the size of enlarged prostate glands, strengthens the immune system, decreases asthma and allergy symptoms, speeds wound healing, and strengthens the skin. Some also claim that zinc is an antioxidant, a compound that blocks the action of activated oxygen molecules known as free radicals, which can damage cells. There is no scientific evidence to support these claims.

There are also claims that zinc reduces the severity and duration of the common cold. There is some evidence suggesting that this may be true.

Use: Zinc is obtained through a number of dietary sources, such as lean meat, seafood, soybeans, nuts, pumpkin and sunflower seeds, eggs, cheese, and wheat bran. The recommended daily allowance of zinc is 15 mg per day for most adults and 30 mg per day for pregnant women. Zinc gluconate lozenges are available in most drug stores and pharmacies. Zinc spray or ointment is sometimes applied to wounds to accelerate healing.

Effects: Some researchers have focused on examining zinc levels in the body associated with cancer and other diseases. A few studies found that zinc levels in serum and/or inside white blood cells were frequently lower in patients with head and neck cancer or childhood leukemia. Low zinc levels were also linked to increased size of head or neck tumors, more advanced stage of disease, and a greater number of unplanned hospitalizations. A well-controlled human study in Italy involving patients with head and neck cancer found that zinc sulfate tablets reversed the loss of taste caused by radiation therapy. The results suggest that zinc sulfate supplements could become an important component in the supportive care of these patients.

Another study found a connection between zinc intake (from both food and supplements) and a lower risk of melanoma (the most serious form of skin cancer) and precancerous lesions of the mouth. Protective effects have also been associated with zinc supplements and prostate cancer risk; however, there is no clinical evidence to support the use of zinc supplements to affect the growth or spread of cancer.

In a review of 8 recent clinical trials, researchers concluded that zinc gluconate reduces the duration and severity of the common cold. Another study found that zinc gluconate lozenges were not effective in treating cold symptoms in children and adolescents, and that further study is needed to determine what, if any, role zinc plays in affecting cold symptoms.

An overdose of zinc can lead to a weakened immune system, vomiting, headache, and fatigue. Very high exposure to zinc (which occurs in some industries) may contribute to the development of prostate cancer.

CHAPTER FOUR

DIET AND NUTRITION METHODS

THIS CATEGORY INCLUDES DIETARY approaches and special nutritional programs related to prevention and treatment of disease.

◣ ACIDOPHILUS

OTHER COMMON NAME(S): Lactic Acid Bacteria

There have been no studies with humans on the role of the bacterium Lactobacillus acidophilus *(commonly called acidophilus) in preventing or treating human cancers. Animal studies on acidophilus reducing the occurrence of cancer have shown varying results.*

DESCRIPTION: Acidophilus is a type of bacterium commonly found in the normal gastrointestinal (GI) tract of mammals, mainly in the small intestine. It is also found in many dairy products, especially yogurt. It may be recommended to prevent or treat uncomplicated diarrhea and vaginal infections, lower cholesterol, promote lactose digestion in lactose-sensitive people, and help prevent disease-causing bacteria and yeast from growing.

Acidophilus is promoted to help lower the incidence of cancer by reducing the carcinogens in the diet and by directly killing tumor cells. Other anticancer claims include a reduction in the cholesterol levels that tumor cells need to grow and the production of B vitamins and vitamin K, which are believed to help the immune system fight off cancer (see Vitamin B Complex and Vitamin K). There is no scientific evidence to support these claims.

USE: When taking acidophilus, the dose usually refers to the number of live bacteria. Most sources suggest 1 to 10 billion bacteria as a recommended dose. This amount is available in tablets, capsules, and powder form. Average dosage suggestions vary from 1 to 3 times per day; however, some scientists warn that concentrations of the bacteria in supplemental form vary widely from one manufacturer to another. Yogurt with "live cultures" and milk supplemented with *L. acidophilus* bacteria are another source.

EFFECTS: Studies on the ability of the bacterium *L. acidophilus* to prevent cancer from occurring have been contradictory. In recent animal studies, animals with diets supplemented with *L. acidophilus* were less susceptible to DNA damage in the colon after treatment with known carcinogens, indicating that the bacterium may prevent the occurrence of colon cancer; however, other studies have shown that diets with *L. acidophilus* had no effect on the formation of breast or skin cancers. In either case, controlled human studies have not been done. Further studies are necessary to determine if these animal study results apply to humans.

L. acidophilus has also been investigated in the laboratory as possessing direct antitumor properties. In 2 separate studies using human breast and colon cancer cells grown in the laboratory, milk that was fermented by acidophilus bacteria was able to slow or prevent the growth of cancer cells. Neither animal nor human studies have been reported on the effects of *L. acidophilus* on established tumors in the body. More research is needed to determine what role, if any, *L. acidophilus* may play in cancer treatment and prevention.

In rare cases, acidophilus can cause serious infections that are difficult to treat with antibiotics. People with compromised immune systems, such as those with AIDS, should use acidophilus with caution. The lack of standardization makes it difficult to determine the quality of acidophilus products. Because acidophilus must contain live cultures to be considered effective, proper packaging and storage are essential. Many of these products do not contain adequate levels of the active organisms or may contain other bacteria that are not beneficial.

◾ AMINO ACIDS

OTHER COMMON NAME(S): None

Amino acids are necessary for human growth and development; however, their effects on cancer are not well studied and not completely known. Some amino acid supplements may interfere with the effectiveness of the chemotherapy drug asparaginase.

DESCRIPTION: Amino acids are a group of 20 different chemical compounds that are the basic building blocks of all the proteins in the human body. Proteins are needed for human growth and development. Twelve of the amino acids, called nonessential amino acids, can be produced in the human body by metabolism of other substances. Eight of the amino acids, called essential amino acids, cannot be produced by the human body and must be obtained from dietary sources. The claims for amino acids in regard to cancer are complex and somewhat confusing. Some alternative medicine practitioners maintain that restricting dietary intake of certain amino acids, such as phenylalanine and tyrosine, may stop tumor growth. At the same time, they claim that while dietary restriction of the amino acids methionine and arginine may inhibit the growth of some cancers, supplements of these amino acids and 2 others, tryptophan and glutamine, may stimulate the growth of other cancers.

Some claim the amino acid cysteine may protect people with cancer from the toxic effects of certain chemotherapy drugs, including cyclophosphamide and doxorubicin. Others say the amino acid glutathione may inhibit the development and progression of cancer and protect patients from the damaging side effects of radiation therapy and certain chemotherapy drugs, such as fluorouracil and cisplatin. There is no clinical evidence to support these claims.

USE: Foods high in protein, especially meat and seafood, are excellent sources of amino acids. Once protein is ingested, the human digestive system breaks it down to amino acids, absorbs the amino acids, and then uses the acids to build new proteins.

Amino acid supplements are also available. Some proponents suggest they be taken on an empty stomach with fruit juice to help the body absorb the amino acids.

EFFECTS: The scientific evidence for the various effects of amino acids on cancer is based mostly on limited animal and laboratory studies that have not been confirmed in human studies. The conflicting evidence from these studies makes it difficult to draw definitive conclusions about the effects of amino acids on cancer.

A more recent controlled human study found that glutamine supplements given to 7 patients with advanced esophageal cancer helped maintain their levels of glutamine and preserved their lymphocyte count for a short time. Lymphocytes are a type of white blood cell that help the body fight infection. Other studies are needed.

Amino acids ingested in foods are safe and necessary for human growth and development. Conflicting evidence suggests both possible beneficial and harmful effects from amino acid supplements on the development, progression, and treatment of cancer. There have been reports that amino acid supplements may interfere with the effectiveness of the chemotherapy drug asparaginase. Supplements are not recommended unless advised by a doctor.

BROCCOLI

OTHER COMMON NAME(S): None

Broccoli contains certain chemicals that may reduce the risk of colorectal cancer, although it is not clear which individual compounds are responsible for the protective effects. The best evidence suggests that eating a wide variety of vegetables reduces cancer risk.

DESCRIPTION: Broccoli is a cruciferous vegetable that belongs to the cabbage and mustard families, which also include arugula, cauliflower, collards, bok choy, kale, mustard greens, radishes, turnips, watercress, rutabaga, and Brussels sprouts. It is considered one of the best sources of nutrients because it is rich in vitamin C, beta carotene, fiber, calcium, and folate (see Beta Carotene, Folic Acid, and Vitamin C). It is the source of many phytochemicals, which are thought to stimulate the production of anticancer enzymes and chemicals (see Phytochemicals). Eating a wide variety of plant-based foods is the best way to get the necessary components.

USE: Broccoli can be eaten raw, boiled, or steamed. It can be purchased fresh or frozen in most grocery and organic food stores. Broccoli retains the most nutrients when eaten raw. Cooking reduces some of the benefits of broccoli because the heating process seems to destroy some beneficial anticancer compounds.

EFFECTS: Recent investigations have shown that the frequent consumption of cruciferous vegetables is associated with a decreased risk for cancer. One population-based study found that high levels of the carotenoid lutein (obtained from vegetables such as broccoli, spinach, and lettuce) were associated with fewer cancers of the colon. Another study revealed that eating cruciferous vegetables seemed to reduce bladder cancer risk, while other vegetables and fruits did not appear to have the same benefit; however, more research is needed.

Researchers have suggested that sulforaphane, present in the broccoli sprouts before the vegetable matures, may be the primary cancer-prevention agent. A study showed that cancer development was reduced by 60% to 80% in laboratory animals that were fed sulforaphane. The compound is thought to prompt the body into manufacturing an enzyme that prevents tumor formation.

The effects of broccoli on the growth of specific cancers have also been studied. For example, scientists have found that a chemical component of broccoli, indole-3-carbinol, inhibited the growth of cultured breast cancer cells in a laboratory study. Further studies are necessary to determine if these animal and laboratory study results apply to humans.

Scientists caution that as promising as broccoli may be for preventing cancer, the results of studies cannot be considered in isolation. Strong evidence suggests that people who eat 5 or more servings of fruits and vegetables a day can cut their risk of cancer from 20% to 50% when compared to those who consume 1 serving or less. The chemical composition of cruciferous vegetables is complex, which makes it difficult to determine which compound or combination of compounds may provide protection against cancer. A balanced diet that includes 5 or more servings a day of fruits and vegetables along with foods from a variety of other plant sources is more effective than eating one particular food in large amounts.

Since it is a food high in fiber, eating large amounts of it may cause gas. High-fiber foods should be reduced or avoided in people with diarrhea and some other colon problems.

▧ CASSAVA

OTHER COMMON NAME(S): Cassava Plant, Tapioca, Tapioca Plant, Manioc

There is no scientific evidence that cassava or tapioca is effective in preventing or treating cancer; however, a theory to explain how an enzyme in the cassava plant may possibly treat cancer has been proposed. This approach has not been scientifically tested.

DESCRIPTION: The cassava plant is a staple crop in Africa, Asia, and South America. Tapioca is a starch found in the roots of the plant. Different parts of the plant, such as the root, leaves, and sometimes the whole plant, are used in herbal remedies.

Some researchers have found that through the breakdown of a chemical called linamarin, cassava plants produce hydrogen cyanide. They believe if linamarase (the enzyme that breaks down linamarin to release hydrogen cyanide) could be selectively introduced into cancer cells, it could kill cancer cells by producing cyanide as it does in the cassava plant. Since normal cells cannot convert linamarin into cyanide, only the cancer cells would be killed by this gene therapy, according to this theory.

In folk medicine, the cassava plant is promoted for the treatment of abscesses, snakebites, boils, diarrhea, dysentery, flu, hernia, inflammation, conjunctivitis, sores, and several other problems including cancer and tumors. There is no evidence to support these claims.

USE: In herbal remedies, the roots of the cassava are made into a poultice and applied directly to the skin to alleviate sores. The leaf, root, and flour obtained from the plant can also be used in a wash that is applied to the skin. Tapioca starch made from the cassava plant is used as an oral hydration agent (to help restore body fluids) in developing countries. Tapioca starch or the chemical linamarin are not currently used in the prevention or treatment of cancer.

The parts of cassava used for food are the tubers, which are usually eaten raw, boiled, or fried. A form of flour is also made from the cassava plant. In Western countries, tapioca (a granular sweet pudding made from cassava starch) is usually found in baby foods and eaten as a dessert.

EFFECTS: There is no scientific evidence to support the claims made for the cassava plant. Many scientists around the world are currently developing gene therapy methods for introducing DNA selectively into the tumor cells of cancer patients. More research is needed to determine if the approach using linamarin and linamarase to kill cancer cells is feasible or beneficial for people with cancer.

The cassava plant produces cyanide when it is damaged or improperly harvested for food. It is a serious potential health hazard if not handled correctly. The breakdown of linamarin by linamarase releases hydrogen cyanide, which can be deadly to humans. Some of the signs of cyanide poisoning are headache, vertigo, agitation, confusion, coma, and convulsions. Some people in developing countries have been poisoned by eating parts of the cassava plant that were not harvested or prepared properly. Cyanide poisoning can lead to death.

▨ CORIOLUS VERSICOLOR

OTHER COMMON NAME(S): Turkey Tail, PSK

There is some scientific evidence from clinical trials that suggests a compound found in Coriolus versicolor *called polysaccharide K (PSK) may provide benefit to people with cancer, including increased survival rates and longer disease-free periods, without causing significant side effects.*

DESCRIPTION: *Coriolus versicolor* is a mushroom used in traditional Asian herbal remedies (see Chinese Herbal Medicine). A protein-bound polysaccharide *K* (PSK) from the mushroom is being studied as a possible cancer treatment. (A polysaccharide is a starch-like carbohydrate formed by a large number of sugar molecules.) Proponents claim that PSK, the primary active ingredient in *Coriolus versicolor*, has strong anticancer properties—perhaps equal to the effects of some conventional chemotherapy drugs. Supporters also contend that PSK has antimicrobial and antiviral properties, which stimulate cells in the blood that destroy invading microorganisms. PSK is also believed to be a strong antioxidant, a compound that blocks the action of activated oxygen molecules known as free radicals, which can damage cells. There is some clinical evidence that PSK may be helpful when used in addition to conventional treatments.

Herbalists claim *Coriolus versicolor* and its extracts can be used to stimulate the immune system. The mushroom is also promoted in traditional Asian medicine to treat cancer. There is no evidence that the mushroom itself is effective.

USE: *Coriolus versicolor* can be taken in capsules, as an extract, or as a tea. The dosage ranges from 1000 to 9000 mg per day, depending on the patient's condition. *Coriolus versicolor* can be obtained in herbal medicine shops and through the Internet.

EFFECTS: No human studies with the *Coriolus versicolor* have been reported in peer-reviewed journals; however, there have been many studies assessing the usefulness of PSK, and not the mushroom. Various studies have found that people with colorectal, stomach, and breast cancer benefited from PSK. A review of 8 controlled human studies found that people who received PSK, along with chemotherapy or radiation therapy, generally experienced longer disease-free periods and increased survival rates compared with patients who underwent only chemotherapy or radiation therapy. It was also noted that 2 of the 3 studies found that PSK contributed to significantly better survival times for people with cancer of the esophagus.

No serious risks are associated with the use of PSK. Side effects that occur infrequently include nausea, vomiting, and diarrhea. Even less common are skin pigmentation, anorexia, anemia, liver dysfunction, leukopenia (abnormally low white blood cell count), and thrombocytopenia (abnormally low level of platelets in the blood).

▮ ELLAGIC ACID

OTHER COMMON NAME(S): None

Research in animal and laboratory models has found that ellagic acid inhibits the growth of tumors caused by certain carcinogens. Studies in humans are underway to determine the effect of long-term daily consumption of raspberries on cell activity in the human colon.

DESCRIPTION: Ellagic acid is a compound found in raspberries, strawberries, cranberries, walnuts, pecans, pomegranates, and other plant foods. Ellagic acid has been found to cause apoptosis (cell death) in cancer cells in the laboratory. How it works is not yet well understood. Some also claim it prevents the binding of carcinogens to DNA and strengthens connective tissue, which may keep cancer cells from spreading. Ellagic acid has also been said to reduce heart disease, birth defects, and liver fibrosis and to promote wound healing. Many of these claims are currently under investigation.

USE: The highest levels of ellagic acid are found in raspberries, strawberries, and pomegranates, especially when they are freeze-dried. Red raspberry leaves, which also contain ellagic acid, are available in capsule, powder, or liquid form. The correct dosages of these preparations are not known.

EFFECTS: Ellagic acid has been demonstrated in animal models to inhibit tumor growth caused by carcinogens. Other studies have also found positive effects. A recent animal study found that ellagic acid protected mice against chromosome damage from radiation therapy. A separate study of ellagic acid indicated that it was effective at inhibiting tumor growth from esophageal cancer cells in mice. Further studies are necessary to determine if these animal study results apply to humans.

A balanced diet that includes 5 or more servings a day of fruits and vegetables along with foods from a variety of other plant sources, such as breads, cereals, grain products, rice, pasta, and beans, is more effective than eating one particular food, such as raspberries, in large amounts.

Ellagic acid is not available in supplement form; however, the raspberry leaf, or preparations made from it, should be used with caution during pregnancy because they may initiate labor.

◾ FASTING

OTHER COMMON NAME(S): None

Instead of being beneficial to health, even a short-term fast can produce negative effects. Fasting over a longer period could cause serious health problems.

DESCRIPTION: Fasting involves not consuming any foods and drinking only water or juice for 2 to 5 days (or longer). Sometimes, tea or broth may be part of the fasting process. Metabolic practitioners believe the body contains many toxins and harmful substances that can be removed by fasting or detoxifying the body (see Metabolic Therapy). They claim that fasting allows the body to focus energy on cleansing and healing itself. According to these practitioners, fasting allows the immune system to work more efficiently, more oxygen and white blood cells to flow through the body, more fat to be burned, energy to increase, and other healing functions to improve. They also believe that total body toxicity is reduced because the body decreases the intake of new toxins and eliminates stored toxins in the body.

Diseases and conditions that have been treated by fasting include acne, allergies, arthritis, asthma, cancer, digestive disorders, fever, headaches, glaucoma, heart disease, hypertension, inflammatory diseases, noncancerous tumors, pain, polyps, and ulcers. Fasting is also promoted to rejuvenate the body, help maintain normal body weight, increase longevity and sex drive, and improve mental clarity, self-awareness, and self-esteem. It is also said to be helpful in quitting or cutting back on use of tobacco, alcohol, caffeine, or nonprescription drugs. Some practitioners claim it can heighten spiritual awareness and compassion for the poor. There is no scientific evidence to support any of these claims.

USE: Short fasts, lasting from 2 to 5 days, are done at home. Other than drinking only water or juice, fasting involves a lot of rest periods. Sometimes, an enema is recommended as part of the regimen (see Colon Therapy), as is sun exposure. Longer fasts require professional supervision and take place at a spa, resort, or similar facility.

EFFECTS: There is no medical basis for using fasting as a treatment for any disease or condition. In fact, researchers find that the body cannot distinguish between fasting and starvation. Studies related to cancer suggest that fasting could actually lead to the promotion of tumors.

A brief fast (eg, 8 to 12 hours) is often advised by medical professionals in preparation for certain diagnostic tests. In this case, the fast helps to produce more accurate test results. Fasting may also be necessary for a period following surgery, especially if digestive system organs are involved. As for maintaining proper weight, experts recommend restricting calories instead of fasting.

Even proponents acknowledge that fasting can produce immediate negative effects, such as headaches, dizziness, fatigue, nausea, body odor, and an unpleasant taste in the mouth. Fasting interferes with the immune system and vital bodily functions and can damage vital organs, such as the liver and kidneys, and other organs. Women who are pregnant or breast-feeding should not fast.

▓ GARLIC

OTHER COMMON NAME(S): Garlic Clove, Garlic Powder, Garlic Oil, Allium

The health benefits of the allium compounds contained in garlic and other vegetables in the onion family have been widely publicized. Garlic is currently under study for its ability to reduce cancer risk, but there is insufficient evidence to support a specific role for this vegetable in cancer prevention. It also has the potential to interfere with anesthesia.

DESCRIPTION: Garlic is a member of the lily family and is closely related to onions, leeks, and chives. Extracts and oils made from garlic are sometimes used as herbal remedies. It is promoted for use as a preventive measure against the formation of cancer. Although several compounds in garlic may have anticancer properties, the allyl sulfur compounds are said to play a major role. There have been claims that garlic has certain immune-boosting properties that may help the body fight off diseases, such as colds or the flu, as well as reduce cancer cell growth. These claims are currently under investigation.

Proponents claim garlic also can be used to treat fungal infections, bacterial infections, hyperglycemia, and roundworms. They also say it has medicinal properties that may help stomach and abdominal problems. The use of garlic has also been claimed to reduce the risk of heart disease, lower serum cholesterol, and reduce blood pressure. There is no scientific evidence to support these claims.

USE: There is considerable debate as to how the form and amount of garlic used might influence health. Proponents disagree as to whether garlic is more beneficial when eaten raw or cooked, or if the garlic extracts, powders, and oils that are available in tablet form are more or less effective.

Garlic is on the Commission E (Germany's regulatory agency for herbs) list of approved herbs, and they suggest a dosage of fresh garlic equal to 4 g per day, or about 1 large clove per day. It is sold as a supplement in health food stores, in drug stores, and over the Internet.

EFFECTS: It is difficult to link the exact role of a particular food in the cancer process. It is even more difficult when the food in question is typically used in small amounts, as is garlic. A balanced diet that includes 5 or more servings a day of fruits and vegetables along with foods from a variety of other plant sources is more effective than eating a particular food in large amounts.

Several studies from around the world have found that people who consumed higher levels of garlic had a lower risk of certain types of cancers. Laboratory studies on mice suggest that certain compounds in garlic may be of benefit in reducing tumor growth or possibly killing tumor cells. Controlled studies in humans are needed to make definitive conclusions about the role of garlic in cancer prevention. Research is also needed to identify the specific compounds in garlic that may be of benefit in cancer prevention.

Consumption of large amounts of garlic may lead to irritation of the gastrointestinal tract, causing stomach pain, gas, and vomiting. One study suggests that the use of garlic may increase the risk of bleeding due to its anti–blood-clotting properties. It should not be used by people who are undergoing surgery, especially if given blood thinners or if postoperative bleeding is of concern. People taking blood-thinning medication, such as warfarin, should consult with their doctor before taking garlic supplements.

GERSON THERAPY

OTHER COMMON NAME(S): Gerson Diet, Gerson Method, Gerson Treatment, Gerson Program

There is no scientific evidence that Gerson therapy is effective in treating cancer. Gerson therapy can be harmful to the body. Coffee enemas have been associated with serious infections, dehydration, constipation, colitis (inflammation of the colon), electrolyte (salt and mineral) imbalances, and even death (see Colon Therapy).

DESCRIPTION: Gerson therapy involves coffee enemas and a special diet with supplements claimed to cleanse the body and stimulate metabolism. Gerson therapy is considered a metabolic therapy and is based on the theory that disease is caused by the body's accumulation of toxic substances (see Metabolic Therapy). According to practitioners, people with cancer have an excess amount of sodium, far outweighing the potassium in their bodies. Food processing and cooking also add more sodium, eventually causing cancer. The fruit and vegetable diet (part of Gerson therapy) is used to correct this imbalance and revitalize the liver so that it can begin to rid the body of malignant cells. Coffee enemas are claimed to eliminate dead cancer cells (detoxification) and relieve pain. There is no scientific evidence to support these claims.

USE: Gerson therapy requires following a strict diet that involves eating a low-salt, low-fat, vegetarian diet and drinking juice from approximately 20 pounds of freshly crushed fruits and vegetables. In addition, patients are given 3 or 4 coffee enemas a day. Various other supplemental substances, such as pepsin, potassium, niacin, pancreatin (a digestive enzyme), and thyroid extracts, are ingested to stimulate various organ functions, particularly the liver and thyroid. Sometimes other treatments such as laetrile, hydrogen peroxide, hyperbaric oxygen therapy, and shark cartilage are also recommended (see Lactrile, Hydrogen Peroxide Therapy, Hyperbaric Oxygen Therapy, Shark Cartilage). The Gerson Institute does not own or operate any medical facilities; however, it refers patients to clinics they license.

EFFECTS: There have been no well-controlled studies to support the beliefs and practices of the Gerson therapy. The Gerson Research Organization conducted a retrospective review and reported that survival rates were higher for patients with melanoma, colorectal, and ovarian cancers who participated in the Gerson program compared to those who did not at another institution.

According to a critique in a major peer-reviewed journal, the explanation for how the method is supposed to work does not follow the established scientific principles of basic nutrition, biology, and cancer immunology.

There are a number of significant problems that may develop from the use of this therapy. Serious illness and death have occurred from some of the components of the treatment, such as the coffee enemas that lead to electrolyte imbalances. Continued home use of enemas may cause the colon's normal function to weaken, worsening constipation problems and colitis. Enemas should be given only under medical guidance. Some metabolic diets used in combination with enemas cause dehydration. Serious infections may result from poorly administered liver extracts. Thyroid supplements may cause severe bleeding in patients with liver metastases. This method may be especially hazardous to women who are pregnant or breast-feeding. Relying on this treatment alone, and avoiding conventional medical care, may have serious health consequences.

◣ GRAPES

OTHER COMMON NAME(S): The Grape Diet, The Grape Cure, Grape Seed Extract, Grape Skins

There is no scientific evidence that a grape diet is effective for treating cancer or any other disease. Some evidence suggests that a chemical in grape seed extract may help to promote antioxidant activity and that the skins of red grapes may help prevent cardiovascular disease and cancer; however, more research is needed to confirm these assertions.

DESCRIPTION: Grapes grow wild on vines or are cultivated. They are believed to be native to northwest Asia, although they are currently grown throughout Europe and the United States. The seeds, skin, leaves, stems, and grape itself are used in herbal remedies. Some chemicals found in grape extracts or grape skins are currently being studied for possible uses in the prevention and treatment of cancer and other diseases.

Proponents claim that the chemicals found in grape seed extract called proanthocyanidins contain powerful antioxidants. Some claim that these antioxidants inhibit the development of some types of cancer, protect against heart disease, and are useful for treating a variety of medical conditions. The compound found in the skins of red grapes called resveratrol is being studied to see how it affects the development and progression of heart disease and cancer.

Alternative practitioners recommend the use of grapes and parts of the grape plant internally for high blood pressure, menopause, varicose veins, high cholesterol, rashes, and urination problems. They also claim that it works for inflammation of the gums, throat, eyes, and mouth. There is no scientific evidence to support these claims.

Although now rarely promoted, the grape diet was used as a treatment to flush toxins from the body and protect the body against cancer and virtually all other diseases. Some supporters believed that the diet cured cancer.

USE: Fresh, preserved, and dried grapes are used in the form of liquid extracts, tinctures, gargles, enemas, douches, and compresses. Grape skins are used to make wine. Grape seed extract and resveratrol are available in tablets and capsule supplements. The doses vary depending on the manufacturer. The grape diet begins with a period of fasting and eating only grapes for 1 or 2 weeks, followed by stages of consuming certain foods and following dietary restrictions.

EFFECTS: While grape extracts may hold some positive benefit for people with cancer, there is no scientific evidence that eating grapes or following the grape diet can cure cancer or any other disease. Although studies have shown potential benefits of certain chemicals in grapes, such as the antioxidant activity in grape seed extract and possible inhibition of cardiovascular disease and cancer from resveratrol, more controlled human studies are needed to make definite conclusions.

An exclusive grape diet is unhealthy and does not supply the body with adequate amounts of protein and important nutrients. A balanced diet that includes 5 or more servings a day of fruits and vegetables along with foods from a variety of other plant sources is more effective than eating one particular food in large amounts. Grape seed extract is believed to be safe, but additional research is needed.

The amount of resveratrol in red wine varies greatly, and increased consumption of wine to increase resveratrol intake poses certain health risks. Alcohol is associated with increased risks of cancers of the mouth, esophagus, pharynx, larynx, and liver in both men and women and of breast cancer in women. Cancer risk also increases with the amount of alcohol consumed; however, the cardiovascular benefits of moderate drinking may outweigh the risk of cancer in men aged 50 and older and in women aged 60 and older.

▌ INOSITOL HEXAPHOSPHATE

OTHER COMMON NAME(S): IP6, Inositol, Phytic Acid, Phytate

Animal and laboratory research has found that inositol hexaphosphate (IP6) may be effective in decreasing tumor incidence and growth. Clinical trials are needed to determine the anticancer effects in humans.

DESCRIPTION: Inositol hexaphosphate (IP6) is a chemical found in beans, brown rice, corn, sesame seeds, wheat bran, and other high-fiber foods. It aids in the metabolism of insulin and calcium, hair growth, bone marrow cell metabolism, and eye membrane development and helps the liver transfer fat to other parts of the body.

Proponents call IP6 a "natural cancer fighter" and claim the chemical inhibits or reverses the growth of various forms of cancers, including breast, colon, and prostate cancers. It is thought to be an antioxidant, a compound that blocks the action of activated oxygen molecules known as free radicals, which can damage cells. Some believe that IP6 slows abnormal cell division and can sometimes transform tumor cells into normal cells. Supporters also claim that it effectively prevents kidney stones, high cholesterol, heart disease, and liver disease. These theories have not been scientifically tested in humans.

USE: Many high-fiber food sources contain IP6, and it is also available as a supplement. Scientists do not know enough about the chemical to recommend a standardized dosage. The supplemental pill form is found in a formula that combines inositol and IP6. It is not known if taking a supplement provides the same effect as when eaten from food sources.

EFFECTS: All of the evidence regarding the anticancer effects of IP6 has come from laboratory and animal studies. A recent study found that dietary myo-inositol (a derivative of IP6) significantly reduced the growth of lung cancer in mice. One recent review of 2 tumor model studies concluded that IP6 has the potential to play a role in the treatment of cancer and high cholesterol. Further studies are necessary to determine if these animal and laboratory study results apply to humans.

Inositol hexaphosphate and its derivatives have also been studied for treatment of panic disorders, autism, obsessive-compulsive disorders, Alzheimer's disease, post-traumatic stress disorders, and depression, but researchers have reached no firm conclusions regarding its impact on any of these conditions.

When taken in moderate amounts, IP6 appears to be safe, although no studies have been conducted to determine its safety. Experts advise individuals who wish to increase their intake of IP6 to incorporate inositol-rich foods into their diets before resorting to supplements. Women who are pregnant or breast-feeding should not use IP6.

JUICING

OTHER COMMON NAME(S): Juice Therapy

Juicing involves extracting juices from fresh fruit and uncooked vegetables as a primary part of the diet. Juice extractors grind food into small pieces, which are spun to extract juice from the pulp. It is promoted as a way to prevent and treat a wide variety of conditions by enhancing the immune system. According to practitioners, "unnatural" dietary habits cause imbalances in the body's cell composition, which are corrected and rebalanced with the nutrients that the juice delivers. Proponents claim that juicing can reverse everything from the natural aging process to chronic diseases such as cancer. This treatment method is frequently used to sustain the body during long fasts or as part of the Gerson regimen (see Gerson Therapy).

Juicing can cause severe diarrhea, which is thought to be "cleansing" because toxins are supposedly removed from the body during this process. There is no scientific evidence that extracted juices are healthier than whole foods. Juice extractors remove the fiber-containing pulp from the fruits and vegetables, so it is important to maintain a diet that includes an adequate amount of fiber.

KOMBUCHA TEA

OTHER COMMON NAME(S): Manchurian Tea, Kargasok Tea

There is no scientific evidence that Kombucha tea is effective in treating cancer or any other disease. No data exist showing that it helps promote good health or prevents any ailments. There have been some serious side effects reported with the consumption of Kombucha tea.

DESCRIPTION: Kombucha tea is made from the flat, pancake-like culture known as the Kombucha mushroom. It is actually not a mushroom but is called one because of its appearance. The culture or mushroom sac used in Kombucha tea consists of several species of yeast and bacteria. Kombucha tea is promoted as a cure-all for a wide variety of conditions, including baldness, insomnia, intestinal disorders, arthritis, chronic fatigue syndrome, multiple sclerosis, AIDS, and cancer. Supporters assert that the tea can boost the immune system and reverse the aging process. Kombucha tea is said to contain antioxidants, compounds that block the action of activated oxygen molecules known as free radicals, which can damage cells. For people with cancer, proponents claim the tea can detoxify (cleanse) the body and enhance the immune system, thereby improving the body's defenses, especially in the early stages of cancer. After the body is cleansed, the tea is said to help repair and balance the body and fight off disease. There is no scientific evidence to support these claims.

USE: Kombucha tea is made by steeping the mushroom culture in tea and sugar for about a week. During this process, the original mushroom floats in the tea and produces a "baby" mushroom on its surface. These new mushrooms can be passed along to other people for starting their own cultures or be kept to make new batches of the tea when the original mushroom goes bad (turns dark brown).

To increase the detoxifying abilities of the tea, people are told to remove chemicals from their diets and eat only fresh fruits and vegetables. They are also told to avoid caffeine, soft drinks, alcohol, hormone-fed meat, fertilized or sprayed foods, preservatives, and artificial coloring and flavoring and to quit smoking.

Kombucha mushroom cultures can be obtained from commercial manufacturers in the United States; however, many people have obtained Kombucha mushrooms from friends because they are easily passed along.

EFFECTS: There is no scientific evidence to support any of the claims made for Kombucha tea. There have been reports of some serious complications associated with the tea because it is highly acidic. Drinking excessive amounts of the tea is not recommended. Deaths have been reported from acidosis linked with the tea, and the Food and Drug Administration has warned consumers to use caution when making and drinking the tea. Several experts warn that since home-brewing facilities vary significantly, the tea could become contaminated with harmful bacteria that could be especially detrimental to people with HIV or other immune disorders. Because the acid in the tea could absorb harmful toxins, it should not be brewed in ceramic, lead crystal, or painted containers. Since the potential health risks of Kombucha tea are unknown, anyone with a preexisting medical condition should consult a doctor before consuming the tea. Women who are pregnant or breast-feeding should not use this tea.

■ LYCOPENE

OTHER COMMON NAME(S): None

People who have diets rich in tomatoes, which contain lycopene, appear to have a lower risk of certain types of cancer. Further research is needed to determine what role, if any, lycopene has in the prevention or treatment of cancer. It is currently thought that the preventive effect of diets high in fruits and vegetables cannot be explained by just one single component in the diet.

DESCRIPTION: Lycopene is the compound that gives tomatoes and certain other fruits and vegetables their color. Proponents claim that lycopene may lower cholesterol and the risk of heart disease, enhance the body's defenses, and protect enzymes, DNA, and cellular lipids. A major claim for lycopene's benefits is in the treatment of cancers of the lung, prostate, stomach, bladder, cervix, and skin. These claims are currently under investigation.

Some researchers believe lycopene may be valuable in the prevention and growth of cancers of the prostate, lung, and stomach. These scientists believe lycopene to be a powerful antioxidant, a compound that blocks the action of activated oxygen molecules known as free radicals, which can damage cells. The antioxidant activity of lycopene is at least twice as great as beta carotene (see Beta Carotene).

USE: Tomatoes are the best source of lycopene, although apricots, guava, watermelon, papaya, and pink grapefruit are also significant sources. Initial studies have suggested that cooked tomatoes (ie, tomato sauce or paste) are a better source of available lycopene than raw tomato juice because the heating action allows the body to quickly absorb the lycopene. Lycopene can also be taken in the form of soft-gel capsule supplements. Doses vary according to manufacturer.

EFFECTS: Since interest in lycopene is relatively recent, there have only been a few experimental studies on the role of lycopene in preventing or treating cancer. Several animal studies found that lycopene treatment reduced the growth of brain and breast tumors, as well as cancer cells. Further studies are necessary to determine if these animal study results apply to humans.

Research does suggest that diets rich in tomatoes may account for a reduction in the risk of several different types of cancer, particularly lung, stomach, and prostate gland cancer. There may also be a protective benefit against cancers of the cervix, breast, oral cavity, pancreas, colorectum, and esophagus. Population studies from many countries have shown that the risk of developing some cancers are lower in people who either have diets high in tomato products or have higher levels of lycopene in their blood. Other compounds in tomatoes or those diets high in tomato products, either acting alone or with lycopene, may be responsible for the protective effects currently associated with lycopene.

Eating a balanced diet that includes 5 or more servings a day of fruits and vegetables along with foods from a variety of other plant sources is more effective than eating one particular food in large amounts. The potential side effects of lycopene supplements are not known.

◾ MACROBIOTIC DIET

OTHER COMMON NAME(S): Macrobiotics

There is no scientific evidence that a macrobiotic diet is effective in treating cancer. It can lower fat intake and increase fiber, so it can provide general health benefits associated with low-fat/high-fiber diets. Macrobiotic diets can lead to poor nutrition if not properly planned. Some earlier versions of the diet may actually pose a danger to health. Research is underway to determine whether a macrobiotic diet may play a role in preventing cancer.

DESCRIPTION: A macrobiotic diet is generally vegetarian and consists largely of whole grains, cereals, and cooked vegetables. Proponents of the macrobiotic diet claim that it can prevent and cure disease, including cancer, and enhance spiritual and physical well-being. A macrobiotic diet is considered a comprehensive way of life, rather than just a diet.

USE: A macrobiotic diet combines elements of Buddhism with dietary principles based on simplicity and avoidance of "toxins" that come from eating dairy products, meats, and oily foods. Older versions of the macrobiotic diet were quite restrictive. One variation allowed only the consumption of whole grains.

A specific macrobiotic diet prescription is determined by a person's age, sex, level of physical activity, and native climate. The standard macrobiotic diet of today consists of 50% to 60% organically grown whole grains, 20% to 25% locally and organically grown fruits and vegetables, and 5% to 10% soups made with vegetables, seaweed, grains, beans, and miso (a fermented soy product). Other elements may include occasional helpings of fresh whitemeat fish, nuts, seeds, pickles, Asian condiments, and nonstimulating and nonaromatic teas. In some cases, the consumption of animal products, certain vegetables, tropical fruits, and other products such as eggs, coffee, and sugar is discouraged.

Macrobiotic principles also prescribe specific ways of cooking food using pots, pans, and utensils made only from certain materials. People who practice the diet do not usually cook with microwaves or electricity, nor do they consume vitamin or mineral supplements or heavily processed foods. The food is chewed until it is fluid to help with digestion. Since food is thought to be sacred, it is prepared in a peaceful setting.

EFFECTS: There have been no controlled human studies to show the macrobiotic diet can be used to prevent or cure cancer. Diets that consist primarily of plant products that are low in fat and high in fiber are believed to reduce the risk of cardiovascular disease and some forms of cancer. One review concluded that dietary macro- and micronutrients play an important role in estrogen metabolism. This may have an impact on hormone-related cancers.

Strict macrobiotic diets that include no animal products may result in nutritional deficiencies, such as inadequate intake of protein, vitamin D, zinc, calcium, iron, and vitamin B_{12} (see Calcium, Vitamin B Complex, Vitamin D, and Zinc). The danger may be magnified for people with cancer who often have increased nutritional and caloric requirements. Relying on this type of treatment alone, and avoiding conventional medical care, may have serious health consequences.

One of the earlier macrobiotic diets, which calls for eating 100% grains, has been associated with severe nutritional deficiencies and even death. Children may be particularly vulnerable to nutritional deficiencies resulting from a macrobiotic diet. Women who are pregnant or breast-feeding should not use this diet.

▧ MAITAKE MUSHROOM

OTHER COMMON NAME(S): Maitake, Maitake Extract, Maitake D-Fraction®

Research has shown that a maitake extract (maitake D-fraction) has some immune system effects in animal and laboratory studies. There is no scientific evidence that the maitake mushroom is effective in treating or preventing cancer in humans.

DESCRIPTION: Maitake is an edible mushroom from the species *Grifola frondosa*. Maitake D-fraction is an extract of the mushroom marketed as a food supplement in the United States and Japan. D-fraction is a polysaccharide that is found in several mushrooms used in Asian medicine. A polysaccharide is a large and complex molecule made up of smaller sugar molecules. Promoters claim that maitake mushroom extract boosts the human immune system and limits or reverses tumor growth. It is also thought to enhance the benefits of chemotherapy and lessen some side effects of anticancer drugs, such as hair loss, pain, and nausea. There is no scientific evidence to support these claims.

USE: Maitake D-fraction is one of the only medicinal mushroom extracts said to be effective when taken orally. It is available in liquid, tablet, and capsule form in health food stores. Maitake mushrooms are available in grocery stores.

EFFECTS: There is little research on maitake mushrooms or the extract (maitake D-fraction). Most of the research on maitake D-fraction has been done in Japan in mice and laboratory studies using an injectable form of the extract. Researchers have found that maitake D-fraction extract enhanced the immune system and inhibited the spread of tumors in mice that had been implanted with breast and liver cancer. Further studies are necessary to determine if these animal and laboratory study results apply to humans. Human studies are underway in Japan and the United States to determine the extract's effects on breast and prostate cancer. More studies are needed to determine maitake's potential usefulness in preventing or treating cancer.

The mushroom itself has been used in cooking and herbal medicine without harm for centuries. So far, studies have not shown any adverse effects from maitake D-fraction, but human studies have not yet been completed.

▌ METABOLIC THERAPY

OTHER COMMON NAME(S): Kelley's Treatment, Gerson Therapy, Gonzalez Treatment, Issels' Whole Body Therapy

There is no scientific evidence that metabolic therapy is effective in treating cancer or any other disease. Some aspects of metabolic therapy may be harmful.

DESCRIPTION: Metabolic therapy uses a combination of special diets and nutritional supplements in an attempt to remove "toxins" from the body and strengthen the body's defenses against disease. Metabolic therapists believe toxic substances in food and the environment create chemical imbalances that lead to diseases such as cancer, arthritis, and multiple sclerosis. They say that metabolic therapy eliminates these toxins and strengthens the body's resistance to invading microorganisms. Some practitioners claim that a special diet can cure serious diseases, including cancer. Others claim that by evaluating a patient's metabolism they can diagnose cancer before symptoms appear, locate tumors, and assess a tumor's size and growth rate. There is no scientific evidence to support these claims.

USE: Metabolic therapy varies a great deal depending on the practitioner, but all are based on special diets that usually emphasize fruits, vegetables, vitamins, and mineral supplements. Other components may include coffee enemas, enzyme supplements, visualization, and stress-reduction exercises (see Colon Therapy, Enzyme Therapy, and Imagery). At least 1 metabolic therapy system also includes the drug laetrile (see Laetrile).

Among the better-known types of metabolic therapy are Gerson therapy, Kelley's treatment, the Gonzalez treatment, and Issels' whole body therapy (see Gerson therapy). The focus is on detoxifying the body and bringing it into balance, as well as strengthening the body's natural defenses. Some metabolic therapies may also involve additional alternative treatments, such as biological dentistry, or complementary treatments, such as psychotherapy.

EFFECTS: There is general agreement that there are differences in the metabolism of cells in people with cancer compared to people without cancer; however, there is no evidence published in peer-reviewed medical journals that supports the claims made for metabolic therapy or any of its components. The treatment has not been shown to have any positive effects for patients with serious diseases.

Some aspects of metabolic therapy may, in fact, be harmful. There are reports of complications related to liver cell injections and diets that contained too little salt. Several deaths have been directly linked to injecting live cells from animals (see Cell Therapy). Also, a number of deaths have been linked to coffee enemas. The drug laetrile may cause nausea, vomiting, headache, dizziness, and even cyanide poisoning, which can be fatal. Care should be taken to make sure that any diet containing raw meat or raw meat juice is free from bacterial contamination. Women who are pregnant or breast-feeding should not use this method. Relying on this type of treatment alone, and avoiding conventional medical care, may have serious health consequences.

▨ MODIFIED CITRUS PECTIN

OTHER COMMON NAME(S): MCP, Citrus Pectin, Pecta-Sol®

Animal studies have found that modified citrus pectin (MCP) inhibits the spread of prostate cancer and melanoma to other organs; however, there have been no clinical studies done to determine whether MCP has the same effect in humans.

DESCRIPTION: Modified citrus pectin (MCP) is a form of pectin that has been altered so that it can be more easily absorbed by the digestive tract. Pectin is a carbohydrate found in most plants and is particularly plentiful in fruits such as apples, grapefruits, and plums. Proponents claim that MCP slows or stops the growth of metastatic prostate cancer (prostate cancer that has spread) and melanoma, a dangerous form of skin cancer. Some also claim that a compound found in MCP strengthens the cancer cell-killing ability of T cells (cells that also protect against viruses).

USE: Modified citrus pectin is available in capsules or a powder. The dosage suggested by manufacturers for the powder is 5 g mixed with water or juice taken 3 times per day with meals. For capsules, the suggested dosage is 800 mg taken 3 times per day with meals.

EFFECTS: One animal study found that MCP inhibits the spread of prostate cancer in rats. The rats with prostate cancer received MCP orally and were found to have a much lower risk of the tumor spreading to the lungs. A second study examined the effects of MCP on lung metastases from melanoma cells. Researchers found that they developed significantly fewer metastatic lung tumors than mice that didn't receive the drug. The results from these 2 studies appear to show that MCP makes it difficult for cancer cells that break off from the main tumor to join together and form colonies in other organs in the very early stages of development. Further studies are necessary to determine if these animal and laboratory study results apply to humans.

Modified citrus pectin is generally considered safe by the Food and Drug Administration. Side effects rarely occur; however, people who are allergic or sensitive to MCP may experience stomach discomfort after taking it.

◾ NONI PLANT

OTHER COMMON NAME(S): Noni Fruit, Noni Juice, Indian Mulberry, Morinda, Hog Apple, Meng Koedoe, Mora De La India, Ruibarbo Caribe, Wild Pine

There is no scientific evidence that the noni plant or noni products are effective in preventing or treating cancer or any other disease. Although animal and laboratory studies have shown some positive effects, there have been no studies done in humans. Research is underway to study various compounds found in the noni plant to determine if they produce useful effects on body tissues.

DESCRIPTION: The noni or morinda plant is an evergreen tree that grows 10 to 20 feet tall in open coastal regions and in forests with altitudes up to 1300 feet. It is commonly found in Tahiti and other Pacific Islands, as well as in parts of Asia and Australia. The juice and whole fruit are used in herbal remedies. Proponents claim that the noni fruit and its juice can be used to treat cancer, diabetes, heart disease, cholesterol, high blood pressure, HIV, rheumatism, psoriasis, allergies, infection, and inflammation and a wide range of other conditions. In India, proponents use noni as a remedy for asthma and dysentery. Some noni juice distributors also promote it as a general tonic, stress reliever, facial and body cleanser, and a dietary and nutritional aid. There is no scientific evidence to support these claims.

USE: Parts of the noni plant are used as a juice, a tonic, a poultice, and in tea. Tea made from leaves of the plant is used as a remedy for tuberculosis, arthritis, rheumatism, and anti-aging. The leaves and bark are sometimes made into a liquid tonic for urinary complaints and muscle or joint pain. The juice, which has an unpleasant taste and odor, is used on the scalp as a treatment for head lice. Unripe noni fruit is mashed together with salt and applied on cuts and broken bones. Ripe fruit is used as a poultice for facial blemishes or as a remedy for skin sores, boils, or infections. Noni products are sold in various forms, including juice, extract, powder, capsules (nutritional supplements and diet aids), facial cleansers, bath gels, and soaps.

EFFECTS: A group of Hawaiian researchers investigated noni juice in the treatment of mice with tumors. Mice who received the treatment survived 123% longer than the untreated mice. Another team of investigators reported that a compound removed from the root of the noni plant may inhibit a chemical process that turns normal cells into cancer cells. Other scientists studying an extract from the roots of the plant found that the substance appeared to prevent pain and induce sleep in mice. Further studies are necessary to determine if these animal and laboratory study results apply to humans. More research is needed before it can be determined what role, if any, noni plant compounds may play in the treatment of cancer or any other health condition.

A balanced diet that includes 5 or more servings a day of fruits and vegetables along with foods from a variety of other plant sources is more effective than consuming one particular food or juice in large amounts. The safety and long-term effects of noni juice and other noni products are not known. Relying on this type of treatment alone, and avoiding conventional medical care, may have serious health consequences.

■ OMEGA-3 FATTY ACIDS

OTHER COMMON NAME(S): None

Studies in animals have found that fish fats rich in omega-3 fatty acids suppress cancer formation. There is no direct evidence that they have similar protective effects in humans.

DESCRIPTION: Omega-3 fatty acids are important nutrients involved in many human biological processes. The body cannot make these chemicals and must obtain them from dietary sources or from supplements. Some clinicians believe that omega-3 fatty acids protect against the spread of solid-tumor cancers that are related to hormone production, particularly breast cancer, and that they inhibit the growth of colon, pancreatic, and prostate cancers. Omega-3s may reduce cachexia, the physical wasting and malnourishment that can occur during later stages of some cancers.

USE: Diet is the best source of omega-3 fatty acids. Oils from some cold-water fish have high concentrations of omega-3s. Oil from flaxseed contains more alpha-linolenic acid (one of the 3 omega-3 fatty acids) than any other known plant source (see Flaxseed Oil). Other plant sources of omega-3 fatty acids include different kinds of beans.

Omega-3 supplements, such as salmon oil, are available at pharmacies and natural food stores. Some nutritionists recommend eating a diet rich in fish containing omega-3 fatty acids, eating 1 to 2 teaspoons of flaxseed or flaxseed oil daily, or taking daily supplements containing 1 to 2 g of omega-3s. Omega-3 fatty acids are unstable and spoil easily, so food manufacturers often remove them from foods to increase shelf life.

EFFECTS: Although some research supports the anticancer claims made for omega-3 fatty acids, far more investigation is needed before researchers reach any conclusions. The relationship between omega-3 fatty acids and cancer or other diseases is not known.

The evidence from the few human studies published in peer-reviewed medical journals is mixed. For example, one study suggested that one of the omega-3 fatty acids limited the recurrence of colon cancer, while another study indicated that clinical findings didn't prove that fish oil containing omega-3 fatty acids prevented cancer or its recurrence. In societies that consume a lot of fish, researchers have noticed links between high intake of omega-3s and lower rates of breast cancer; however, other laboratory evidence shows that the balance between 2 different types of omega fatty acid levels plays a role in the formation of breast cancer. Eating a balanced diet that includes 5 or more servings a day of fruits and vegetables along with foods from a variety of other plant sources is more effective than consuming one particular type of food in large amounts.

Not enough is known about omega-3 fatty acids to determine if they are safe in large quantities or in the presence of other drugs. Omega-3s may increase total blood cholesterol and inhibit blood clotting. People who take anticoagulant drugs or aspirin should not consume additional amounts of omega-3 due to the risk of excessive bleeding. The source of omega-3 fatty acids also may be a health concern. Because of pollution, many fish caught in the wild contain toxins absorbed from pollution. Experts recommend varying the type of fish eaten to reduce the chances of ingesting poisonous substances, such as mercury. Farm-raised fish tend to carry fewer toxins than fish in the wild.

Supplements may cause fishy breath odor, belching, or abdominal bloating. They may also increase a tendency toward anemia in menstruating women. Women who are pregnant or breast-feeding should consult their doctor before adding extra omega-3 to their diets.

▌ SELECTED VEGETABLE SOUP

OTHER COMMON NAME(S): SV, Sun Soup

Selected vegetable soup (SV) is promoted as a treatment for cancer. It is a freeze-dried brown powder that contains a specific selection of vegetables and herbs, including soybean, mushroom (shiitake), red date, scallion, garlic, lentil bean, leek, mung bean, hawthorn fruit, onion, American ginseng, angelica root, licorice, dandelion root, senegal root, ginger, olive, sesame seed, and parsley (see Garlic, Ginger, Ginseng, Licorice, Shiitake Mushroom, and Soybean). A recent controlled human study found daily consumption of SV, along with conventional cancer treatment, to be nontoxic and associated with improvement in weight maintenance and survival of patients with advanced non-small cell lung cancer. The study involved a small sample size (eg, 12 patients). More research is needed to determine the effectiveness of SV.

▌ SHIITAKE MUSHROOM

OTHER COMMON NAME(S): Japanese Mushroom

Animal studies have found antitumor, cholesterol-lowering, and virus-inhibiting effects of the active compounds in shiitake mushrooms. Clinical studies are needed to determine if these effects can be beneficial for people with cancer and other diseases.

DESCRIPTION: A shiitake mushroom is an edible fungus native to Asia and grown in forests. Shiitake mushrooms are the second most commonly cultivated edible mushrooms in the world. Extracts from the mushroom, and sometimes the whole mushroom itself, are used in herbal remedies. Shiitake mushrooms are promoted to fight the development and progression of cancer and AIDS by boosting the body's immune system. These mushrooms are also said to help prevent heart disease by lowering cholesterol levels in the blood and treating infections by producing interferon (a group of natural proteins that inhibits viruses from multiplying). Promoters claim that eating the whole mushroom (cap and stem) may have therapeutic value, but they do not say how much must be eaten to have an effect. They say the content and activity of the compounds depend on how the mushroom is prepared and consumed.

A compound contained in shiitake mushrooms, lentinan, is believed to stop or slow tumor growth. Another component, called activated hexose-containing compound, is also said to reduce tumor activity and lessen the side effects of cancer treatment. The mushrooms also contain the compound eritadenine, which is thought to lower cholesterol. These claims are currently under investigation.

USE: The natural mushroom is widely available in grocery stores, while extracts of the mushroom are sold in capsule form in health food stores and on the Internet. The extracts of the active compounds in shiitake mushrooms are usually used for medicinal purposes, rather than the natural mushroom itself. Extracts of the active compounds, such as lentinan and eritadenine, are mainly sold in Japan. Activated hexose-containing compound is sold in the United States, Europe, and Japan as a nutritional supplement.

EFFECTS: Animal studies have found some positive results regarding the antitumor, cholesterol-lowering, and virus-inhibiting effects of the active compounds in shiitake mushrooms. At least 1 controlled human study of lentinan has shown it to be effective against advanced and recurrent stomach and colorectal cancer. Researchers are studying 1 of the compounds extracted from the mushroom to see if it can reduce tumor activity in men with prostate cancer. More human trials are necessary to confirm the health claims made for shiitake mushrooms and to understand which compounds have antitumor effects for which type of cancers and at what dosages.

Research shows that eating a balanced diet that includes 5 or more servings a day of fruits and vegetables along with foods from a variety of other plant sources is more effective than consuming one particular food in large amounts. Shiitake mushrooms and their extracts are generally considered safe, but some people have been known to develop allergic reactions affecting the skin, nose, throat, and lungs.

▌ SOYBEAN

OTHER COMMON NAME(S): Soy, Soy Protein, Soy Powder

Isoflavones in soy have been found to have protective effects against breast and prostate cancer in laboratory, animal, population, and case control studies. Well-controlled human studies are needed to understand how these findings apply to cancer prevention in humans. Results of research on the effects of consuming isoflavones on colon cancer risk have been mixed. Human studies on individual soy components are currently underway.

DESCRIPTION: The soybean plant is an annual plant that is indigenous to East Asia. It has oblong pods that contain 2 to 4 seeds. Soy lecithin is the part that is extracted from the soya bean, soya oil, and soya seed. Soybean products are promoted for their protective properties against breast, prostate, colon, and lung cancer. As a protein source, soybean products are promoted as a healthier protein alternative to eating meat, as useful to lower cholesterol, and as an aid to weight loss.

USE: Soybean can be consumed in many forms—tofu, soy milk, and soy powder being 3 of the most popular. The amount of isoflavones varies between different types of tofu and soy milk products. Soy is also available in the form of dietary supplements. Soy protein powders and bars are available in nutrition stores and health food markets. The powders can be added to liquids and are also used in cooking. Soy lecithin, an extract from the seeds of the soya bean, has been approved by Commission E (Germany's regulatory agency for herbs) for use in lowering cholesterol.

EFFECTS: A number of laboratory and animal experiments and population studies have found that soy isoflavones have the potential to reduce the risk of developing several types of cancer, including breast, prostate, and colon cancer. The effects of soy are considered to be due to the isoflavones that many soy products contain. Isoflavones, sometimes called phytoestrogens or plant estrogens, act like weak forms of estrogens naturally produced in the body. Genistein and daidzein, both soy isoflavones, are thought to be responsible for the protective benefits of soy. Well-controlled clinical studies are needed to understand how these findings apply to cancer prevention in humans.

Because isoflavones have weak estrogen-like activity, it remains uncertain how this affects the growth of estrogen receptor-positive breast cancers. Some researchers suggest they may act as antiestrogens and reduce cancer growth, while others suggest their estrogenic activity could actually cause cancers to grow faster. Until this issue is resolved, many oncologists recommend that people who take tamoxifen or people with estrogen-sensitive breast tumors should avoid the addition of large amounts of soy to their diets.

Soy products are also used to lower cholesterol and blood pressure and to relieve symptoms of menopause and osteoporosis. Research suggests that including soy protein in a diet low in saturated fat and cholesterol may help reduce the risk of heart disease.

The consumption of soybeans is generally considered safe; however, eating a balanced diet that includes 5 or more servings a day of fruits and vegetables along with foods from a variety of other plant sources is more effective than consuming one particular food in large amounts. Side effects are rare but may include occasional gastrointestinal problems such as stomach pain, loose stool, and diarrhea.

▨ VEGETARIANISM

OTHER COMMON NAME(S): Lactovegetarian, Lacto-Ovo-Vegetarian, Semivegetarian, Vegan

Some studies have linked vegetarian diets to lower risk for heart disease, diabetes, high blood pressure, obesity, and certain types of cancer (ie, colon cancer). Doctors point out that a totally vegetarian diet may not provide all the necessary nutrients if it is not well planned.

DESCRIPTION: Vegetarianism is the practice of eating a diet consisting mainly or entirely of food from plant sources such as fruits and vegetables. Vegetarian diets vary widely. Some include no animal products, while others include dairy products, eggs, and fish. The nutrition guidelines of the American Cancer Society (ACS) recommend including 5 or more servings a day of fruits and vegetables along with regular consumption of breads, cereals, grain products, rice, pasta, and beans. The ACS recommends limiting intake of high-fat foods, particularly from animal sources. The National Cancer Institute also recommends a diet low in fat and high in plant foods in order to decrease cancer risk. The American Dietetic Association states that when planned properly, vegetarian diets are healthy and nutritionally sound and offer health benefits for preventing and treating certain diseases.

USE: All vegetarian diets include plant-based foods, such as grains, legumes, seeds, nuts, vegetables, and fruits, but vary according to the kinds of animal products consumed. For example, a vegan (total vegetarian) diet excludes all animal products, including meat, fowl, fish, dairy, and eggs. A lacto-ovo-vegetarian diet is similar to the vegan diet but includes dairy products and eggs; a lacto-vegetarian diet is also similar to the vegan diet but includes dairy products. One small group of vegetarians called fruitarians eat only raw fruits and fruit vegetables (like tomatoes) because they believe that cooking fruit damages its nutritional properties.

EFFECTS: Population studies have linked vegetarian diets with a decreased risk of heart disease, diabetes, high blood pressure, obesity, and colon cancer. A review of research on the effects of vegetarian diets among Seventh-Day Adventists, whose religious doctrine advises against eating animal flesh, stated that Seventh-Day Adventists experienced less heart disease and fewer cases of some cancers than the general population. The report cautioned that abstinence from tobacco and alcohol may have contributed to some of the health effects associated with vegetarian diets in the Seventh-Day Adventist community. A population study in Germany found the death rate for colon cancer to be lower among moderate and strict vegetarians compared with that of the general population. Another population study found that a diet rich in grains, cereals, and nuts protected against prostate cancer.

Two nutritionists studying the benefits and risks of vegetarian diets reported that vegetarians are not necessarily healthier than nonvegetarians and that well-planned omnivorous diets (animal and vegetable products) can provide health benefits as well. They also pointed out that since many vegetarians adopt a healthier lifestyle—more physical exercise and no smoking—this factor may help improve their overall health.

Strict vegetarians (those who eat no animal products at all) must be careful to consume adequate amounts of protein. Other nutrients that may be missing from vegetarian and vegan diets include vitamin B₁₂, vitamin D, calcium, zinc, and iron (see Calcium, Vitamin B Complex, Vitamin D, and Zinc). Many health care professionals consider vegan diets risky, especially for infants and toddlers. Switching to a vegetarian diet may increase the amount of dietary fiber consumed, which could cause intestinal problems. Dietitians suggest a gradual rather than quick change in diet.

▨ WHEATGRASS

OTHER COMMON NAME(S): Wheatgrass Diet

There have been no scientific studies in humans to support any of the claims made for wheatgrass or wheatgrass diet programs.

DESCRIPTION: Wheatgrass is a member of the genus *Agropyron*, which includes a wide variety of wheat-like grasses. Wheatgrass is a tall grass (12 to 40 inches) commonly found in temperate regions of Europe and the United States. It is a perennial and can be grown outdoors or indoors. The roots and rhizomes (underground stems) are used in herbal remedies.

Wheatgrass is promoted for oral use to treat a number of conditions, including the common cold, coughs, bronchitis, fevers, infections, and inflammation of the mouth and pharynx. Proponents also use wheatgrass liquid preparations to irrigate inflammatory disease of the urinary tract and to prevent kidney stones.

Proponents further claim that a dietary program based on wheatgrass commonly called "the wheatgrass diet" can cause cancer to go into remission and extend the life of people with cancer. They believe that the wheatgrass diet strengthens the immune system, kills harmful bacteria in the digestive system, and rids the body of toxins and waste matter. There is no scientific evidence to support these claims.

USE: Wheatgrass is available in its natural state and in tablets, capsules, liquid extracts, tinctures, and juices. It can also be used to make tea. The wheatgrass diet excludes all meat, dairy products, and cooked foods. It emphasizes "live foods," such as uncooked sprouts, raw vegetables and fruits, nuts, and seeds.

EFFECTS: There is no scientific evidence to suggest that wheatgrass or the wheatgrass diet can cure or prevent disease. There are only anecdotal reports that describe tumor regression and extended survival among people with cancer who followed the wheatgrass diet. Eating a balanced diet that includes 5 or more servings a day of fruits and vegetables along with foods from a variety of other plant sources, such as breads, cereals, grain products, rice, pasta, and beans, is more effective than consuming one particular food in large amounts.

Wheatgrass is generally considered safe. Wheatgrass should not be used to flush out the urinary tract if the patient has swelling caused by heart or kidney insufficiency. Women who are pregnant or breast-feeding should not use wheatgrass.

◼ WILLARD WATER

OTHER COMMON NAME(S): None

Manufacturers describe Willard Water as "catalyst-altered water," meaning that it is a diluted water solution. Proponents claim that Willard Water eases the burning caused by radiation therapy, relieves sores in the mouth and on the lips, eliminates bad breath, removes plaque from teeth, heals minor skin irritations (eg, scrapes, bruises, cuts, insect bites, burns), prevents hangovers, and eases pain from arthritis and muscle sprains. They also claim it flushes toxins from the body and eliminates harmful free radical molecules. The liquid can be swallowed, sprayed directly on the skin or in the mouth, added to herbal remedies or bath water, or used as an ointment.

Since no scientific studies have been conducted on Willard Water, there is no evidence to support these claims. It has not been proven useful for any medical condition, and the exact contents are not known. Not enough is known about Willard Water to know whether it is safe.

CHAPTER FIVE

PHARMACOLOGICAL AND BIOLOGICAL TREATMENT METHODS

THIS CATEGORY PROVIDES INFORMATION about substances that are synthesized and produced from chemicals or concentrated from plants and other living things. Extracted chemicals are not the same as the raw plant or a plant in its natural state.

◣ ANTINEOPLASTON THERAPY

OTHER COMMON NAME(S): Antineoplastons

There is no scientific evidence that antineoplaston therapy is effective in treating cancer or any other disease. The treatment is currently under investigation.

DESCRIPTION: Antineoplaston therapy is an alternative form of cancer treatment that involves using a group of synthetic chemicals called antineoplastons to protect the body from disease. Antineoplastons are made up mostly of peptides and amino acids originally taken from human blood and urine. Supporters claim they are a part of something called "the body's natural biochemical defense system." This system is said to operate independently from the body's immune system and protect against diseases like cancer, which involve a breakdown in the chemistry of the body's cells. Proponents claim antineoplaston therapy has been successful in treating many forms of cancer. They claim people with cancer have a deficiency of naturally occurring antineoplastons, and that this therapy replenishes the body's supply allowing the biochemical defense system of the body to convert cancer cells into normal cells. There is no scientific evidence to support these claims.

USE: Antineoplastons are given orally or by injection into a vein. The duration of treatment ranges from 4 to 12 months. A year of treatment can cost from $36,000 to $60,000, depending on the type of treatment, the number of consultations, and the need for surgery to implant a catheter for drug delivery.

EFFECTS: There is no scientific evidence showing that antineoplaston therapy cures cancer. Although a recent review of 17 small human studies found some promising results, most of the studies were directed by the developer of antineoplaston therapy, Stanislaw Burzynski, MD, PhD, a Polish doctor and researcher. During the 1980s, the National Cancer Institute (NCI) reviewed cases of cancer patients that Dr. Burzynski had treated with antineoplaston therapy. The NCI found no evidence that these patients benefited in any way from the therapy. In 1991, the NCI again reviewed several of Burzynski's cases and concluded that the results warranted further investigation through clinical trials. But, for various reasons, the clinical trials were canceled in 1995. Due to the lack of scientific evidence and the popularity of this therapy among some people with cancer, the Food and Drug Administration has recently granted Dr. Burzynski permission to conduct clinical trials of antineoplaston therapy at his clinic. The NCI is also conducting laboratory experiments on the peptides involved in antineoplaston therapy. Proponents claim that antineoplaston therapy is nontoxic. Side effects may include stomach gas, slight rashes, chills, fever, change in blood pressure, and unpleasant body odor during treatment. High levels of blood sodium can also be a significant problem with this therapy. Relying on this type of treatment alone, and avoiding conventional medical care, may have serious health consequences.

APITHERAPY

OTHER COMMON NAME(S): Bee Venom Therapy, Bee Venom, Venom Immunotherapy

While research is being performed on the antitumor properties of some of the active ingredients in bee products, there have been no studies in humans showing that bee venom or other honeybee components are effective in preventing or treating cancer.

DESCRIPTION: Apitherapy refers to the use of various products of the common honeybee in alternative remedies. These include venom, propolis (a waxy substance produced by honeybees that is used to solidify hives), raw honey, royal jelly, and pollen. Some researchers believe some of the active ingredients in bee products may have possible anticancer effects; however, there is no clinical evidence to support these claims.

Practitioners claim bee venom relieves chronic pain, and can be used to treat various rheumatic diseases, including several types of arthritis, neurological diseases (multiple sclerosis, low back pain, and migraine), and skin conditions (eczema, psoriasis, and herpes). Other proponents claim raw honey has antifungal, antibacterial, anti-inflammatory, and antitumor properties. They say it is an energy-building source, with minerals and 7 vitamins from the B complex group (see Vitamin B Complex); however, this has not been scientifically proven. Pieces of honeycomb containing pollen are said to be successful for treating allergies. Ingesting bee pollen is also claimed to increase endurance, energy, and overall performance. There is no scientific evidence to support these claims.

USE: The usual application of bee venom involves using a live bee to sting the patient at a specific site, such as a joint with arthritis, and repeating this procedure over a period of time. Injections can also be used. The 2 most popular forms of delivery for other apitherapy applications (ie, honey and pollen) are pills and injections. In China, raw honey is applied directly to burns as an antiseptic and painkiller. Bee products are widely available in pharmacies, health food stores, and shops that specialize in bee products.

EFFECTS: Most research in this area has focused on preventing allergic reactions to bee venom; however, several animal and laboratory studies have examined the anticancer effects of some active ingredients contained in bee products (mellitin and propolis). Propolis, a natural resin produced by honeybees, has been found to contain ingredients that may inhibit the development of colon cancer in rats. In the laboratory, mellitin has been combined with certain antibodies to target cancer cells. Further studies are necessary to determine if these animal study results apply to humans.

Some people have extreme allergic reactions to bee stings, the most severe of which can prove fatal. Asthmatic attacks and the death of a young girl have been attributed to the use of royal jelly.

▧ BOVINE CARTILAGE

OTHER COMMON NAME(S): None

Bovine cartilage is cartilage that has been extracted from various parts of a cow, such as the trachea. It is promoted as a treatment for cancer, osteoporosis, and other conditions. The therapeutic potential of various types of cartilage has been studied for more than 40 years (see Shark Cartilage). It has been proposed that bovine cartilage boosts the immune system and inhibits tumor cell growth. Some claim it contains a protein that inhibits angiogenesis (the development of blood vessels), which in theory involves stopping the blood supply to cancer cells. There is no scientific evidence to support these claims. Clinical trials are currently underway to evaluate the effectiveness of bovine cartilage in many types of solid tumors.

▌ CANCELL

OTHER COMMON NAME(S): Entelev, Cantron, Sheridan's Formula, Jim's Juice, Crocinic Acid, Radic

There is no scientific evidence that cancell has any effect on cancer or any other disease. The Food and Drug Administration received a permanent injunction against its manufacturers making it illegal to sell cancell across state lines.

DESCRIPTION: Cancell is a dark liquid made up of common chemicals, including nitric acid, sodium sulfite, potassium hydroxide, sulfuric acid, inositol, and catechol (see Inositol Hexaphosphate). Cancell is promoted as a cure for all forms of cancer and a wide variety of other diseases. According to its manufacturers, it is supposed to cause cancer cells to self-destruct by depriving them of the ability to receive energy.

Cancell has also been promoted to be effective against AIDS, herpes, chronic fatigue syndrome, lupus, endometriosis, Crohn's disease, fibromyalgia, diabetes, emphysema, scleroderma, Lou Gehrig's disease, multiple sclerosis, cystic fibrosis, muscular dystrophy, Parkinson's disease, Alzheimer's disease, hemophilia, high and low blood pressure, mental illness, and some forms of epilepsy. There is no scientific evidence to support these claims.

USE: Cancell is promoted for both internal and external use. Manufacturers typically recommend administration by both routes at the same time for 45 days or until all signs of the disease disappear. Cancell and similar products are available for purchase in some health food stores or on the Internet.

For internal use, cancell is administered either orally or rectally. Orally, one-quarter teaspoon is held under the tongue for 5 minutes before swallowing. Rectally, one-quarter teaspoon is injected into the rectum with a medicine dropper. Both of these procedures must be repeated every 6 hours. For external use, a solvent is first swabbed on the inside of a clean area on the wrist or the ball of the foot, and the dose of cancell is applied to a cotton pad. The cotton pad is then secured to the area with tape.

The promoters of cancell also recommend lifestyle and dietary changes including quitting smoking and avoiding high concentrations of certain vitamins. They also strongly discourage patients from using cancell with any other conventional cancer treatment.

EFFECTS: There is no evidence that cancell is effective in treating cancer. Animal studies conducted by the National Cancer Institute (NCI) more than 20 years ago found no anticancer activity. The NCI performed another series of tests in the early 1990s using human cancer cells and again found no response. The claims that cancell is effective against other diseases have not been scientifically proven.

People may experience temporary, moderate fatigue and flu-like symptoms after taking the product. Ingredients and strength of the mixtures may vary. Cancell is not produced in conformity with good manufacturing practices. Relying on this type of treatment alone, and avoiding conventional medical care, may have serious health consequences.

CELL THERAPY

OTHER COMMON NAME(S): Cellular Therapy, Fresh Cell Therapy, Live Cell Therapy

There is no scientific evidence that cell therapy is effective in treating cancer or any other disease. Serious side effects can result from cell therapy. In fact, it may be lethal and several deaths have been reported.

DESCRIPTION: Cell therapy involves the injection of living tissue from animal organs, embryos, or fetuses into patients. In cell therapy, live or freeze-dried cellular material from the healthy organs, fetuses, or embryos of animals (such as sheep or cows) are injected into patients to supposedly repair cellular damage and heal sick or failing organs. Cell therapy is promoted as an alternative therapy for cancer, arthritis, atherosclerosis, and Parkinson's disease. Cell therapy is also used to counter the effects of aging, to reverse degenerative disease processes, and to improve general health, increase vitality and stamina, and enhance sexual function. Some practitioners have proposed using cell therapy to treat AIDS patients. There is no scientific evidence to support these claims.

USE: First, healthy live cells are harvested from the organs of juvenile or adult live animals, animal embryos, or animal fetuses. (Most cell therapists today use cells derived from embryonic animal tissue.) These cells may be harvested from the brain, pituitary gland, thyroid gland, thymus gland, liver, kidney, pancreas, spleen, heart, ovary, and testis. Patients might receive one or several types of the animal cells. Some cell therapists inject fresh cells into their patients. Others freeze the cells first. Frozen cells have a longer "shelf life" and can be screened for disease.

A course of cell therapy to address a specific disease might require several injections over a short time, whereas cell therapy designed to treat the effects of aging and increase vitality may involve injections received over many months.

Animal organ cells are also sold in pill form as dietary supplements, usually called glandular supplements. These too are alleged to go to the aid of organs of the same kind in the body to promote healing.

EFFECTS: None of the therapeutic successes claimed by cell therapists have ever been proven through scientific testing. They are all based on anecdotal reports, testimonials, and publicity issued by practitioners of the therapy. Proponents of cell therapy admit they don't know how cell therapy works within the body. There are no scientific peer-reviewed publications in medical journals to support the claims of cell therapy.

Cell therapy may be dangerous and several cases have been reported in the medical literature of patient deaths directly linked to the therapy. Patients may contract bacterial and viral infections carried by the animal cells, and have experienced life-threatening and even fatal allergic reactions. Animal cells may seriously compromise the immune system. Other reports list complications such as immune vasculitis, encephalitis, and polyradiculitis (nerve inflammation) following cellular treatment. Serious immunological reactions resulting in death have also been reported.

This treatment should be avoided, especially by women who are pregnant or breast-feeding. Relying on this type of treatment alone, and avoiding conventional medical care, may have serious health consequences.

◾ CHELATION THERAPY

OTHER COMMON NAME(S): None

Chelation therapy is one of several effective treatments for lead poisoning; however, there is no scientific evidence that it is effective for treating other conditions such as cancer. Chelation therapy can be toxic and has the potential to cause kidney damage, irregular heartbeat, and even death.

DESCRIPTION: Chelation therapy involves the injection of ethylene diamine tetra-acetic acid (EDTA), a chemical that chelates (binds) heavy metals, which include iron, lead, mercury, cadmium, and zinc. Chelating drugs remove poisonous buildups of metals by circulating in the bloodstream and attaching to the heavy metal molecules, helping to remove them from the body in the urine. Chelation therapy has been approved by the Food and Drug Administration as a treatment for lead poisoning for more than 40 years.

It is promoted as an alternative treatment for many unrelated conditions, such as multiple sclerosis, muscular dystrophy, high cholesterol, hardening of the arteries, and others. Alternative methods practitioners further claim chelation therapy acts as an antioxidant, a compound that blocks the action of activated oxygen molecules known as free radicals, which can damage cells. There is no scientific evidence to support these claims.

USE: Chelation therapy is given intravenously. Sometimes it is administered as an infusion that drips into the vein over a period of 3 or 4 hours. A typical treatment cycle may include 20 injections or infusions applied over 10 to 12 weeks. Chelation therapy can also be given orally. Because the therapy removes some important minerals from the body, patients often receive vitamin and mineral supplements during treatment. Practitioners recommend a minimum of 20 to 40 treatments initially; however, some may recommend continued therapy for up to 100 treatments over several years.

EFFECTS: Chelation therapy is a proven treatment for poisoning from lead and other heavy metals. There is no evidence that the treatment benefits patients with any other medical problems, such as cancer or heart disease. Several well-respected national and government organizations have found no scientific evidence that chelation therapy is an effective treatment for any medical condition except heavy metal poisoning.

Chelation therapy may produce toxic effects, including kidney damage, irregular heartbeat, and inflammation of the veins. Since the therapy involves the removal of minerals from the body, there is also a risk of hypocalcemia (low calcium) and bone damage. It may also compromise the immune system and decrease the body's ability to produce insulin. People may experience pain at the site of EDTA injection.

Chelation therapy is often accompanied by the infusion of large doses of vitamins and other minerals, which may actually contribute to the processes that produce harmful free radicals in the body. Loss of zinc can also lead to mutations in cells. For this reason, chelation therapy may actually increase the risk of cancer. Women who are pregnant or breast-feeding should not use this method. Relying on this type of treatment alone, and avoiding conventional medical care, may have serious health consequences.

▮ COENZYME Q10

OTHER COMMON NAME(S): CoQ10

Dietary or supplemental Coenzyme Q10 (CoQ10) may promote health and fight some diseases, but more research is needed to determine the role of supplements in health and disease. Results from small studies need to be verified by larger human studies to determine CoQ10's role in reducing heart problems resulting from chemotherapy drugs and in treating cancer.

DESCRIPTION: CoQ10 is an enzyme that regulates numerous chemical reactions in the body. It occurs naturally in the body and can also be obtained from a number of foods, such as mackerel, salmon, sardines, beef, soybeans, peanuts, and spinach (see Enzyme Therapy and Soybean). Scientists believe CoQ10 is an antioxidant. An antioxidant is a compound that blocks the action of activated oxygen molecules known as free radicals, which can damage cells. Deficiencies of CoQ10 are thought to contribute to disease. Some studies have found CoQ10 deficiency in people with cancer.

Coenzyme Q10 is promoted as a treatment for cancer, heart disease, stroke, gum disease, and immune deficiencies. Some claim that CoQ10 can reduce pain and weight loss among people with cancer. Supporters also claim CoQ10 supplements protect against the toxic side effects of chemotherapy drugs, such as adriamycin, which can harm the heart. These claims are currently under investigation.

USE: Coenzyme Q10 occurs naturally in the body. It can also be obtained from a number of foods or as a supplement. The usual supplement dosage found in the literature is 90 to 400 mg per day. Supplements are available in tablets, capsules, and gelcaps.

EFFECTS: Although preliminary studies involving small numbers of patients suggest certain anticancer benefits of CoQ10 supplements, the amount of evidence is minimal. Low levels of CoQ10 have been associated with heart damage and chemotherapy treatment for cancer. Research has found that for people who received CoQ10, there were some protective effects against heart damage related to chemotherapy. No scientific clinical research was found related to pain, weight loss, or increased appetite. More studies are needed with larger groups of patients to compare with conventional cancer treatments.

Few serious reactions to CoQ10 have been reported. Side effects may include headache, heartburn, and fatigue. Very high doses may cause involuntary muscle movements. Some users report mild diarrhea and skin reactions. Little is known about dosage or consequences of long-term use of CoQ10 supplements. There have been reports that CoQ10 may interact with blood-thinning medications and pose a risk for prolonged bleeding.

▌ COLEY TOXINS

OTHER COMMON NAME(S): Coley's Toxins, Mixed Bacterial Vaccines, Issels' Fever Therapy

There is no scientific evidence that Coley toxins alone are effective in treating cancer. Some research has examined combining this immunotherapy with conventional cancer treatments. Some studies found this combined treatment approach to be more effective than conventional treatment alone, while other studies did not find any significant benefit to the combined approach. Modern immunotherapy is likely to be more effective.

DESCRIPTION: Treatment using Coley toxins is an alternative form of cancer immunotherapy that involves injections of inactive bacterial cultures (*Streptococcus pyogenes* and *Serratia marcescens*). Immunotherapy is a method of treatment in which a person receives various biologic substances designed to stimulate the immune system and help the body fight off diseases such as cancer. Proponents claim Coley toxins stimulate the immune system in people with cancer, which helps to fight off disease. Proponents believe the high fever caused by Coley toxins helps to rid the body of cancer because tumor cells are more sensitive to heat than normal cells.

USE: Coley toxins are injected into the bloodstream in increasing doses and continued for at least 3 to 4 months. Patients are monitored closely for side effects and to control fevers if they develop. The original formula for Coley toxins is no longer used in the United States. Coley toxins are used in Central America, Germany, and China; however, it is not clear if they are using the original Coley toxins or a combination of Coley toxins and other bacteria.

EFFECTS: Scientific evidence suggests Coley toxins or mixed bacterial vaccines (MBV) may have a therapeutic role in the treatment of cancer in a combined treatment approach, although results have been mixed. One review found that people who received Coley toxins or a MBV, in combination with conventional treatment, tended to have higher survival rates than patients who received conventional treatment alone. A more recent review compared patients treated with surgery and Coley toxins to patients treated with conventional methods. Results suggested that survival rates for Coley patients did not vary significantly from those treated with conventional methods. More research is needed to determine what benefit, if any, this therapy might have for people with cancer.

Although Coley toxins are often regarded historically as a key step that has led to modern immunotherapy, much has been learned about the science of immunology and practice of immunotherapy since that time. Modern immunotherapy is likely to be of greater value, especially in treating certain cancers, such as renal cell (kidney) cancer, melanoma, and lymphoma.

The inactive bacteria in Coley toxins can produce fever and nausea. Less common side effects include headache, back pain, chills, chest pain, and shock-like reactions. There may be a danger that the administration of Coley toxins could produce serious infections among patients with weakened immune systems. Women who are pregnant or breast-feeding should not use these toxins.

▨ DHEA

OTHER COMMON NAME(S): None

There is no scientific evidence that dehydroepiandrosterone, called DHEA, is safe or effective. It should not be used for treating cancer, especially in hormone-responsive cancers. DHEA may have some usefulness in treating mood and memory problems of older age. People aged 30 years and younger run the risk of suppressing the body's production of DHEA if they take supplemental DHEA.

DESCRIPTION: Dehydroepiandrosterone (DHEA) is a steroid hormone produced by the adrenal gland and is broken down into other important hormones, such as estrogen and testosterone. It is found naturally in humans, plants, and animals. Advocates claim that DHEA supplements can prevent the growth and recurrence of some cancers, protect against heart disease, improve memory, reduce the risk of osteoporosis in women, and help prevent other diseases such as diabetes, Parkinson's, and Alzheimer's. Since levels of DHEA usually begin to decline after a person reaches 30 years, proponents claim that the supplements can help slow the aging process. Proponents also contend that DHEA stimulates the immune system, reduces fat, builds muscle, promotes sleep, increases a person's overall sense of well-being, and increases sex drive. Some practitioners say that DHEA is an effective treatment for colitis and depression. There is no scientific evidence to support these claims.

USE: The dietary supplements sold in the United States are likely to be made from an extract of the yam plant. DHEA is taken orally and applied topically. It is formulated in tablets, capsules, and creams, and can also be made into a tea. There are no widely accepted dosage guidelines for DHEA.

EFFECTS: There is no scientific evidence that DHEA can slow or prevent the growth of cancer, or that the extract from the yam plant will increase DHEA levels in the body. The few clinical research studies that link DHEA with improved health are not considered scientifically valid.

An analysis of published research found that there was little association with levels of DHEA and heart disease in men or women. Various studies have also concluded that DHEA had no influence on cancer, life span, increased muscle mass, reduced body fat, or disease prevention; however, a recent study in humans suggests that DHEA supplements may help treat the autoimmune disease lupus. DHEA may also be helpful in improving mood, energy, sex drive, and in some cases, memory performance in aging adults. This raises the question of DHEA's usefulness in older individuals with depression. More studies are currently underway.

It is not known whether DHEA is safe for long-term use. Some researchers believe DHEA supplements might actually increase the risk of breast cancer, prostate cancer, heart disease, diabetes, and stroke. Dehydroepiandrosterone may stimulate tumor growth in women with cancers related to estrogen, such as breast cancer and uterine cancer, and men with prostate cancer. Men with benign prostatic hypertrophy (an enlarged prostate gland) should avoid DHEA because it could increase swelling.

High doses of DHEA may cause aggressiveness, irritability, insomnia, and the growth of body or facial hair on women. It also may stop menstruation and decrease the levels of HDL cholesterol ("good cholesterol"), which increases the risk of heart disease. Other reported side effects include acne, heart rhythm disturbances, hepatitis, scalp hair loss, and oily skin. Women who are pregnant or breast-feeding should not use DHEA.

▌ DI BELLA THERAPY

OTHER COMMON NAME(S): Di Bella Multitherapy

There is no scientific evidence that Di Bella therapy is effective in treating cancer. It can cause serious and harmful side effects.

DESCRIPTION: Di Bella therapy consists of a mixture of the drugs somatostatin, bromocriptine, as well as vitamins, melatonin, and other substances combined in varying amounts depending on the patient (see Melatonin and the section on Herbs, Vitamins, and Minerals). Proponents of Di Bella therapy claim the drug mixture stimulates the body's self-healing properties and can shrink tumors and even cure cancer. The inventor claims he has treated and cured thousands of people who have had a variety of cancers, and that his formula causes no side effects.

USE: Patients undergoing Di Bella therapy consume the custom-made drug mixture daily. The potency of the mixture and which drugs are involved depends on the type of cancer under treatment.

EFFECTS: Research has shown that Di Bella therapy is not effective in treating cancer. Italy's Health Ministry conducted a study involving nearly 400 patients with various forms of advanced cancers. The researchers concluded that Di Bella therapy did not deserve further clinical testing in patients with advanced cancer.

Bromocriptine (Parlodel®), one of the ingredients in the Di Bella formula, is approved by the Food and Drug Administration for use in addition to conventional treatment to reduce the size of some pituitary tumors before surgery and during radiation. It is also used to treat Parkinson's disease and fertility problems.

Some of the side effects of Di Bella therapy include nausea, vomiting, diarrhea, and neurological symptoms. Women who are pregnant or breast-feeding should not use this method. Relying on this type of treatment alone, and avoiding conventional medical care, may have serious health consequences.

▌ DMSO

OTHER COMMON NAME(S): None

There is no scientific evidence that dimethyl sulfoxide, commonly known as DMSO, is effective in treating cancer. It is currently under study as a drug carrier used to increase the effectiveness of some chemotherapy agents for the treatment of bladder cancer. If administered in high concentrations, DMSO can cause death.

DESCRIPTION: DMSO is an industrial solvent produced as a byproduct of paper manufacturing that has been promoted as an alternative cancer treatment. Proponents say that DMSO causes malignant cells to become benign, and slows or halts the progress of cancers in the bladder, colon, ovary, breast, and skin. Some claim that it is effective in treating leukemia, and it has also been used as a component of some metabolic cancer therapies. It has also been used as a cream or ointment applied to the skin to reduce pain, decrease swelling, treat arthritis, and promote healing in normal tissue. Some people have promoted DMSO as a cancer preventative agent. They claim it works by "cleaning" the cell membrane and decreasing the effect of cancer-causing substances; however, these claims have not been proven.

DMSO is also promoted to reduce the side effects of chemotherapy and radiation treatments in people with cancer. In addition, it has been promoted as a way to control "withdrawal symptoms" experienced by cancer patients when taken off conventional cancer treatment. There is no scientific evidence to support these claims.

USE: As an alternative therapy for cancer, DMSO is available in many health food stores and mail order outlets. It is typically taken either orally or in an intravenous injection, in many cases with other drugs. For topical applications, DMSO is available in gel, liquid, and roll-on forms. The dosage used varies widely, from 3 times a day to once every other day.

EFFECTS: Previous research did not find that DMSO was useful in the treatment of cancer; however, more recent research in rats has shown that DMSO deserves further evaluation as a drug carrier to enhance the effectiveness of some chemotherapy agents for the treatment of bladder cancer. Dimethyl sulfoxide is approved by the Food and Drug Administration to treat a single type of bladder disorder (interstitial cystitis) in humans.

Dimethyl sulfoxide is a common chemical used in the laboratory. It is sometimes used to help tumor cells mature and/or differentiate; however, the concentrations used in the lab would be fatal to a human being. A small amount of DMSO is sometimes also used to dissolve drugs and to deliver them through the skin. In these cases, it is the drug, not DMSO that has biological activity.

Human studies with DMSO were halted due to questions about its safety, especially with regard to its ability to affect the eye. The most commonly reported side effects include burning and itching upon contact with the skin. It can also cause a powerful garlic-like odor on the breath and skin. In high concentrations, DMSO can be fatal to humans. Women who are pregnant or breast-feeding should not use this treatment.

▌ ENZYME THERAPY

OTHER COMMON NAME(S): Digestive Enzyme Therapy, Pancreatic Enzyme Therapy, Systemic Enzyme Therapy

There is no scientific evidence that enzyme supplements are effective in treating cancer or any other disease. There is no information to determine the safety of the supplements.

DESCRIPTION: Enzyme therapy involves the consumption of enzyme supplements as an alternative form of treatment. Enzymes are proteins that stimulate and accelerate numerous biological reactions in the body. Digestive enzymes, many of which are produced in the pancreas, break down food and assist with the absorption of nutrients into the bloodstream. Metabolic enzymes build new cells and repair damaged ones in the blood, tissues, and organs.

Enzymes are sometimes used in conventional medicine. For example, the approved chemotherapy drug asparaginase is an enzyme. Some enzymes are also important in gene therapy research, which is a new but promising treatment for cancer and other serious diseases. Pancreatic enzymes may be given to treat digestive problems resulting from surgical removal of the pancreas or certain diseases of the pancreas.

Enzyme therapy, however, involves the use of enzyme supplements by alternative medicine practitioners to fight disease. Digestive enzyme supplements are claimed to relieve digestive problems such as ulcers and food allergies, and also to strengthen the immune system, help to destroy viruses, ease the discomfort of sore throats, aid weight loss, and relieve hay fever, ulcers, and rheumatoid arthritis. Proponents also claim certain enzyme supplements remove the protective coating from cancer cells, allowing white blood cells to identify and attack the intruders.

Use: Human cells naturally produce about 10,000 different enzymes that are essential in normal metabolism. Enzyme supplements are extracted from animal organs and some plants. Among the most popular enzyme supplements are pancreatic enzymes, which come from animal pancreas.

Enzyme supplements are available in pills, capsules, and powders. Supplements often consist of combinations of several different enzymes. Enzyme therapy is a component of some forms of metabolic therapy, particularly the Kelley and Gonzalez programs (see Metabolic Therapy). There is currently no established safe or effective dosage.

Effects: There have been no well-controlled human studies showing the effectiveness of enzyme supplements in treating cancer, improving digestion, or curing any other disease. According to experts, enzymes, regardless of their source, are eventually broken down into amino acids and absorbed in the digestive tract. One small, uncontrolled study reported that large doses of pancreatic enzymes increased survival times among patients with inoperable pancreatic cancer. A controlled human study sponsored by the National Cancer Institute is underway to evaluate the use of pancreatic enzymes with nutritional support for treating pancreatic cancer.

Some enzymes, like Coenzyme Q10, have been reported to cause side effects (see Coenzyme Q10). There is not enough information to determine the safety of enzyme supplements.

GAMMA LINOLENIC ACID

OTHER COMMON NAME(S): GLA, Borage Seed Oil, Black Currant Oil

Some studies have shown that gamma linolenic acid (GLA) can inhibit the growth of some cancer cell lines in tissue cultures in the laboratory; however, there is no evidence that it is effective in preventing or treating cancer in humans. Human studies are currently being done to evaluate the effect of essential fatty acids on the growth of cancer cells (see Omega-3 Fatty Acids). There is some evidence that GLA may be useful in treating neurological problems related to diabetes. A recent study suggests a promising role for the use of GLA in acute respiratory distress syndrome.

DESCRIPTION: GLA is a highly unsaturated fatty acid made in the human body from other essential fatty acids. The main sources of GLA are oils of evening primrose, borage, and black currant plants (see Evening Primrose). Many commercial preparations sell these extracts as GLA. It is also found in human breast milk. Gamma linolenic acid is used in the production of prostaglandins (hormone-like substances made in the body). Prostaglandins are believed to be involved in many processes in the body, including regulation of the immune system. It has been proposed that GLA supplements may inhibit the growth of cancer cells. This claim is currently under investigation.

Gamma linolenic acid has been promoted as a fatty acid that also helps people with a variety of diseases, such as rheumatoid arthritis, cardiovascular disease, diabetes, and others.

USE: GLA supplements are available in liquid and capsules. Gamma linolenic acid is usually found in combination with other ingredients (eg, evening primrose supplements contain about 10% GLA). An injectable form of GLA is under study in the United Kingdom. Dosages vary according to manufacturer.

EFFECTS: Most of the research on GLA has been done using evening primrose oil. This makes it difficult to credit the effects to GLA, linolenic acid, Vitamin E, or other components of the oil. A well-controlled human study found that GLA had a beneficial effect on neurological problems related to diabetes, especially in patients whose condition was under control. Neither evening primrose oil nor GLA has been shown to be effective in preventing or treating cancer in humans.

Dietary GLA can contribute to prostaglandin synthesis and regulation; however, the types of prostaglandins and their exact role in fighting cancer are still unknown. GLA can inhibit the growth of certain human tumor cells in the laboratory. Animal and human studies have found that dietary GLA has no effect on established tumors. A new injectable form of GLA has been developed and has been used in a single human study with limited success.

GLA does not appear to be toxic; however, it has been reported to aggravate temporal lobe epilepsy and should not be used by people who take anticonvulsant medication. Long-term use of GLA may lead to inflammation, blood clots, or decreased immune system functioning.

▌ GLUCARATE

OTHER COMMON NAME(S): Calcium Glucarate, D-Glucarate™

Several laboratory and animal studies found that glucarate has some preventive and anticancer effects; however, it has not yet been found to be effective in humans.

DESCRIPTION: Glucarate is a phytochemical (plant compound) found primarily in apples, grapefruit, broccoli, Brussels sprouts, and bean sprouts (see Broccoli and Phytochemicals). It also occurs naturally in the body in very small amounts. Proponents claim that glucarate supplements reduce the risk of colon, lung, liver, skin, and prostate cancer by increasing the body's ability to eliminate cancer-causing toxins that come from diet and the environment. Supporters also say that glucarate hinders the formation of breast and uterine cancers by removing excess estrogen and other hormones that promote these diseases from the body. These claims are under investigation.

USE: Glucarate supplements are available in capsules and tablets. There is no standardized dosage.

EFFECTS: Glucarate may have potential as an anticancer agent; however, there is no evidence yet to show that the supplement is effective in treating cancer or lowering cancer risk in humans. A number of animal studies published in peer-reviewed medical journals found that dietary glucarate caused rats to develop fewer breast cancer tumors, and shrank some existing tumors. Animal studies also found that dietary glucarate inhibited the development of tumors in the colon, lung, liver, skin, and prostate. These results suggest that dietary glucarate is worthy of further investigation to evaluate its possible role in preventing and treating cancer in humans. There are no known side effects associated with the use of glucarate.

GREEK CANCER CURE

OTHER COMMON NAME(S): METBAL®, Cellbal®

There is no scientific evidence that the Greek Cancer Cure is effective in preventing or treating cancer. There is no information to determine the safety of this method.

DESCRIPTION: This treatment consists of a blood test reportedly used to diagnose cancer, and intravenous therapy designed to cure the disease. The injections are said to contain a combination of organic substances such as sugars, vitamins, amino acids, and other ingredients. Practitioners of the Greek Cancer Cure claim the regular use of a special intravenous injection, which they refer to as a serum, boosts the patient's immune system, enabling it to fight and destroy tumor cells. The inventor of the Greek Cancer Cure claimed to have cured a high percentage of patients who had cancers of the skin, bone, uterus, stomach, and lymph system.

USE: The first stage of the Greek Cancer Cure is a blood test that claims to determine the nature, location, and seriousness of a patient's tumor. The second stage involves daily intravenous injections of the serum. Treatment lasts from 6 to 30 days. The secret formula is believed to consist of brown sugar, nicotinic acid (also known as niacin or vitamin B_3), vitamin C, and alanine, an amino acid (see Amino Acids, Vitamin B Complex, and Vitamin C). An oral supplement is also available. Patients are also advised to limit their intake of salts and acids, limit physical activities, and avoid drugs such as aspirin and laxatives. They are also asked to stop chemotherapy or radiation therapy before beginning the treatment program.

EFFECTS: There is no scientific evidence that the Greek Cancer Cure has any effect on cancer. No studies have shown that either the blood tests or the injections used in the Greek Cancer Cure result in any measurable benefit in the treatment of people with cancer. The safety of this treatment has not been proven. The intravenous serum can contain levels of nicotinic acid high enough to cause burning at the injection site. Relying on this type of treatment alone, and avoiding conventional medical care, may have serious health consequences.

■ HOMEOPATHY

OTHER COMMON NAME(S): Homeopathic Medicine

There is no scientific evidence that homeopathic remedies are effective in treating cancer. Many advocates of homeopathy admit that they do not know how the treatments work, but insist that future research will unlock the mystery.

DESCRIPTION: Homeopathic remedies are water (and sometimes alcohol) solutions containing tiny amounts of various naturally occurring plants, minerals, animal products, or chemicals. Proponents claim that homeopathic solutions, even though they may contain minuscule quantities of the original ingredient, contain a "memory" of the substance that somehow interacts with the body to cure disease. Homeopathy is promoted to treat problems such as arthritis, asthma, colds, flu, and allergies. There are some advocates who believe that homeopathy can be used to treat and cure cancer. Some practitioners claim homeopathy can help cancer patients by decreasing pain, improving vitality and well being, stopping the spread of cancer, strengthening the immune system, and alleviating certain symptoms and side effects from radiation and chemotherapy. There is no scientific evidence to support any of these claims.

USE: Homeopathy is based largely on the notion that "like cures like." In other words, a substance that causes symptoms of disease can relieve those same symptoms when administered in very small amounts. A patient complaining of vomiting and diarrhea might receive a solution containing tiny amounts of thorn apple, since larger amounts of that herb cause those symptoms.

When a patient complains of certain symptoms, the homeopath consults a reference guide that lists thousands of individual symptoms, and searches for an entry that matches the patient's description. The practitioner then takes an extract of the plant, mineral, animal product, or chemical remedy that matches the patient's symptoms and repeatedly dilutes it in water. Every time the extract is diluted in water, a part of the diluted water is then added to another sample of water and so on until the final solution contains virtually none of the original extract. Each solution may go through the dilution process as many as 30 to 50 times. After the dilution process is complete, the patient is then given the remedy.

EFFECTS: There is no scientific evidence showing that homeopathic remedies possess any therapeutic value. Some researchers suggest that homeopathy may result in beneficial effects for patients who believe the treatment is working—a phenomenon known as the placebo effect. A placebo is an inactive substance or treatment. For example, one study investigating the use of complementary therapies (including homeopathy) by people with cancer showed that while certain complementary therapies had no actual antitumor effect, patients reported psychological improvement including increased hope and optimism.

Although some homeopathic solutions contain toxic chemicals, they are typically present in amounts too small to present any danger. Relying on this type of treatment alone, and avoiding conventional medical care, may have serious health consequences.

▌ HYDRAZINE SULFATE

OTHER COMMON NAME(S): None

There is some conflicting research on hydrazine sulfate; however, most carefully designed studies have shown it does not help people with cancer live longer or feel better. It may also cause potentially serious side effects.

DESCRIPTION: Hydrazine sulfate is a chemical commonly used in industrial processes. It is used as an alternative method to treat some symptoms of advanced cancer. It is usually produced in a laboratory, but does occur naturally in tobacco plants, tobacco smoke, and in some mushrooms. Proponents claim hydrazine sulfate may relieve cachexia, a condition that occurs when cancer disrupts the body's metabolism, leading to progressive loss of appetite, weight loss, weakness, and muscle atrophy (wasting away). Cachexia affects about half of all cancer patients, especially those with advanced cancer of the lung, pancreas, or gastrointestinal system. It is responsible for 10% to 22% of all cancer deaths.

USE: Hydrazine sulfate is usually given in pills or capsules. It can also be injected. A common dosage is 60 mg 4 times a day for several days, then from 2 to 3 times a day for 35 to 40 days. Treatment is then stopped for 2 to 6 weeks, and is sometimes repeated for up to 40 times.

Hydrazine sulfate is not approved for use with cancer patients in the United States. It can be obtained by doctors through the investigational new drug program of the Food and Drug Administration. In Canada, hydrazine sulfate is available by prescription. It is widely used in Europe, and in Russia, where it is known as Sehydrin.

EFFECTS: Research on hydrazine sulfate has produced conflicting results. Several well-controlled human studies found that hydrazine sulfate treatment did not reduce the size of tumors or increase patient survival time; however, some patients reported feeling better for brief periods during treatment with hydrazine sulfate, such as experiencing less pain, lower fever, and increased appetite. Other studies reported that patients treated with the chemical had more normal glucose metabolism, weight gain, and improved appetite.

One study of patients with inoperable lung cancer found that after adding hydrazine sulfate to a combination chemotherapy treatment, patients were able to consume more calories and showed other positive metabolic changes. Among patients who started the study in better condition, those given hydrazine sulfate lived longer than those taking a placebo. Among those who started in worse condition, hydrazine sulfate did not improve survival. Based on this study, the National Cancer Institute felt that additional studies involving more patients were needed.

Well-controlled studies of treatment involving patients who had advanced lung cancer, colon cancer, or leukemia and who received hydrazine sulfate along with their chemotherapy regimen showed that hydrazine sulfate did not provide any benefit to cancer patients. Nerve damage occurred more often and the quality of life was significantly worse among the group receiving hydrazine sulfate.

Side effects are uncommon, but include mild to moderate levels of nausea, vomiting, itching, dizziness, poor motor coordination, and/or tingling or numbness in the hands and feet. Hydrazine sulfate should not be taken with tranquilizers, barbiturates, alcohol, or foods high in tyramine (eg, aged cheeses and fermented products). Liver damage can be caused by high doses (ie, more than 20 times the regular dose). Women who are pregnant or breast-feeding should not use this therapy.

▨ HYDROGEN PEROXIDE THERAPY

OTHER COMMON NAME(S): Hydrogen Peroxide

Although hydrogen peroxide is well known for its antiseptic properties, there is no evidence that it has value as a treatment for cancer or other diseases. It can be toxic at concentrations above 10%.

DESCRIPTION: Hydrogen peroxide is a clear, odorless solution that is widely available for use in cleaning and disinfecting wounds. In high concentrations (eg, 35%), hydrogen peroxide is used by alternative practitioners as a treatment for cancer and other diseases. Proponents claim that hydrogen peroxide therapy can be used to oxidize toxins, kill bacteria and viruses, and stimulate the immune system. It is promoted for everything from cleansing the digestive tract to curing cancer and other diseases such as arthritis. Some people advocate cleaning foods with it prior to eating. Supporters of hydrogen peroxide therapy believe that cancer cells grow rapidly if they are deprived of oxygen. They claim that hydrogen peroxide can cure cancer by bombarding cancer cells with more oxygen than they can handle (see Oxygen Therapy).

USE: Hydrogen peroxide is used internally or injected. Some practitioners promote it for use rectally, vaginally, as a nasal spray, and as eardrops. It is often used to soak affected parts of the body. The more concentrated solution recommended by alternative medicine practitioners is sold in some health food stores.

Because of its antiseptic and whitening properties, hydrogen peroxide is found in some toothpastes and mouthwashes, usually in a 3% (or less) solution. In stronger solutions of about 10%, it is used as hair bleach, and in industry to bleach paper and cloth, to manufacture other chemicals, and as an ingredient in some rocket fuels.

EFFECTS: Medical researchers have studied hydrogen peroxide for more than a century to determine if it can cure various diseases. Many researchers have studied the effects of hydrogen peroxide on tumors in laboratory animals. When used alone, hydrogen peroxide was not effective. Some have investigated it as an addition to radiation therapy. Although some patients appeared to benefit, many did not. Attempts to treat patients with hydrogen peroxide injections directly into solid tumors or into the blood system have generally been ineffective. There is currently no scientific evidence that hydrogen peroxide therapy is effective for treating any of the conditions that have been claimed.

Hydrogen peroxide can be harmful if swallowed. Drinking the concentrated solutions sold in some health food stores (35%) can cause vomiting, severe burns of the throat and stomach, and even death. Direct skin contact or breathing the vapors of hydrogen peroxide can also be harmful. Hydrogen peroxide injections can have dangerous side effects. High blood levels of hydrogen peroxide create oxygen bubbles that can block blood flow and cause gangrene and death. Acute hemolytic crisis (destruction of blood cells) has also been reported following intravenous injection of hydrogen peroxide. Women who are pregnant or breast-feeding should not use this method.

▮ IMMUNO-AUGMENTATIVE THERAPY

OTHER COMMON NAME(S): IAT

There is no scientific evidence that immuno-augmentative therapy (IAT) is effective in treating cancer. The IAT serum has not been tested for safety according to widely accepted medical standards.

DESCRIPTION: Immuno-augmentative therapy (IAT) is promoted as an alternative form of cancer treatment involving daily injections of a protein mixture made from blood in an attempt to restore normal immune function. Proponents claim IAT causes cancer to stabilize or go into remission. It is not promoted as a cure for cancer, but as a life-long treatment of daily injections. Like diabetic patients, IAT patients are told that they can live normal lives as long as they continue their daily injections.

Practitioners of IAT believe that cancer cells begin to grow and multiply when a person's immune system is weakened or out of balance. Components of the blood products are claimed to contain 3 tumor antibodies and "deblocking" proteins, all from healthy donors. Tumor antibodies are said to attack the cancer, and the deblocking proteins remove a "blocking factor" that prevents the patient's immune system from detecting the cancer. Proponents further claim IAT is a safe, nontoxic, and effective treatment for all types of cancer. There is no scientific evidence to support these claims.

USE: This therapy involves daily self-injections of a protein mixture made from human blood. At a special IAT facility, a patient is given a physical examination, blood tests, and urinalysis. Once the patient's immune system status is determined, the IAT treatment begins. Patients are given IAT drugs according to their particular situation. Treatment continues until the practitioner determines that the patient's cancer is controlled. The average stay is 10 to 12 weeks. The patient is then shown how to self-inject and is sent home to continue treatment.

EFFECTS: There is no evidence to support claims that IAT has any beneficial effects for people with cancer. Success stories associated with the treatment are based on anecdotal reports provided by the creator's clinics, and they include little or no supporting evidence.

The concept that cancer can be treated by enhancing activity of the immune system is reasonable, and is the basis for conventional immunotherapy. Unlike IAT, conventional immunotherapy, founded on scientific principles of immunology and evaluated by well-controlled human studies, has been useful in treating melanoma, lymphoma, kidney cancer, bladder cancer, and other types of cancer.

The safety of IAT has not been established. Based on personal reports from patients who have received IAT, side effects appear to be minor and include fatigue, pain at the injection site, and flu-like symptoms. Some medical professionals fear infectious agents, such as HIV and hepatitis, may contaminate the unregulated compounds used in IAT, which come from human blood. Relying on this type of treatment, and avoiding conventional medical care, may have serious health consequences.

▨ INOSINE PRANOBEX

OTHER COMMON NAME(S): Isoprinosine®, Methisoprinol, Inosiplex, Imunovir®

There is no scientific evidence that inosine pranobex is effective in treating cancer. Experimental data suggests that it may help boost the immune system; however, more studies in humans are needed to determine the benefits. The drug cannot be sold legally in the United States.

DESCRIPTION: Inosine pranobex is a substance that may mimic the actions of immune-stimulating hormones produced in the thymus gland. Proponents claim inosine pranobex strengthens the immune system and fights viral infections. They also say it decreases the risk of infection in people with cancer who undergo chemotherapy, radiation therapy, or surgery, all of which suppress the immune system. Some assert that inosine pranobex intensifies the effects of the anticancer drug interferon and increases the activity of natural killer cells (a type of white blood cell), which may inhibit the growth of tumors. Some practitioners recommend it as an alternative to conventional cancer therapy. It is also used to treat people with AIDS and other viral diseases, including herpes, shingles, viral hepatitis, influenza, the common cold, and viral encephalitis, although there is not enough clinical evidence to prove its effectiveness.

USE: Inosine pranobex is administered in 500 mg capsules. Some studies have used a dosage of 3 g per day for 28 days.

EFFECTS: A number of animal and laboratory studies conducted mostly in Europe have found that inosine pranobex increases T-helper lympho-cytes and natural killer cell activity, which may inhibit the growth of tumors. Further studies are necessary to determine if these animal and laboratory study results apply to humans.

One study found no differences in survival or recurrence rates between patients treated with surgery alone and patients treated with surgery plus inosine pranobex. In another, much smaller study, researchers concluded that inosine pranobex combined with the chemotherapy drug 5-fluorouracil was not effective in the treatment of metastatic colorectal cancer.

Not enough is known about inosine pranobex to make conclusions about its safety. Possible side effects include stomach upset and heartburn.

▚ KREBIOZEN

OTHER COMMON NAME(S): Carcalon, Creatine

There is no scientific evidence that Krebiozen is effective in treating cancer or any other disease. According to the Food and Drug Administration, creatine has been associated with several dangerous side effects.

DESCRIPTION: Krebiozen (pronounced kree-bee-ozen) is the commercial name of an alternative cancer formula originally prepared from the blood of horses that have been injected with bacteria. An analysis by several federal agencies later found Krebiozen to contain mineral oil and a form of creatine. Creatine is a substance that naturally occurs in the human body and is sold as a dietary supplement. Proponents have claimed that Krebiozen cures cancer. They have cited private experiments claiming that Krebiozen stops tumor growth in mice and induces recovery in some people with advanced cancer.

USE: Krebiozen has been manufactured in powder and liquid forms. The liquid form of Krebiozen is combined with mineral oil and delivered through injection.

EFFECTS: Federal government agencies that conducted a thorough investigation of Krebiozen concluded that it had no anticancer activity in humans. This conclusion was drawn by a committee of 24 scientists, who studied the completed medical records of 504 cases submitted by the Krebiozen Research Foundation. Following the investigation, the National Cancer Institute agreed, saying that it saw no justification for a clinical trial, and that from a scientific standpoint the case was "closed."

There is no information on the safety of Krebiozen; however, creatine supplements have been associated with some adverse reactions including vomiting, diarrhea, seizure, anxiety, myopathy (muscle tissue disorder), irregular heartbeat, blood clots, and even death.

▌ LAETRILE

OTHER COMMON NAME(S): Amygdalin, Vitamin B$_{17}$

There is no scientific evidence that Laetrile is effective in treating cancer or any other disease. It contains a small percentage of cyanide and several cases of cyanide poisoning have been linked to its use. The Food and Drug Administration has not issued approval for Laetrile as a medical treatment and its use is illegal in the United States.

DESCRIPTION: Laetrile is a compound produced from amygdalin, a naturally occurring substance found primarily in the kernels of apricots, peaches, and almonds. Laetrile was once called "the perfect chemotherapeutic agent" since it was alleged to selectively kill cancer cells while being nontoxic to normal cells. Supporters say that Laetrile can prevent cancer from occurring, can help patients' cancer stay in remission, and can provide pain relief to people with cancer.

There are 2 proposed explanations for Laetrile's use. Proponents claim that cancer cells trigger the release of the cyanide found in Laetrile, causing the death of the cancer cells due to cyanide poisoning. The second theory proposed for Laetrile's effectiveness is that cancer is really a "vitamin deficiency" and that Laetrile is the missing "vitamin B$_{17}$." Other reported uses for Laetrile have been in the prevention and treatment of high blood pressure and arthritis. There is no scientific evidence to support these claims.

USE: Laetrile is most commonly extracted from apricot pits. It is usually taken as part of a metabolic therapy involving a specific diet with high doses of other vitamins (see Metabolic Therapy). Although no standard therapy for Laetrile exists, a typical treatment consists of daily intravenous administration for 2 to 3 weeks, followed by the use of oral tablets as a maintenance therapy. Laetrile is also used in enemas, and in solutions applied directly to skin lesions. Laetrile treatments may cost thousands of dollars per week and can only be obtained from some hospitals in Mexico because it is illegal in the United States.

EFFECTS: During the 1970s, Laetrile achieved great popularity in the United States as an alternative anticancer therapy. For this reason, despite the lack of scientific evidence for the efficacy of Laetrile, the National Cancer Institute (NCI) evaluated it through a retrospective case review. A human study was also performed at medical centers around the country. Both studies found that Laetrile provided no significant benefit to people with cancer. In contrast to the findings by the NCI, one of the leading proponents of Laetrile claims to have treated nearly 30,000 cancer patients in various stages of clinical trials of the drug with promising results. These results have not been reviewed nor repeated by the scientific medical community.

There is no scientific evidence that Laetrile is effective as an anticancer treatment. Cancer cells do not trigger the release of cyanide making them more susceptible to the effects of Laetrile. All of the successes claimed by its supporters are based on anecdotal reports, testimonials, and publicity issued by promoters.

The use of Laetrile has been directly linked to cyanide toxicity and death in a few cases. This treatment should be avoided, especially by women who are pregnant or breast-feeding. Relying on this type of treatment alone, and avoiding conventional medical care, may have serious health consequences.

▌ LIPOIC ACID

OTHER COMMON NAME(S): Alpha-Lipoic Acid

Lipoic acid is an antioxidant that plays an important role in metabolism. Recent research has shown that it is beneficial in treating nerve damage in people with diabetes. There is currently no evidence that lipoic acid prevents the development or spread of cancer.

DESCRIPTION: Lipoic acid is an antioxidant found in certain foods, including red meat, spinach, broccoli (see Broccoli), potatoes, yams, carrots, beets, and yeast. An antioxidant is a compound that blocks the action of activated oxygen molecules known as free radicals, which can damage cells. Oxidation may also play a role in causing poor health as people age, and some researchers claim that lipoic acid is beneficial to maintaining good health in old age. It is promoted to protect the body against cancer and other diseases. The nutrient has been used to treat diabetic polyneuropathy, a nerve disease found in many diabetic patients that causes pain and numbness in the hands and feet. In addition to treating nerve damage in people with diabetes, researchers claim lipoic acid also lowers blood sugar levels.

Promoted as the most powerful and versatile of all the antioxidants, including vitamin E and vitamin C, lipoic acid is claimed to strengthen the effects of other antioxidants and regenerate antioxidants used up in the fight against free radicals (see Vitamin C and Vitamin E). Some proponents believe that lipoic acid may inhibit the gene that triggers cancer cells to grow; however, there is no scientific evidence to support these claims.

USE: A healthy diet that includes meat and vegetables containing lipoic acid is the best source of this nutrient. The body also produces lipoic acid naturally, but as one ages, the body produces less lipoic acid. Supplements are available in health food stores and on the Internet, but high doses of any antioxidant supplement may actually cause cell damage. A safe and effective dosage of this supplement has not been established.

EFFECTS: In a recent review article, researchers reported that a number of experimental studies and clinical trials during the past 5 years have found alpha-lipoic acid to be useful in treating nerve problems in diabetic patients and can improve insulin sensitivity in people with type 2 diabetes. They also suggested that it might be useful in treating liver disease as well. Laboratory and animal studies have found that alpha-lipoic acid is beneficial in treating stroke, cataract formation, HIV infection, nerve degeneration, and radiation injury; however, there are no scientific studies showing that lipoic acid supplements will directly prevent the development or progression of cancer.

Lipoic acid found naturally in foods is safe. Research has shown that 300 to 600 mg of lipoic acid a day may be safely taken with no side effects. Extremely high doses of lipoic acid supplements, however, may damage cells and should be avoided.

▨ LIVER FLUSH

OTHER COMMON NAME(S): None

A liver flush involves eating or drinking a combination of specially selected herbs, enzymes, juices, and oils to detoxify or drive "harmful" chemicals from the liver. Liver flush formulas vary widely by practitioner and are also available commercially. Some practitioners advise combining liver flushes with fasting (see Fasting). Proponents claim that liver flushing rids the organ of unwanted food by-products, fats, and toxins, therefore inhibiting the formation of diseases, including cancer. They also claim that because the liver is an important hormone regulator, cleansing it will aid conditions caused by hormone imbalances. There is no scientific evidence to support any of the claims made for liver flushes. Individual components of the herbal mixtures used in a liver flush may present health hazards. Relying on this type of treatment alone, and avoiding conventional medical care, may have serious health consequences.

LIVINGSTON-WHEELER THERAPY

OTHER COMMON NAME(S): None

There is no scientific evidence that Livingston-Wheeler therapy is effective in treating cancer or any other disease. There is no information to determine the safety of this method.

DESCRIPTION: Livingston-Wheeler therapy is an alternative cancer method that includes vaccines, antibiotics, vitamin and mineral supplements, digestive enzymes, cleansing enemas, and a vegetarian diet (see Colon Therapy, Enzyme Therapy, Vegetarianism, and the Chapter on Herbs, Vitamins, and Minerals).

Livingston-Wheeler therapy is promoted primarily for use in the treatment of cancer, but it is also used to treat lupus, arthritis, and other chronic conditions. In the case of cancer, proponents believe that when the body's immune system weakens, it allows the spread of a bacterium named *Progenitor cryptocides* to cause cancer. Because practitioners claim Livingston-Wheeler therapy is a form of immunotherapy (a treatment that stimulates a person's immune system), they claim it can boost the immune system to help a person fight off serious diseases like cancer. There is no evidence to support these claims.

USE: Patients enter a 10-day treatment program, which can be very expensive and requires home treatment as well. Follow-up visits to the clinic are also encouraged. At the clinic, patients are evaluated and given standard blood and urine tests. Special hormone, liver function, and tumor marker tests are also done. The patient's immune system is also tested in order to design a personalized immune-enhancement vaccine. In addition to the vaccine, the patient may be given antibiotics, nutritional supplements, digestive enzymes, bile salts, enemas, laxatives, and blood transfusions. A strict vegetarian diet is enforced and the patient participates in group or support therapy (see Support Groups).

EFFECTS: Based on the studies and research currently available, there is no evidence that Livingston-Wheeler therapy has any beneficial effects for people with cancer. Few studies have evaluated the Livingston-Wheeler therapy. One investigation involving seriously ill cancer patients found no difference in survival rates between patients receiving conventional treatment and those undergoing Livingston-Wheeler therapy. In fact, those patients receiving Livingston-Wheeler seemed to experience a lower quality of life.

One report on the bacteria *Progenitor cryptocides*, which proponents claim causes cancer, found that the bacteria does not exist. It is actually a mixture of several different types of bacteria mislabeled as one. The other components of this type of therapy have also been criticized for lack of scientific evidence.

The safety of Livingston-Wheeler therapy has never been firmly established. Some reported reactions to the vaccine given in the therapy include aching, slight fever, and tenderness at the injection site.

LYPRINOL™

OTHER COMMON NAME(S): Lyprinex™

Lyprinol is a fatty acid extracted from Perna canaliculus, *a green-lipped mussel (shellfish) native to New Zealand. Lyprinol is promoted in New Zealand as a dietary supplement that can kill cancer cells and treat arthritis and asthma. Today, the extract is sold in capsule form in pharmacies and supermarkets in New Zealand and on the Internet.*

Although the researcher who promotes Lyprinol claims that it inhibits 2 cell pathways that may cause inflammation and possibly cancer in animals and humans, another New Zealand researcher warned that Lyprinol might, in fact, promote tumor growth rather than kill cancer cells. No human studies have been conducted to support the researcher's claims. Relying on this type of treatment alone, and avoiding conventional medical care, may have serious health consequences.

MELATONIN

OTHER COMMON NAME(S): None

Research suggests that melatonin, which is naturally produced by the body, plays a large role in the daily rhythms of sleeping and waking. The melatonin supplement is popular as a sleeping aid, but studies documenting safe dosage, risks, and benefits are lacking. There have been mixed study results regarding the use of melatonin in people with cancer for increasing survival and improving quality of life.

DESCRIPTION: Melatonin is a hormone produced by the pineal gland, which is located just beneath the center of the brain. There is evidence that melatonin may have a role in the regulation of circadian rhythms (daily body cycles), sleep patterns, mood, reproduction, tumor growth, and aging. Melatonin is also manufactured synthetically and used as a supplement, which is promoted primarily as a sleep aid. Melatonin is also promoted to help people adjust to odd or irregular work schedules and to counter the effects of jet lag because it may restore normal sleeping and waking schedules.

Because of melatonin's suspected antioxidant properties, proponents believe it has the ability to suppress the growth of some types of cancer cells, especially when combined with other anticancer drugs. It has also been proposed that melatonin can decrease the toxic effects of radiation therapy and chemotherapy. Some practitioners also believe that melatonin influences hormones in the body that regulate reproduction, the timing of ovulation, and aging. Many of these claims are currently under investigation.

USE: Melatonin is sold as a supplement and is available in drugstores, in health food stores, and on the Internet. There are no widely accepted recommendations for dosage or duration of use. Melatonin can also be found in many foods, such as milk, peanuts, almonds, turkey, and chicken, but in such small amounts that someone would have to eat large volumes to obtain a measurable dose.

EFFECTS: There is evidence that melatonin supplements can influence sleep and fatigue; however, the exact connection is not well understood. Numerous human studies of melatonin and its effects on cancer have been conducted, and the results were mixed and inconclusive. Some found that melatonin increased survival time, while others indicated that melatonin caused little or no response in tumors. Some studies reported that cancer went into total or partial regression in a few patients. A study of melatonin's ability to ease the side effects of chemotherapy drugs found that high doses of the hormone had little effect. Melatonin combined with interleukin-2 has been studied as an anticancer treatment.

The effects of long-term use of melatonin and how it interacts with other medications or supplements are unknown. Research has not yet shown the most effective way to use melatonin supplements (ie, for patients with sleep disorders or for people with occasional insomnia). They have also been shown to cause insomnia or nightmares in some people. Since melatonin may affect ovulation, women who are trying to conceive, are pregnant, or are breast-feeding should not use this supplement. The National Institute on Aging has also warned that melatonin supplements may lead to high blood pressure, diabetes, and even cancer.

Some practitioners believe that children and adults younger than 40 years should not take melatonin because they produce enough of the hormone naturally. They also state that people with immune-system disorders (eg, severe allergies), autoimmune diseases (eg, rheumatoid arthritis), or immune-system cancers (eg, lymphoma) should not take melatonin because it may further stimulate the immune system and worsen these conditions. Practitioners also caution people with severe mental illness and those taking steroid medications against using melatonin.

▌OXYGEN THERAPY

OTHER COMMON NAME(S): Hyperoxygenation, Bio-oxidative Therapy, Oxidative Therapy, Ozone Therapy, Oxidology, Oxymedicine

There is no evidence that oxygen therapy is effective in treating cancer or any other disease. It may even be dangerous. There have been reports of patient deaths from this method.

DESCRIPTION: Oxygen therapy consists of one or more chemicals that are supposed to release oxygen after they are put into the body. The extra oxygen theoretically increases the body's ability to destroy disease-causing cells. Two of the most common compounds used in oxygen therapy are ozone (a chemically active form of oxygen) and hydrogen peroxide (see Hydrogen Peroxide Therapy). Oxygen therapy, as described here, is very different from hyperbaric oxygen, which involves the use of pressurized oxygen (see Hyperbaric Oxygen Therapy).

Oxygen therapy is promoted as a treatment for many diseases, including certain cancers, asthma, emphysema, AIDS, arthritis, cardio-vascular disease, and Alzheimer's disease. Some proponents claim that cancer cells, and the microorganisms that cause cancer, thrive in low-oxygen environments. They believe adding oxygen to the body creates an oxygen-rich condition in which cancer cells cannot survive. Oxygen therapy advocates claim that it increases the efficiency of all cells in the body and increases energy production, stimulates the production of antioxidants, and enhances the immune system. There is no scientific evidence to support these claims.

USE: Ozone gas may be introduced under pressure into the rectum or injected into a muscle. Some practitioners use a special device to force ozone into a pint of blood that has been drawn from the patient. The blood is then returned to the patient's body. For hydrogen peroxide therapy, the liquid is first diluted and then given to patients orally, rectally, intravenously, or vaginally. Sometimes less frequently used oxygen therapy compounds are injected into muscles. The frequency of treatments varies widely, from 3 times a day for several weeks, to once a week for several months.

EFFECTS: There is no evidence that "bathing" cancer cells in oxygen will harm or kill the cancer cells. The medical literature contains several accounts of patient deaths attributed directly to oxygen therapy.

Large amounts of injected hydrogen peroxide can result in a condition called arterial gas embolism, which can lead to irreversible lung damage and death. Relying on this type of treatment alone, and avoiding conventional medical care, may have serious health consequences.

▨ POLY-MVA

OTHER COMMON NAME(S): None

Poly-MVA is a compound that contains various minerals, vitamins, and amino acids such as lipoic acid, palladium, B₁₂, and other B complex vitamins (see Amino Acids, Lipoic Acid, and Vitamin B Complex). Poly-MVA is a reddish-brown liquid that is mixed with water or juice. It is not licensed for use in the United States.

Poly-MVA is promoted as a nutritional supplement that is a nontoxic alternative to chemotherapy. The development of Poly-MVA is rooted in the theory that cancer is a systematic disease related to many factors, including irreparable gene damage due to cancer-causing substances. Makers of Poly-MVA say that it demonstrates antitumor activity. There are claims that it is effective against tumors in the brain, lung, ovaries, and breast and that it boosts the immune system, reduces pain, and helps people regain energy and appetite. Some even claim that it can lead to longer survival. According to its manufacturers, the compound attacks cancerous cells and protects DNA and RNA. They contend that the lipoic acid allows the various minerals, vitamins, and amino acids to be easily absorbed into the system where they can kill cancerous cells.

There is no scientific evidence that Poly-MVA is effective in preventing or treating cancer. Most of the reports of successful use of Poly-MVA are anecdotal or represent small studies that have not been published in scientific journals. There have been no well-controlled studies of the compound. The potential risks and side effects are currently unknown.

█ PREGNENOLONE

OTHER COMMON NAME(S): None

Pregnenolone is a steroid the body produces that plays a role in the synthesis of several hormones, such as progesterone and DHEA (see DHEA). It is primarily promoted as an alternative treatment that improves memory and alertness and reduces stress and fatigue. Some promoters claim it also helps treat a variety of other conditions such as arthritis, cancer, osteoporosis, multiple sclerosis, PMS, and menopause. There is no scientific evidence to support these claims. Pregnenolone supplements are sold in capsule form, and there is no standardized dosage. Very little is known about the safety of the supplements or the effects of long-term use.

█ REVICI'S GUIDED CHEMOTHERAPY

OTHER COMMON NAME(S): Revici's Biologically Guided Chemotherapy, Revici Cancer Control, Lipid Therapy, Revici's Method

There is no scientific evidence that Revici's guided chemotherapy is effective in treating cancer or any other disease. It may also cause potentially serious side effects.

DESCRIPTION: Revici's guided chemotherapy is a chemical therapy promoted as an alternative cancer treatment. The therapy varies for every patient but can include a chemical formulation consisting of lipid alcohols, caffeine, zinc, and iron or a formulation consisting of fatty acids, selenium, magnesium, and sulfur (see Selenium and Zinc).

Revici's guided chemotherapy is promoted for the treatment of various cancers, including colon, bone, lung, and brain cancers, as well as Alzheimer's disease, arthritis, AIDS, chronic pain, drug addiction, injury from radiation, and schizophrenia. Proponents believe that cancer and other diseases can be remedied by formulating nontoxic chemotherapeutic medicines to restore the proper balance of lipids.

USE: Emanuel Revici, MD, the inventor of the therapy, used blood and urine tests to detect lipid imbalances and then developed a chemical formula of lipids and lipid-based substances that were unique to each patient. Revici's guided chemotherapy is administered by mouth or injection in dosages that are tailored to each patient. After the initial treatment, patients are taught to test their urine at home and monitor the lipid imbalance. If there are changes, the patient is given a new formula. This therapy is available at a few clinics started by Revici associates.

EFFECTS: The only published clinical evaluation of Revici's guided chemotherapy appeared in the *Journal of the American Medical Association* in 1965. Of the 33 cancer patients referred to Revici for treatment after conventional therapy failed, 22 of the patients died of cancer while on Revici's therapy, 8 showed no improvement, and the remaining 3 showed signs of cancer progression. The group concluded that Revici's method was without value. Studies of Revici's chemotherapy are hampered in that each formulation is different. A number of scientists who have offered to evaluate his methods were not able to reach agreement with Revici about a study protocol.

Revici's guided chemotherapy for cancer has never been proven to be safe or effective. Revici himself said that his treatment might cause the area around a cancerous tumor to become inflamed, and the tumor itself may grow larger and more painful before it shrank or disappeared. Selenium compounds, sometimes used in this therapy, can be toxic. This treatment should be avoided, especially by women who are pregnant or breast-feeding. Relying on this type of treatment alone, and avoiding conventional medical care, may have serious health consequences.

▎ SEA CUCUMBER

OTHER COMMON NAME(S): None

Sea cucumbers are marine animals that have a soft, dark body with the shape and texture of a cucumber. They range in size from 1 inch to 6 ½ feet long and about a half inch thick and are found in all oceans, especially the Indian and the western Pacific. Promoters claim sea cucumbers release poisons that fight conditions such as cancer, arthritis, sports injuries, tendonitis, and other inflammatory diseases. There is no scientific evidence to support these claims. Research is currently underway to determine the active ingredients in these poisons and evaluate their effectiveness in interfering with cancer progression in animal studies.

■ SHARK CARTILAGE

OTHER COMMON NAME(S): None

There is no scientific evidence that shark cartilage, sold as a food supplement, is an effective treatment for cancer, osteoporosis, or any other disease. Although some laboratory and animal studies have shown that components isolated from shark cartilage possess a modest ability to inhibit the growth of new blood vessels, these effects have not been proven in humans. Human studies are currently underway.

DESCRIPTION: Shark cartilage is extracted from the heads and fins of sharks. Cartilage is a type of elastic tissue found in the skeletal systems of many animals, including humans. Sharks have no bones, so cartilage is the primary component of their skeletal system.

Proponents believe that shark cartilage supplements or cartilage from other animals, such as cows, slow or stop the growth of cancer (see Bovine Cartilage). Shark cartilage, according to supporters, contains a protein that inhibits angiogenesis, the process of blood vessel development. Tumors require a network of blood vessels to survive and grow, so cutting off the tumor's blood supply starves it of nutrients it needs to live, causing it to shrink or disappear. Some proponents also claim that shark cartilage reverses bone diseases such as osteoporosis, arthritis, psoriasis, and inflammation of the intestinal tract.

USE: Shark cartilage is available as a capsule, powder, or liquid extract. It can be applied directly to the skin or injected by needle into the bloodstream, under the skin, into the lining of the abdomen, or directly into the muscle. It is also sometimes used as an enema (see Colon Therapy). The dose and length of treatment vary widely. There is no assurance, however, that the supplements sold contain the cartilage or its main compounds.

EFFECTS: There is no reliable evidence that shark cartilage is an effective treatment for cancer, osteoporosis, or other conditions. The scientific validity of most bovine and shark cartilage studies in people is questionable because the researchers do not describe how treatment was administered, how patients were assessed, long-term survival outcomes, or information about the components of the cartilage and how it was used.

Some laboratory and animal experiments have shown that shark cartilage possesses a modest ability to inhibit the growth of new blood vessels. These effects have not been conclusively shown in humans; however, one study concluded that orally administered liquid shark cartilage effectively inhibited the growth of new blood vessels in healthy men. In a recent study involving 47 patients, researchers concluded that shark cartilage had no effect on patients with advanced-stage cancers. A study using liquid shark cartilage extract for the treatment of lung cancer along with conventional therapies is underway.

Shark cartilage is not thought to be toxic, although it has been known to cause nausea, indigestion, fatigue, fever, and dizziness in some people. It may also slow down the healing process for people recovering from surgery. People with low white blood cell counts should not take shark cartilage enemas because there is a risk of life-threatening infection. Children should not take it because it could interfere with body growth and development. Women who are pregnant or breast-feeding should also avoid these supplements. Relying on this type of treatment alone, and avoiding conventional medical care, may have serious health consequences.

◼ SHARK LIVER OIL

OTHER COMMON NAME(S): None

Shark liver oil is widely used in addition to conventional cancer treatment in Europe. There has been no scientific evidence showing the effectiveness of alkylglycerols, a component in shark liver oil, in humans. More recent research has focused on one component of shark liver oil called squalamine. *Laboratory research suggests that it has antitumor effects in animal models; however, its effects in humans are not yet known. Human studies are currently being conducted.*

DESCRIPTION: Shark liver oil is one of the richest sources of alkylglycerols, natural chemicals formed by the combination of a fatty acid and an alcohol molecule. Alkylglycerols are also found in significant amounts in the liver, spleen, bone marrow, and breast milk (both cow and human). They are thought to be beneficial in several ways. They are promoted to fight cancer by killing tumor cells indirectly. Proponents claim that alkylglycerols activate the immune system by stimulating macrophages (immune system cells that attack and consume invading organisms) and inhibiting protein kinase A (a protein that is a key regulator of cell growth). Additionally, proponents claim that alkylglycerols reduce the side effects of chemotherapy and radiation treatment. This activity is supposedly due to the ability of alkylglycerols to protect cell membranes from oxidative stress.

Due to their proposed immune stimulatory effect, alkylglycerols are also claimed to be effective against colds, flu, chronic infections, asthma, psoriasis, arthritis, and AIDS. Since macrophages are also a key cell in wound healing, alkylglycerols are said to have healing effects. There is no scientific evidence to support these claims. Other compounds in shark liver oil, such as squalamine, have also been promoted to have beneficial anticancer effects.

USE: Shark liver oil is commercially available in capsule and liquid forms. A commonly used dosage is 1 to 2 capsules (250 mg) daily as a preventative measure and up to 6 capsules per day to prevent some of the side effects of radiation therapy. These supplements are available at health food stores and on the Internet.

EFFECTS: The claims for the activities of alkylglycerols have never been widely accepted. There does not appear to be any recent clinical research on the benefits of alkylglycerols in preventing or treating cancer. More recently, research has focused on squalamine, an antimicrobial substance found in shark liver oil that fights bacteria, yeasts, and fungi. Independent researchers discovered that squalamine had antitumor effects in different animals and found that squalamine decreased the number of lung metastases found in laboratory animals. Squalamine, which has been extracted from the oil, is being tested in various clinical trials.

Although many people have taken shark liver oil, the issue of potential toxicity at normal doses has not been well studied. Some mild gastrointestinal disturbances, such as nausea, indigestion, and diarrhea, have been reported to occur with the ingestion of shark liver oil in its liquid form.

▌ UROTHERAPY

OTHER COMMON NAME(S): Urine Therapy, Urea

There have been no well-controlled studies to support the claims that urotherapy can control or reverse the spread of cancer.

DESCRIPTION: Urotherapy is an alternative method that involves the use of a patient's own urine to treat himself or herself for cancer. Advocates of urotherapy propose several ways by which the treatment can slow or stop the growth of cancer. One is that urine can stimulate the body's immune system. Cancer and other diseases release chemicals called antigens into the bloodstream. When the immune system detects them, it responds by producing antibodies to fight the invading disease. Some of the antigens produced by cancer cells appear in the urine, so practitioners have hypothesized that if they give urine to cancer patients, the immune system would react more vigorously by producing more antibodies, thereby increasing its capacity to kill tumor cells. Other practitioners have speculated that urine inhibits the ability of cancer cells to crowd together, which disrupts the flow of nutrients and waste excretion. Without any way to feed or eliminate waste products, the tumor cells die.

One proponent asserts that certain components in urine establish a biochemical defense system that operates independently of the body's immune system. It is claimed that these chemicals don't destroy cancer cells, but "correct" their defects and prevent them from spreading. There is no scientific evidence to support these claims.

USE: Patients undergoing urotherapy may drink their own urine, use it as an enema, or have it injected directly into the bloodstream or into tumors. In powdered form, urea, the byproduct of protein metabolism and the primary component of urine, has been applied directly to tumors appearing on the skin. Urea may also be packed into capsules or dissolved in a flavored drink. There are no established guidelines for determining how much urine or urea is required for this method.

EFFECTS: There are some anecdotal reports of urotherapy's ability to stop cancer growth; however, there is no scientific evidence that shows urotherapy to be an effective cancer treatment. There is no valid evidence that urine or urea administered in any form has any beneficial effect for cancer patients. Drinking or injecting urine or applying it directly to the skin is reported to be safe and not associated with harmful side effects, but the safety of these practices have not been established by scientific studies.

714-X

None

There is no scientific evidence that 714-X is effective in treating any type of cancer. It has not been proven to be safe or effective for any use.

DESCRIPTION: 714-X is a substance containing camphor, nitrogen, ammonium salts, sodium chloride, and ethanol. It is used as an alternative method in North America, Western Europe, and Mexico to treat cancer and AIDS. It is not available in the United States.

According to proponents, people with serious diseases, such as cancer, carry tiny living particles in their bloodstream called somatids. They claim that disease can be diagnosed and monitored by noting the number and forms of somatids in a person's blood. 714-X is said to cure cancer and AIDS by interfering with the flow of somatids through the bloodstream. This interference is said to cause the immune system to grow stronger and diseases to regress.

It is claimed that cancer cells produce a substance called cocancerogenic K factor (CKF) that protects cancer cells from the immune system. 714-X supposedly strips CKF by supplying the body with nitrogen and leaves tumor cells vulnerable to attack by the immune system. There is no evidence to support these claims.

USE: 714-X is prepared as a sterile solution and injected into a lymph node in the groin. Ice packs are used to cool the area of injection both before and after. A course of treatment involves daily injections for 21 days, followed by 3 days of rest. The cycle is typically repeated a total of 3 times.

In Canada, 714-X is available by prescription under the Emergency Drug Release Program of Health Canada. It is not approved, however, for general therapeutic use. 714-X is not approved for use in the United States.

EFFECTS: One component of 714-X, camphor, is being researched in animals for potential anticancer activity. There are also some anecdotal reports of successful treatment with 714-X, although extensive research is needed in order to substantiate these reports. Some patients have reported beneficial effects after taking 714-X, but no scientific evidence supports any claims about the existence of somatids or that 714-X can cure cancer or AIDS. No formal clinical studies have been conducted on 714-X.

Resource Guide

Health Information on the Internet

THERE IS A VAST AMOUNT OF information about cancer and uncon-ventional methods on the Internet. Mass communication makes it possible for people to share ideas and information quickly. There is much information on the Internet, however, written by promoters of unproven treatments. Since any group or individual can publish on the Internet, it is important to consider the credentials and reputation of the organization providing the information.

The Health on the Net Foundation (HON) established a Code of Conduct for medical and health care related sites, providing guidelines for choosing and creating sites that are ethical and contain reliable information. Sites that adhere to these 8 principles are considered to demonstrate ethical behavior.

HON CODE OF CONDUCT

1. Any medical/health advice provided and hosted on the site will only be given by medically/health trained and qualified professionals unless a clear statement is made that a piece of advice offered is from a nonmedically/health qualified individual/organization.

2. The information provided on the site is designed to support, not replace, the relationship that exists between a patient/site visitor and his/her existing physician.

---

3. Confidentiality of data relating to individual patients and visitors to a medical/health web site, including their identity, is respected by this web site. The web site owners undertake to honor or exceed the legal requirements of medical/health information privacy that apply in the country and state where the web site and mirror sites are located.

4. Where appropriate, information contained on this site will be supported by clear references to source data and, where possible, have specific HTML links to that data. The date when a clinical page was last modified will be clearly displayed (eg, at the bottom of the page).

5. Any claims relating to the benefits/performance of a specific treatment, commercial product or service will be supported by appropriate, balanced evidence in the manner outlined above in Principle 4.

6. The designers of this web site will seek to provide information in the clearest possible manner and provide contact addresses for visitors that seek further information or support. The webmaster will display his/her e-mail address clearly throughout the web site.

7. Support for this web site will be clearly identified, including the identities of commercial and noncommercial organizations that have contributed funding, services, or material for the site.

8. If advertising is a source of funding, it will be clearly stated. A brief description of the advertising policy adopted by the web site owners will be displayed on the site. Advertising and other promotional material will be presented to viewers in a manner and context that facilitates differentiation between it and the original material created by the institution operating the site.

Reprinted with permission from the Health on the Net Foundation. The Health on the Net Foundation (HON: http://www.hon.ch) is a not-for-profit organization headquartered in Geneva, Switzerland. According to its mission statement, HON is dedicated to realizing the benefits of the Internet and related technologies in the fields of health and medicine.

Listing of Organizations

ALTERNATIVE MEDICINE HOMEPAGE

http://www.pitt.edu/~cbw/altm.html

Created and maintained by a University of Pittsburgh librarian, the Alternative Medicine HomePage is a point of reference to complementary and alternative medicine (CAM) information. It provides an organized index for Internet links to related databases, mailing lists, directories, and other resources.

AMERICAN BOTANICAL COUNCIL (ABC)

http://www.herbalgram.org

512-926-4900

ABC was founded and incorporated in 1988 as a nonprofit research and education organization. They publish a journal called HerbalGram, and they offer an online herb reference guide and selections from the Commission E monographs.

AMERICAN CANCER SOCIETY (ACS)

http://www.cancer.org

800-ACS-2345

ACS offers comprehensive, up-to-date cancer information 24 hours a day, 7 days a week. An online daily news magazine provides information on recent news events and research. A wide variety of educational programs, services, and referrals are offered, as well as information related to complementary and alternative methods.

CANADIAN BREAST CANCER RESEARCH INITIATIVE (CBCRI)

http://www.breast.cancer.ca

416-961-9406

CBCRI is a partnership of 7 Canadian breast cancer organizations and governmental bodies that encourages and supports research related to the prevention and treatment of breast cancer. They offer extensive reviews of scientifically credible and methodologically rigorous research on several unconventional therapies.

CANCERNET PDQ®

http://cancernet.nci.nih.gov/pdq.html

CancerNet is a web site that provides recent and accurate cancer information from the National Cancer Institute (NCI), which is the US Government's cancer research agency. PDQ contains treatment information on more than 80 types of adult and childhood cancers and is beginning to include summaries on complementary and alternative medicine.

FDA CENTER FOR FOOD SAFETY AND APPLIED NUTRITION (CFSAN)

http://vm.cfsan.fda.gov

Outreach and Information Center: 888-SAFEFOOD (888-723-3366)

CFSAN is an office of the US Food and Drug Administration. It regulates domestic food, imported foods, and cosmetics sold across state lines. The center promotes and protects public health interest by ensuring that food is safe, nutritious, and wholesome, and that it is honestly, accurately, and informatively labeled. They offer information on dietary supplements and the Special Nutritionals Adverse Monitoring System.

HEALTHSCOUT

http://www.healthscout.com

HealthScout is a general health web site that provides health care news and medical information, including information about complementary and alternative medicine. Connections to other health resources are also provided.

National Agricultural Library Food and Nutrition Information Center (FNIC)

http://www.nal.usda.gov/fnic

301-504-5719; TYY: 301-504-6856

FNIC is one of several information centers at the National Agricultural Library (NAL), part of the US Department of Agriculture's (USDA) Agricultural Research Service. The NAL is a major international source for agriculture and related information. FNIC provides information on dietary supplements, including vitamins, minerals, and herbs.

National Institutes of Health (NIH) National Center for Complementary and Alternative Medicine (NCCAM)

http://nccam.nih.gov

Toll Free: 888-644-6226

Outside the US: 301-519-3153

TTY: 866-464-3615 (toll free)

NCCAM evaluates alternative medicine practices to determine their effectiveness, to serve as a public information clearinghouse, and to provide a research-training program. The NCCAM facilitates and conducts research but does not serve as a referral agency for individual practitioners or treatments.

NIH Office of Dietary Supplements (ODS)

http://ods.od.nih.gov

301-435-2920

This office has an extensive International Bibliographic Information on Dietary Supplements (IBIDS) database. It contains articles and abstracts from scientific journals, information about dietary supplements, and a search engine that allows users to search for specific vitamins, minerals, and herbal products. The information in this database is limited to the top 85 to 100 most popular vitamins, minerals, and herbal ingredients.

OncoLink

http://www.oncolink.org

OncoLink is a web site founded by the University of Pennsylvania in 1994 to help cancer patients, families, health care professionals, and the general public obtain accurate cancer-related information free of charge. OncoLink provides comprehensive information about research advances, specific types of cancer, cancer treatment, and information about complementary and alternative medicine.

Quackwatch

http://www.quackwatch.com

Quackwatch, Inc. is a nonprofit corporation whose purpose is to combat health-related frauds, myths, fads, and fallacies. The Quackwatch web site is a comprehensive source of information regarding fraudulent claims.

US Pharmacopeia (USP)

http://www.usp.org

800-822-8772

The USP establishes and publishes standards for the strength, quality, and purity of drugs and dietary supplements for human and veterinary use in the United States Pharmacopeia and the National Formulary (USP-NF). National health care practitioner reporting programs support USP standards and information programs. In addition, USP supports many public service programs.

Index

Absinthe, 191–192
Absinthium, 191–192
Acidophilus, 196–197
Aconite, 95
Actibine, 192–194
Acumoxa, 78–80
Acupuncture, 55–56, 68, 93. *See also* Asian healing therapies
Acupuncture therapy, 55–56
Ai ye, 154–155
AK, 57–58
Alexander technique, 59–60
All heal, 151–152
Allium, 205–206
Aloe, 95–97
Aloe vera gel, 95–97
Alpha-lipoic acid, 254–255
Alsihum, 97
Alternative Medicine HomePage, 270
Alzium, 97
Amber, 173–174
American Botanical Council (ABC), 270
American Cancer Society (ACS), 13–14, 270
American larch, 146–147
American nightshade, 162–163
Amino acids, 197–199
Amygdalin, 253–254
Anesthesia, 8, 81–83
Antineoplaston therapy, 228–229

Antineoplastons, 228–229
Antioxidants, 160–162, 254–255
Anvirzel, 155–156
Aphrodyne, 192–194
Apitherapy, 229–230
Applied kinesiology, 57–58
Arborvitae, 177–178
Arnica, 97–98
Arnica flowers, 97–98
Arnica root, 97–98
Aromatherapy, 15–16
Aromatic medicine, 15–16
Art therapy, 16–17
Asian healing therapies. *See* Acupuncture; Ayurveda; Chinese herbal medicine; Electroacupuncture; Feng shui; Moxibustion; Ohashiatsu; Qigong; Reflexology; Reiki; Tai chi; Tui-na; Watsu; Yoga
Astragalus, 99
Auricular moxibustion, 78–80
Australian tea tree oil, 175–177
Aveloz, 100
Ayurveda, 18–19. *See also* Asian healing therapies
Ayurvedic medicine, 18–19

Bach remedies, 129–130
Balm mint, 159–160

Bear's grape, 162–163
Bee venom, 229–230
Bee venom therapy, 229–230
Bet A, 102–103
β-carotene, 100–102
Beta carotene, 100–102
Betulinic acid, 102–103
Bio-oxidative therapy, 259–260
Bioelectricity, 68–69
Bioenergetic analysis, 19–20
Bioenergetic medicine, 19–20
Bioenergetic therapy, 19–20
Bioenergetics, 19–20
Biofeedback, 20–22. *See also* Relaxation methods
Biofield therapy, 91–92
Biological dentistry, 58–59
Bio-oxidative therapy, 259–260
BioResonance tumor therapy, 68–69
Bird lime, 151–152
Black boxes, 68–69
Black cohosh, 103–104
Black currant oil, 243
Black salve, 60–61
Black sampson, 124–126
Black snakeroot, 103–104
Black tea, 138–140
Black walnut, 105
Black walnut hulls, 105
Blackwort, 122–123
Body vacuuming, 66–67

Bodywork, 59–60, 90
Borage seed oil, 243
Botanical salve, 60–61
Botanicals as medicine, 5, 7, 60–61
Bovine cartilage, 230–231
Brandy mint, 159–160
Breast-feeding, 12
Breathwork, 22. *See also* Relaxation methods
Broccoli, 199–200
Bromelain, 105–107
Bruisewort, 122–123
Bugbane, 103–104
Bugwort, 103–104
Butalin, 102–103
Butternut, 105

Calcium
    carbonate, 107–108
    glucarate, 244
Canadian Breast Cancer Research Initiative (CBCRI), 270
Cancell, 231–232
Cancer root, 162–163
Cancer salves, 60–61
CancerNet PDQ, 270
Cannabis, 148–150
Cantron, 231–232
Capsaicin, 109–110
Capsicum, 109–110
Carcalon, 252–253
Carnivora, 181–182
Carotenoids, 160–162
Cartilage
    bovine, 230–231
    shark, 263–264
Cassava, 200–201
Cassava plant, 200–201
Castor, 61–62
Castor bean, 61–62
Castor oil, 61–62
Categories of methods, vii–viii
Cat's claw, 110–111
Celandine, 112–113
Celandine poppy, 112–113
Cell com system, 68–69

Cell therapy, 232–233
Cellbal, 245
Cellular therapy, 232–233
Centella, 113–114
Cesium chloride, 114–115
Chamomile, 115–116
Chaparral, 116–117
Chelation therapy, 234–235
Chi-kung, 45–46
Chili pepper, 109–110
Chinese herbal medicine, 118–119
Chinese herbs, 118–119
Chinese tea, 138–140
Chinese yam, 190–191
Chiropractic, 63–64
Chiropractic techniques, 63–64
Chlorella, 119–120
Chromatotherapy, 74–76
Citrus pectin, 217–218
Clove oil, 121–122
Cloves, 121–122
Coenzyme Q10, 235–236
Coffee enemas, 64–65, 206–208
Cold laser therapy, 64
Coley toxins, 236–237
Coley's toxins, 236–237
Colic root, 190–191
Colon hydrotherapy, 64–65
Colon therapy, 64–65
Colored light therapy, 74–76
Comfrey, 122–123
Common arnica, 97–98
Common celandine, 112–113
Common larch, 146–147
Common pokeweed, 162–163
Complementary and alternative therapies
    American Cancer Society (ACS) stance on, 13–14
    commonly used terms in, 2–3
    defining, 1

    and dietary supplements, 5–7
    evaluating claims about, 3–5
    and fraudulent products, 4, 12
    guidelines for using, 9
    and health care teams, 11–13
    and the Internet, 268–269
    organizations, 270–271
    potential dangers of, 7–10
    side effects of, 4
    and surgery, 10
Copper, 123–124
CoQ10, 235–236
Coriolus versicolor, 201–203
Counseling, 43–45
Cranial balancing, 65–66
Cranial osteopathy, 65–66
Cranial sacral manipulation, 65–66
Craniopathy, 65–66
Craniosacral therapy, 65–66
Creatine, 252–253
Creative therapies. *See* Art therapy; Dance therapy; Music therapy
Creosote bush, 116–117
Crocinic acid, 231–232
Crowberry, 162–163
Crystal healing, 22–23
Crystals, 22–23
Cupping, 66–67
Curaderm, 60–61
Curanderismo, 24–25
Curanderos, 24–25
Cymatic therapy, 25

D-Glucarate, 244
Dance therapy, 25–26
Dangers of complementary and alternative methods, 8–10
Defining complementary and alternative methods, 1–3
Detoxification therapy, 64–65

Devil's fuge, 151–152
DHEA, 237–239, 261
Di Bella multitherapy, 239–240
Di Bella therapy, 239–240
Diet and nutrition methods, viii, 196–227
Dietary supplements, 5–7, 271. *See also* Vitamins guidelines for safe use of, 6, 12
labels, 7–8
and surgery, 10
Digestive enzyme therapy, 241–242
DMSO, 240–241
Dogbane, 155–156

Eastern white cedar, 177–178
Echinacea, 124–126
Effectiveness of therapies, evaluating, 3–5
Electrical devices, 68–69
Electroacupuncture, 68. *See also* Asian healing therapies
Electrodermal screening, 68. *See also* Asian healing therapies
Electromagnetic therapy, 68–69
Electromagnetism, 68–69
Electronic devices, 68–69
Ellagic acid, 203
Enema irrigation, 64–65, 206–208
Energy field therapy, 91–92
Energy medicine, 68–69
English walnut, 105
Entelev, 231–232
Enzyme therapy, 241–242
Escharotic therapy, 60–61
Escharotics, 60–61
Essential oils, 15–16
Essiac, 126–127
Essiac tea, 126–127
European larch, 146–147
Evaluating claims, 3–5

Evening primrose, 127–128
Eye balm, 137–138
Eye root, 137–138

Faith healing, 27–28. *See also* Religion
Fasting, 204–205
Feldenkrais method, 59–60
Felon herb, 154–155
Feng shui, 28–29. *See also* Asian healing therapies
Fire cupping, 66–67
Fish fats, 220–221
Flavonoids, 160–162
Flaxseed, 128–129
Flaxseed oil, 128–129
Flor Essence, 126–127
Flower remedies, 129–130
Folacin, 130–131
Folate, 130–131
Folic acid, 130–131
Food and Drug Administration (FDA), 5
Center for Food Safety and Applied Nutrition (CFSAN), 270
Fragrances, 15–16
Fraudulent products, 4, 12
Fresh cell therapy, 232–233
Fu-Tzu, 95
Fu Zhen therapy, 132

Gamma linoleic acid, 243–244
Garlic, 205–206
Garlic clove, 205–206
Garlic oil, 205–206
Garlic powder, 205–206
German chamomile, 115–116
Germanium, 132–133
Germanium sesquioxide, 132–133
Gerson diet, 206–208
Gerson method, 206–208
Gerson program, 206–208
Gerson therapy, 206–208, 211, 216–217. *See also* Metabolic therapy

Gerson treatment, 206–208, 216–217
Ginger, 133–134
Ginger root, 133–134
Ginkgo, 134–135
Ginkgo Biloba, 134–135
Ginseng, 136–137, 172
GLA. *See* Gamma linoleic acid
Glucarate, 244
Goatweed, 173–174
Gold book tea, 173
Golden bough, 151–152
Goldenseal, 137–138
Goldsiegel, 137–138
Gonzalez treatment, 216–217
Gotu Kola, 113–114
Grape cure, the, 208–209
Grape diet, the, 208–209
Grape seed extract, 208–209
Grape skins, 208–209
Grapes, 208–209
Grass, 148–150
Greasewood, 116–117
Greater celandine, 112–113
Greek cancer cure, 245
Green algae, 119–120
Green mint, 159–160
Green tea, 138–140
Ground raspberry, 137–138
Group therapy, 49–51
Guided imagery, 33–35

Hackmatack, 177–178
Hansi, 140
Hatha yoga, 53–54
Health care teams, 11–13
Health on the Net Foundation (HON), 268–269
HealthScout, 270
Heat therapy, 69–71
Heat treatment, 69–71
Hemp, 148–150
Herb, vitamin, and mineral methods, viii, 95–195
Herbal Essence, 126–127
Herbal medicine. *See* Chinese herbal medicine

High colonic, 64–65
High enema, 64–65
High pH therapy, 114–115
Hochu-ekki-to, 143–144
Hog apple, 218–219
Holism, 29–30
Holistic aromatherapy,
  15–16
Holistic health, 29–30
Holistic medicine, 29–30.
  See also Spiritual
  healing
Holy thistle, 150–151
Homeopathic medicine,
  246–247
Homeopathy, 246–247
Horn method, the, 66–67
Hot pepper, 109–110
Hoxsey formula, 140–142
Hoxsey herbal treatment,
  140–142
Hoxsey herbs, 140–142
Hoxsey method, 140–142
Hoxsey treatment, 140–142
Huang ch'i, 99
Huang qi, 99
Humor therapy, 31
Hungarian chamomile,
  115–116
Hydrazine sulfate, 247–248
Hydro-colon therapy, 64–65
Hydrocotyle, 113–114
Hydrogen peroxide,
  248–249
Hydrogen peroxide therapy,
  248–249
Hydrotherapy, 71–72
Hyperbaric oxygen therapy,
  72–74. *See also* Oxygen
  therapy
Hypercalm, 173–174
Hyperoxygenation, 259–260
Hyperthermia, 69–71
Hypnosis, 32–33. *See also*
  Relaxation methods
Hypnotherapy, 32–33
Hypnotic therapy, 32–33

IAT, 250–251

Imagery, 33–35. *See also*
  Meditation; Relaxation
  methods
Immuno-augmentative
  therapy, 250–251
Imunovir, 251–252
Indian dye, 137–138
Indian mulberry, 218–219
Indian saffron, 178–179
Indian snakeroot, 142–143
Indian turmeric, 137–138
Indian valerian, 178–179
Inkberry, 162–163
Inosine pranobex, 251–252
Inosiplex, 251–252
Inositol, 209–210
Inositol hexaphosphate,
  209–210
Integrative therapy, 2
Internet, the, 268–269
Interventions
  psychological, 43–45
  psychosocial, 49–51
IP6, 209–210
Ipe roxo, 156–157
Ipes, 156–157
Isapgol, 165–166
Isoflavones, 223–224
Isoprinosine, 251–252
Isphagula, 165–166
Issels' fever therapy,
  236–237
Issels' whole body therapy,
  216–217

Japanese mushroom,
  221–223
Jaundice root, 137–138
Jiang huang, 178–179
Jim's juice, 231–232
Jin gui shen qi, 173
Juice therapy, 210–211
Juicing, 210–211
Juzen-taiho-to, 143–144

Kampo, 143–144
Kampoyaku, 143–144
Kansas snakeroot, 124–126
Kargasok tea, 211–212

Kava, 144–146
Kava-kava, 144–146
Kavalactones, 144–146
Kelley's treatment, 216–217
Killwart, 100
Kira, 173–174
Kirlian photography, 35–36
Klamath weed, 173–174
Knitbone, 122–123
Kombucha tea, 211–212
Krebiozen, 252–253

Labels, dietary supplement,
  7–8
Labyrinth walking, 36. *See
  also* Relaxation methods
Labyrinths, 36
Lactic acid bacteria,
  196–197
Lacto-ovo-vegetarian,
  224–226
Lactovegetarian, 224–226
Lady thistle, 150–151
Laetrile, 253–254
Lapacho, 156–157
Lapacho Colorado, 156–157
Lapacho Morado, 156–157
Lapachol, 156–157
Larch, 146–147
Larch Arabinogalactan,
  146–147
Latin American Healing,
  24–25
Laugh therapy, 31
Laurier rose, 155–156
Leopardsbane, 97–98
Licorice, 147–148
Licorice root, 147–148
Light boxes, 74–76
Light therapy, 74–76
Linseed, 128–129
Lint bells, 128–129
Linum, 128–129
Lipid therapy, 261–262
Lipoic acid, 254–255
Liu wei di huang, 173
Live cell therapy, 232–233
Liver flush, 255–256

Livingston-Wheeler therapy, 256–257
Lycopene, 212–214
Lyprinex, 257
Lyprinol, 257

Macrobiotic diet, 214–215
Macrobiotics, 214–215
Magnet therapy, 76–77
Magnetic field therapy, 76–77
Magnetic therapy, 76–77
Maitake, 215–216
Maitake D-fraction, 215–216
Maitake extract, 215–216
Maitake mushroom, 215–216
Manchurian tea, 211–212
Manioc, 200–201
Manual healing and physical touch methods, vii–viii, 55–94
Marian thistle, 150–151
Marijuana, 148–150
Mary thistle, 150–151
Massage, 77–78. See also Relaxation methods
Massage therapy, 77–78
MCP. See Modified citrus pectin
Meditation, 36–38. See also Breathwork; Imagery; Relaxation methods
Melaleuca oil, 175–177
Melatonin, 257–259
Meng koedoe, 218–219
Metabolic therapy, 216–217. See also Gerson therapy
METBAL, 245
Methisoprinol, 251–252
Milk thistle, 150–151
Milk vetch, 99
Milkbush, 100
Mind, body, spirit methods, 15–54
Mint, 159–160
Mistletoe, 151–152

Mixed bacterial vaccines, 236–237
Modified citrus pectin, 217–218
Molybdenum, 152–153
Monkshood, 95
Mora de la India, 218–219
Morinda, 218–219
Mountain arnica, 97–98
Mountain tobacco, 97–98
Movement therapy, 25–26, 59–60
Moxibustion, 78–80. See also Asian healing therapies
Mugwort, 154–155
Muscle testing, 57–58
Mushrooms
    Coriolus versicolor, 201–203
    Maitake, 215–216
    Shitake, 221–223
Music therapy, 25, 38–39
Myofascial release, 80
Myotherapy, 80–81. See also Relaxation methods

National Agricultural Library Food and Nutrition Information Center (FNIC), 271
National Institutes of Health (NIH), 271
Native American healing, 39–40
Natural medicine, 41–42
Naturopathic medicine, 41–42
Naturopathy, 41–42
Neural therapy, 81–83
Neuro-linguistic programming, 42–43. See also Relaxation methods
NLP, 42–43
Noni fruit, 218–219
Noni juice, 218–219
Noni plant, 218–219
Nontraditional therapies, 3

Ohashiatsu, 83. See also Asian healing therapies
Oil of cloves, 121–122
Oilnut, 105
Oleander, 155–156
Oleander leaf, 155–156
Omega-3 fatty acids, 220–221
OncoLink, 271
Organizations, 270–271
Orthomolecular medicine, 156
Osteopathic medicine, 83–85
Osteopathy, 83–85
Overview of complementary and alternative methods, 1–14
Oxidative therapy, 259–260
Oxidology, 259–260
Oxygen therapy, 259–260. See also Hyperbaric oxygen therapy
Oxymedicine, 259–260
Ozone therapy, 259–260

Palma christi, 61–62
Pancreatic enzyme therapy, 241–242
Paprika, 109–110
Pau d'arco, 156–157
PC-SPES, 158–159
Pecta-Sol, 217–218
Pencil tree, 100
Pennywort, 113–114
Peppermint, 159–160
Peppermint oil, 159–160
Pharmacological and biological treatment methods, viii, 228–267
Phytate, 209–210
Phytic acid, 209–210
Phytochemicals, 160–162
Pigeon berry, 162–163
Pinebark extract, 167
Plumbagin, 181–182
Poison nut, 174–175
Poke, 162–163
Poke salad, 162–163

Pokeberry, 162–163
Pokeroot, 162–163
Pokeweed, 162–163
Polarity balancing, 85–86
Polarity energy balancing, 85–86
Polarity therapy, 85–86. *See also* Relaxation methods
Poly-MVA, 260–261
Polyphenols, 160–162
Pot, 148–150
Potassium, 164–165
Prayer and spirituality, 48–49
Pregnancy, 12
Pregnenolone, 261
Pressure point therapy, 80–81
Proven treatments, 2
Provitamin A, 100–102
PSK, 201–203
Psychic surgery, 86–87
Psychological intervention, 43–45
Psychosocial interventions, 49–51
Psychosocial treatment, 49–51
Psychotherapeutic treatment, 43–45
Psychotherapy, 43–45. *See also* Support groups
Psyllium, 165–166
Psyllium seed husk, 165–166
Purple clover, 168–169
Purple cone flower, 124–126
Pycnogenol, 167

Qigong, 45–46. *See also* Asian healing therapies
Quackery, 3
Quackwatch, Inc., 271
Quaker buttons, 174–175

Rabdosia rubescens, 168
Radic, 231–232
Radix, 178–179

Rauwolfia, 142–143
Red clover, 168–169
Red pepper, 109–110
Red valerian, 178–179
Reflexology, 87–88. *See also* Asian healing therapies; Relaxation methods
Reiki, 88–90. *See also* Relaxation methods
Reiki healing, 88–90
Reiki system, 88–90
Relaxation methods. *See* Biofeedback; Body-work; Breathwork; Hypnosis; Imagery; Labyrinth walking; Massage; Meditation; Myotherapy; Neuro-linguistic program-ming; Polarity therapy; Reflexology; Reiki
Religion, 27–28, 46–49, 88–90. *See also* Faith healing; Shamanism; Spiritual healing; Spirituality and prayer
Remifemin, 103–104
Remission, 3
Research, 2
Reserpine, 142–143
Resource Guide, 268–271
Revici's biologically guided chemotherapy, 261–262
Revici's cancer control, 261–262
Revici's guided chemo-therapy, 261–262
Revici's method, 261–262
Rheumatism root, 190–191
Rife machine, 68–69
Rolfing, 59–60
Rose bay, 155–156
Rosen method, 90
Rubenfeld synergy method, 90
Ruibarbo caribe, 218–219

Saw palmetto, 169–170

Sea cucumber, 262–263
Selected vegetable soup, 221
Selenium, 170–172
Semivegetarian, 224–226
Serpentwood, 142–143
714-X, 267
Shadow boxing, 51–52
Shaman, 46–48
Shamanism, 46–48. *See also* Religion
Shark cartilage, 263–264
Shark liver oil, 264–265
Sheridan's formula, 231–232
Shiatsu, 83
Shiatsu massage, 59–60, 94. *See also* Massage
Shitake mushroom, 221–223
Sho-saiko, 143–144
Siberian ginseng, 172
Side effects of alternative therapies, 4
Silymarin, 150–151
Six flavor tea, 173
Slippery root, 122–123
Snakeroot, 142–143
Sonopuncture, 90
Sound therapy, 25, 38–39
Soy, 223–224
Soy powder, 223–224
Soy protein, 223–224
Soybean, 223–224
Spinal manipulation, 63–64
Spiritual healing, 27–28
Spirituality and prayer, 48–49
St. John's plant, 154–155
St. John's wort, 173–174
Strychnos nux-vomica, 174–175
Strychnos seed, 174–175
Sulfides, 160–162
Sun chlorella, 119–120
Sun soup, 221
Supplements. *See* Dietary supplements
Support groups, 49–51. *See also* Psychotherapy

Surgery
  psychic, 86–87
  and supplements, 10
SV, 221
Swamp cedar, 177–178
Sweet root, 147–148
Systemic enzyme therapy,
  241–242

T-UP, 95–97
Taheebo, 156–157
Tahuari, 156–157
T'ai chi, 51–52
Tai chi, 51–52
Tai chi chih, 51–52
Tai chi chuan, 51–52
Tai ji, 51–52
Tai ji juan, 51–52
Tai ji quan, 51–52
Talepetrako, 113–114
Tapioca, 200–201
Tapioca plant, 200–201
Tea of life, 126–127
Tea tree oil, 175–177
TENS, 92–93
Tension tamer, 173–174
Tetterwort, 112–113
Therapeutic touch, 91–92
Therapy, 43–45
Thuja, 177–178
Tipton weed, 173–174
Tofu, 223–224
Traditional Chinese
    Medicine, 118–119.
    See also Asian healing
    therapies
Trager approach, 59–60
Transcendental meditation,
    36–38
Transcutaneous electrical
    nerve stimulation,
    92–93
Tree of life, 177–178
Trefoil, 168–169

Trigger point injections,
    80–81
Trigger point therapy, 80–81
Trumpet bush, 156–157
Trumpet tree, 156–157
TT, 91–92
Tui-na, 93. See also Asian
    healing therapies
Turkey tail, 201–203
Turmeric, 178–179

Ukrain, 112–113
Ultraviolet blood
    irradiation, 74–76
Ultraviolet light therapy,
    74–76
Una de Gato, 110–111
Urea, 265–266
Urine therapy, 265–266
Urotherapy, 265–266
US Pharmacopeia (USP),
    271
Usui system of reiki, 88–90

Valerian, 179–181
Valerian extract, 179–181
Valerian root, 179–181
Valerian tea, 179–181
Vegan, 224–226
Vegetarianism, 224–226
Venom immunotherapy,
    229–230
Venus flytrap, 181–182
Virginia poke, 162–163
Visualization, 33–35
Vitae elixxir, 182
Vitalitea, 126–127
Vitamins. See also Dietary
    supplements
  A, 182–184
  B complex, 130–131,
    184–185
  B17, 253–254
  C, 185–187

E, 187–188
K, 189–190

Water therapy, 71–72, 94
Watsu, 94. See also Asian
    healing therapies
Weed, 148–150
Wheatgrass, 226–227
Wheatgrass diet, 226–227
Wild clover, 168–169
Wild Mexican yam,
    190–191
Wild pine, 218–219
Wild wormwood, 154–155
Wild yam, 190–191
Willard water, 227
Wolfsbane, 95, 97–98
Wormwood, 191–192

Yellow cedar, 177–178
Yellow paint, 137–138
Yellow puccoon, 137–138
Yellow root, 137–138
Yocon, 192–194
Yoga, 53–54. See also Asian
    healing therapies;
    Relaxation methods
Yohimbe, 192–194
Yohimbe bark, 192–194
Yohimbine, 192–194
Yohimbine hydrochloride,
    192–194
Yohimex, 192–194
Yomax, 192–194

Zapping machine, 68–69
Zen Buddhism. See
    Meditation
Zhenjiu, 55–56
Zinc, 194–195
Zinc gluconate, 194–195
Zinc sulfate, 194–195
Zone therapy, 87–88